Family Circle

GUIDE TO BEAUTY

YOUR HAIR · YOUR FACE YOUR FIGURE

**BY MARY MILO
FAMILY CIRCLE BEAUTY EDITOR**

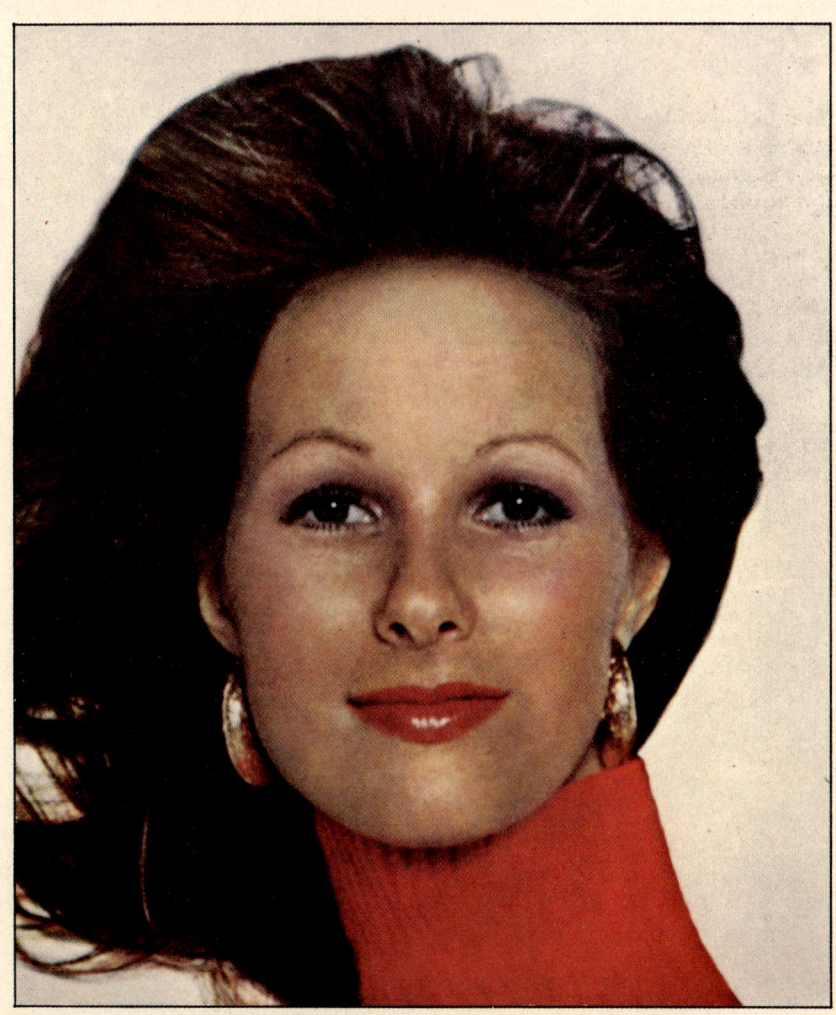

DESIGNED BY DANA NORDHAUSEN
DRAWINGS BY RAY SKIBINSKI

Revised Edition

A New York Times Company Publication

CONTENTS

YOUR HAIR
- 4 Know your hair type
- 8 How to get a good haircut
- 12 A hair style that becomes you
- 14 How-to's
- 17 Grooming your hair
- 18 Secrets of the comb-out
- 18 No-set hairdos
- 20 What length is your hair?
- 20 Long-hair hairdos
- 21 Hairpieces
- 22 Hairpiece hairdos
- 22 Wigs
- 24 What is your face shape?
- 26 Balance your face
- 26 Hairdos that solve problems
- 28 12 best-liked hairdos
- 30 What setting for your hair?
- 31 What care for your hair?
- 32 Hair conditioners
- 33 Protect your hair
- 34 Moneysavers
- 34 What you want in a permanent
- 35 Hair straightening
- 36 Hair-coloring guide

YOUR MAKEUP
- 40 Give your makeup a magic touch
- 43 How to choose and use the new makeups
- 44 How the famous salons do the new makeups
- 46 What cosmetics for your complexion?
- 47 Harmonize your makeup colors
- 49 Look your best in night light
- 50 Party face fresheners
- 51 Quick preparty pickups
- 51 Hair color as a makeup key
- 52 Look your best in daylight
- 54 Daytime makeup that lasts all day
- 54 Beauty for the traveler
- 56 Outdoor beauty
- 58 Choose your makeup colors
- 58 Balance your face with makeup
- 64 Shape your face with makeup
- 66 Face-changers
- 68 If you wear glasses
- 70 What should you do about facial hair?
- 71 Other helps for your looks
- 71 How to get rid of beauty flaws
- 74 Face-saving facial exercises
- 76 Under-eye circles—how to relieve them
- 78 To eliminate crow's feet

Revised Edition published simultaneously in U.S.A. and Canada by The Family Circle, Inc., a subsidiary of The New York Times Media Company, Inc. Copyright © 1972, 1964 by The Family Circle, Inc. Protected under Berne and other international copyright conventions. Title and trademark FAMILY CIRCLE registered U.S. Patent Office, Canada, Great Britain, Australia and other countries. Marca Registrada. All rights reserved. This volume may not be reproduced in whole or in part in any form without written permission from the publisher.

Printed in U.S.A. Library of Congress Catalog Card Number 72-83736. ISBN 0-405-09841-3.

YOUR COMPLEXION
- 80 Skin beauty guide
- 82 Skin-analysis chart and key
- 83 What care for your skin?
- 83 How to clean your face
- 84 Handle your skin with a light touch
- 88 How to do a home facial
- 90 Any-age skin care
- 90 Outdoor skin care
- 91 What goes on in a salon facial?
- 94 What's your skin type?
- 97 Normalize your complexion
- 98 How to tone your skin
- 98 Conditioning treatment
- 99 Skin problems
- 100 How to stroke wrinkles away

YOUR LOOK
- 104 The total look of beauty
- 107 Slim-and-trim eye foolers
- 108 Take your measure
- 108 What's your figure type?
- 110 How to look prettier in a picture
- 112 Beauty for the working wife
- 112 Look pretty at 40-plus
- 114 Use your body gracefully
- 116 Miss Craig's instant-thinning plan

YOUR GROOMING
- 118 Refresh with a bath
- 120 Guide to good grooming
- 122 Grooming aids
- 123 Fragrance
- 124 Nude beauty
- 126 Professional manicure to do at home
- 127 Hand problems
- 127 Arm problems
- 129 Instant beauty aids
- 130 What care for your feet?
- 130 Good-grooming checklist

YOUR FIGURE
- 132 Figure beauty
- 134 How much should you weigh?
- 134 Tested ways to lose weight
- 134 Helps in gaining weight
- 134 What should you eat?
- 135 Basic diet pattern
- 137 Exercise for figure beauty and vitality
- 140 Miss Craig's tension-freeing exercise
- 142 Stretch exercises
- 144 Slim-while-you-sit yoga
- 146 4-week exercise plan
- 148 Bonnie Prudden's four-week shape-up
- 156 Index
- 160 Acknowledgments

KNOW YOUR HAIR TYPE

How do you meet today's beauty challenge? With so many exciting new products and so many delightful ways to use them, it is easier than ever to look like a new woman. And here to help you is a how-to guide to the best of good looks—the kind of lavishly pictured clear-cut information that more than 12,000,000 women look for each month in the beauty pages of Family Circle. Start with your hair. If you want a hair style that becomes you, that keeps its shape, that looks really great from shampoo to shampoo—you have to do more than just set your hair. The care you give your hair, its condition, even its color add to the finished effect. So do the haircut, the base permanent, if any, and the way you use brush, comb, and spray during the comb-out. With all the hair-care preparations now available, it is more important than ever to choose the ones that are right for you. To choose wisely you need to know what kind of hair you really have. Is it oily or dry? Resilient or limp? Treated or damaged? Porous or resistant? Tinted, bleached, or rinsed? Curly or straight? Elastic or easy to break? Manageable or hard to control? Once you know your own hair, you can treat it wisely and you can find a haircut and style that will make your hair easy to handle. We start you off with a guide to your kind of hair, hair styles that solve problems, and suggestions for keeping your hair healthy and beautiful.

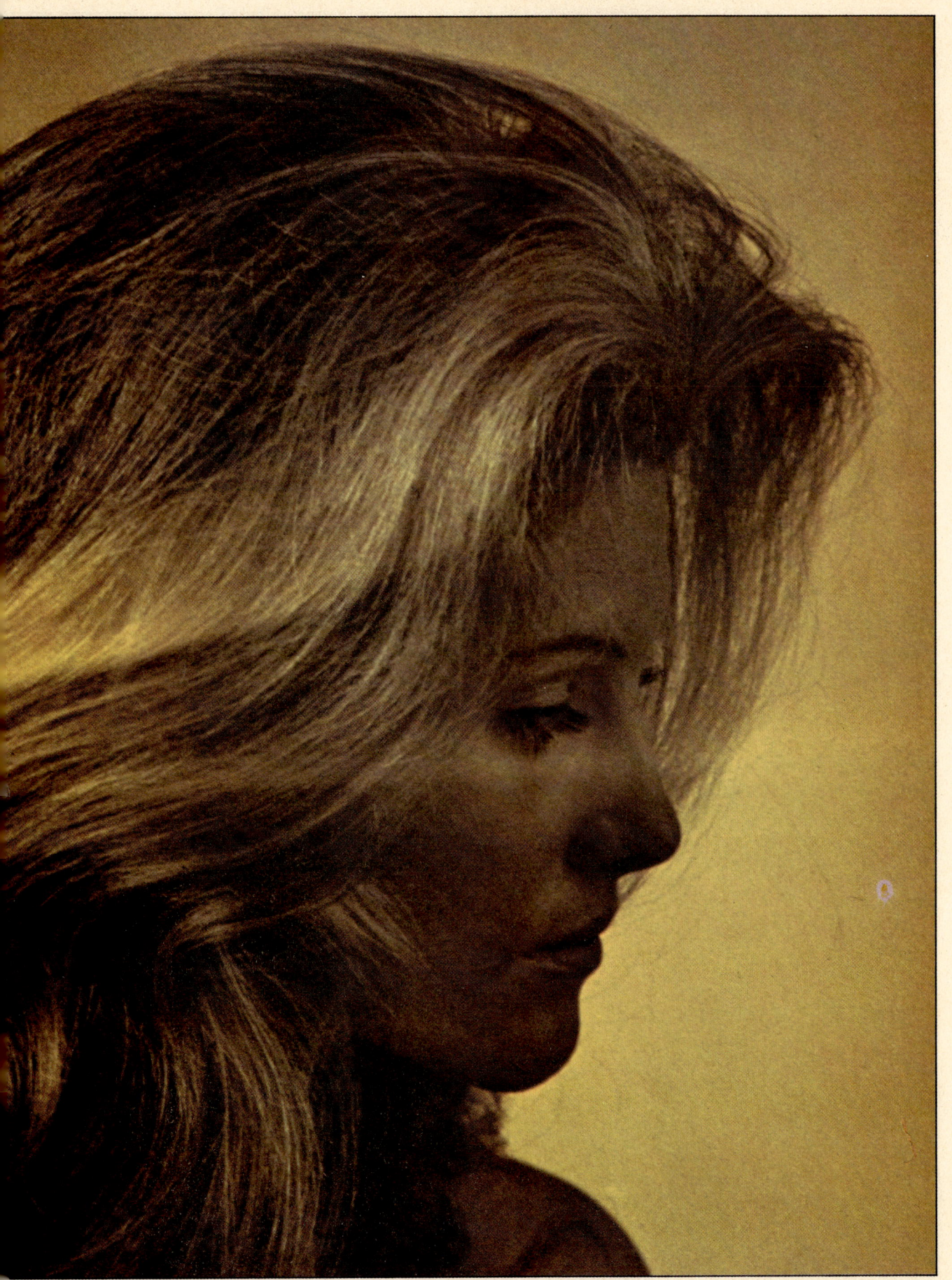

Does your hair have body? Does your hair keep a set easily, have movement and bounce, hold barrettes and ornaments well? If so, it has good body. If not, a permanent wave or even a firm set will give body. Certain colorings, setting lotions and conditioners also add body to the hair. If hair wilts easily, keep it fairly short.

• Sometimes a body permanent and weekly settings on large rollers give the hair all the body it needs. Back-combing also puts body into the hair.

• Hair that is extremely limp and lacking in body needs the tight springy curl of a permanent to become manageable and to be able to hold a set.

Is your hair brittle? Does the hair break easily, have split ends, refuse to hold a curl even with a body wave? This is hair that is brittle or damaged, and special treatment may be needed. To test hair strength, take a single hair and stretch a short section. When a strand is stretched to the breaking point, broken ends of normal hair curl; broken ends remain straight if hair lacks elasticity. This hair needs conditioning treatment.

• Brittle damaged hair may result from overtreatment, such as careless bleaching and permanenting, or from recent illness or general poor health (watch diet and exercise) or from overexposure to sun and wind.

• Handle damaged hair gently; do not wind rollers overtightly and avoid rollers that clamp together.

• Stay away for a while from durable hair coloring, bleaching, and permanents or space these treatments as far apart as possible.

• Use a mild neutral shampoo and a protein hair conditioner after the shampoo to act as a filler and to strengthen the hair and to give it body.

• Protect hair from sun and wind with hat or scarf; watch out for overdry indoor air. Have drier heat at low or medium and hold drying time after a set to the minimum.

• A simple hair style—one of the currently fashionable short cuts to get rid of damaged hair while new healthier hair grows out—may be in order.

Is your hair thin? Sometimes hair thins as one grows older but the thinning is often slight and usually starts on the forehead about an inch above the hairline. If the scalp is visible through the hair, if the part in the hair stands out sharply, if you look "skinned" after a haircut or a shampoo, hair may be considered thin. Fine hair may appear thin because of the delicacy of the strands.

• This kind of hair needs body and therefore needs a permanent. But it is often hard to give lasting wave to this kind of hair. The secret is to use a mild waving solution and leave it on the hair only a short time. If properly done (make a test curl) the permanent swells the hair shaft and gives the hair a spongier quality and a greater willingness to hold a set, providing bulk.

• The styling should emphasize fullness with lots of curls and waves for bouffant effects. Fine hair should not be allowed to grow long, because it gets weaker as it gets longer and ends tend to break off. Besides, long hair seems to thin out because of the downward pull of the hair's weight.

Is hair lustrous? Hair has gloss and sheen because of its natural oils and the firmness of the hair platelets; well-brushed, the hair is polished and meshed and oils are distributed so that the hair gleams and appears beautiful. Color also contributes to luster—the range from lights to darks in hair color gives a shifting pattern of light and shade that emphasizes the lines of the hair style. White hair may lack luster both because of oil deficiency and because color gradations are lacking.

• If hair lacks luster, use a balsam conditioner after your shampoo.

• Hair coloring will add to hair luster; color picks up the lines of the hair style.

Is your hair straight? Does your hair refuse to stay back or up from your face? Will it, however, lie beautifully straight and close to your head? If so, your hair really *is* straight. Straight hair can be made curly with a permanent, but the best styling comes through working with the kind of hair you have and then using a body wave where the curl is actually needed.

• Don't try to make straight hair, if it is short, go up and away from the face as the hair will be hard to handle. The natural movement of straight hair is down and forward.

• Straight hair needs a layered cut to fall to the exact length you want the hair style to be.

• Never curl straight hair too tightly; it needs to be curled only a little to give the ends a turn and perhaps to give a lift at the crown; end curls should make only one complete turn when brushed out.

• The beauty of a straight-hair style is in the cut. Never thin straight hair; when the fullness is left in, there is more chance for any natural curve to develop, and the added weight helps straight hair to hold its shape.

Is your hair curly? Curly hair, natural or resulting from a permanent, can be worn back and up because it is supported by the arch of the curl.

• In styling curly hair needs a blunt cut to bring out the curl and the pattern of hair growth.

• If curly hair is short, brush it in all directions, and the natural pattern will develop; this is the pattern that should be used in the styling.

• Some curly hair will have certain sections that are straight, and these straight areas should also be taken advantage of in the styling.

• Excessively curly hair should be kept all one length and tapered only at the ends. Care must be taken to get the hair just the right length; if cut too short, coarse curly hair will end up as a stiff brush; if hair is too long, it will be hard to style; keep the hair as short as is possible while still having it manageable. For easy handling of overcurly hair, use a hard-hold setting-lotion-conditioner and comb down the hair for five minutes while it is still wet.

• Roll the hair on supersize rollers, choosing a style that can be molded into smooth lines.

• Once hair is dry and curlers are out, use two brushes to brush the hair flat all round the head. Hold the hair in place with the hands to settle it and then go on brushing till a wave pattern appears.

• Use a spray lightly to hold the style in place; too wet a spray will cause the hair to spring back into curls.

• Avoid overcurliness from a permanent by having hair in good condition to start and getting only a body wave.

• Too-curly hair can be straightened by a method similar to the permanent wave that gives straight hair a curl; the new hair at the scalp will, of course, continue to grow out curly and straightening must be repeated.

Do you have a hidden wave? Does your hair seem straight yet refuse to lie flat and close to the head? If so, it has too much wave for a straight hairdo and must have some hidden wave. Many women think their hair is straight when it actually would have a slight tendency to wave if it were short enough. To discover the natural tendencies of your hair, shampoo, rinse, and towel-dry the hair. Then comb it down all around and push it into shape round the head. Is there any tendency for it to fall into certain lines or curves?

• Where definite (though perhaps slight) curves appear, you do have a slight amount of wave that you can work with in your hair styling.

• If hair is short, wave may show quite readily. You may find some sections of hair have wave; some seem to have none. The wave that can best be used in a hair style is that at the temple, the sideburns, and in the top hair.

If hair is long, suggests hair-stylist Victor Vito, you may find any hidden wave by isolating small sections of hair —12 to 24 hairs—in various places over the head. Then, starting about an inch from the tip, snip off a piece of the strand and hold the remainder across the hand. Does hair show a tendency to bend? If not, keep cutting the small strand shorter and shorter till you find a length at which curve forms. When you find a length that shows a slight curve, keep this as the length for your overall hair style.

If you have even a slight wave, you will do better in your hair styling if you work with this tendency rather than trying to force your hair into a direction that is unnatural to it.

Hair with a slight amount of wave will need less time to permanent and to set if you follow the tendency of the wave in the lines of the style. Or you may find that a partial wave is enough.

Does your hair need resetting often? Does your hair need to be reset every day? If so, you are probably working against the natural trends of your hair. When you follow the natural tendency, or movement, of your hair and have the right length of hair to catch the natural wave, the style stays pretty.

Between settings, notice which section of the set loosens first. Only this section need be reset. Or this section may need restyling or shortening to hold its curl. Or here you may need a few permanent curls—or even a little more length to hold the style correctly.

Is your hair porous? Does your hair shed water readily after rinsing and dry quickly? Or does it mat when wet and take a long time to dry? If hair is slow to dry, it probably is very porous and will need careful timing when waving lotions or color tints are applied.

Handle porous hair gently while it is wet; make frequent tests while coloring lightening or waving; use a protein conditioner after the shampoo so hair will be easy to comb.

Towel-dry the hair before setting and avoid overhot air in drying.

Use very gentle wave lotions.

Hair must be made porous if certain treatments—bleaches, color tints, and permanenting—are to be effective. Ends—"old" hair—are usually more porous than new growth.

Is your hair dry? Is your hair flyaway—supercharged with electricity? If so, it probably is baby-fine and dry. Dry hair often means dry scalp—if there is little natural oil in the scalp skin, face and body skin may also be dry. Hair may become dry from treatment—permanent waves, tinting, bleaching, too much cleansing power in the shampoo. Also drying are sun, wind, and overheated indoor air.

Use a dry-hair shampoo; follow shampooing with a creme rinse to reduce the static electricity that makes the hair flyaway.

Is your hair oily? Does hair become stringy within a few days after it's washed? This may indicate an oily scalp—one that needs frequent shampooing.

Normal hair has a certain amount of oil that keeps the hair glossy and the scalp comfortable. But excessively oily hair quickly becomes limp; the strands separate and refuse to hold a curl. Dirt is readily picked up from the air and held by the oil.

Shampoo oily hair twice a week or oftener, even daily to keep down oil.

Wrap your hairbrush in bandaging gauze—it will absorb oil—and brush the hair nightly to remove the excess oil.

A clear medicated lotion, such as is used for oily facial skin, keeps the scalp fresh between shampoos.

Is your hair hard to manage? Does your hair have a mind of its own—refuse to settle into the style you choose? Then your hair is probably wiry, or resistant. It has a great deal of elasticity and, after setting, quickly snaps back into its own willful ways.

Use hot water on the hair to bring it under control before setting and then use a strong-hold setting lotion. Wind only a small amount of hair on the rollers and set the rollers in the natural direction of hair growth. Allow sufficient drying time for the hair to set thoroughly before brushing.

A good haircut and shaping to follow the natural growth pattern of the hair will help make resistant hair easier to manage.

If you have fought a losing battle with a stubborn cowlick, a curved part is the answer. Choose a hair style that swirls the part through the unruly hair at the back or the top of the head; this will subdue the cowlick and make the hair lie flat. When hair is styled in this way, working with the hair's direction of growth, the hair bordering the part will fit the head snugly and neatly. The curved part should follow the natural contour of the head and emphasize the direction in which the hair tends to fall on both sides of the part.

A permanent wave or a hair straightening of some sections of the hair will sometimes help to bring unruly hair under control.

Is your hair color-treated? Often you have to decide whether or not you are dealing with treated or untreated hair. If you use a semipermanent (or six-week) rinse, a tint, a bleach, or even a rinse that leaves color deposits in the hair, you must consider that you have "treated" hair.

This may mean that you have to choose a shampoo for treated hair, have a conditioning treatment before a permanent, or that you should have a metal-remover treatment before you use a different kind of hair color.

You may also need a special shampoo for color-treated hair and a gentle-type permanent. Be careful in timing of coloring and waving, and protect lightened hair from the color-changing effects of sunlight.

Design your hair style so that roots of tinted or bleached hair will show as little as possible between touch-ups. The two important areas for concealment are the hairline and the part. To conceal roots at the hairline, bangs are the best solution. The bangs should be lifted and brought forward enough to cover the hairline. The trick for concealing the roots at the part is to lift the hair on either side—like a cornfield where you don't see the earth, only waving tassels. To achieve the needed height for concealing roots, set the hair on rollers along the part. A partless hairdo is effective. A full bang and a partless hairdo conceal any dark roots. No permanent is necessary if hair has a slight tendency to curve.

What is the texture? Is your hair strong, heavy? Is a single strand easily visible to the eye? Then the hair is probably coarse. Is hair very light, flyaway, barely visible in a single strand? Then it is fine —or even baby-fine. Often there are both fine and coarse hairs on the same head. The crown and forehead hair is usually coarser than neckline, temple, and sideburn hair. Fine hair is usually more resistant to curl than coarse hair. Fine temple hair, however, may be curly; fine neckline hair is often resistant to curl. Coarse hair will usually take a shorter curling time and longer coloring time than fine hair. Coarse hair grows less thickly than fine hair but may appear thicker because of the heaviness of the individual strands. Blond hair is finest, and there are more hairs per square inch; red is next, and black hair is coarsest. Not all blond hair is, however, fine, nor is all dark hair coarse. Color is, just the same, a clue to texture and can help you determine what treatments your hair needs.

How To Get A Good Haircut

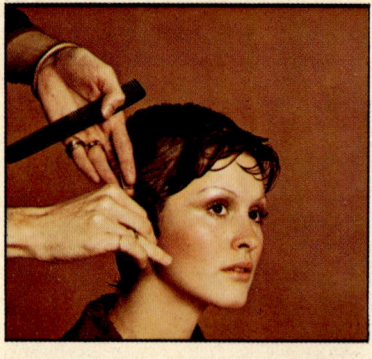 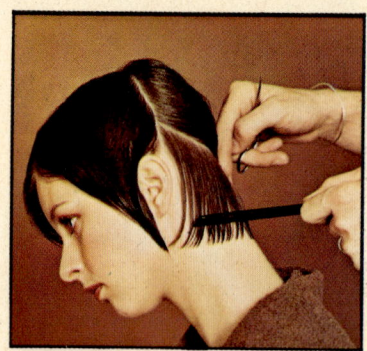
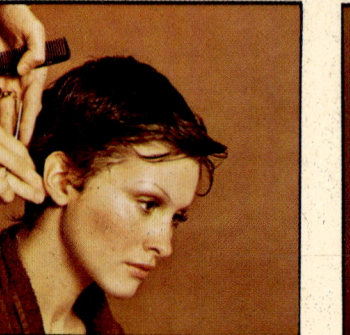 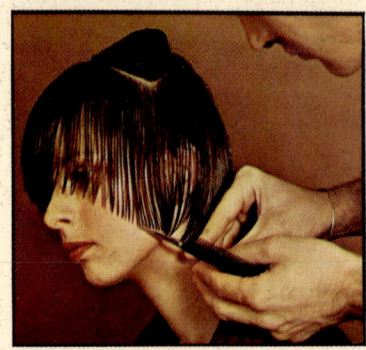
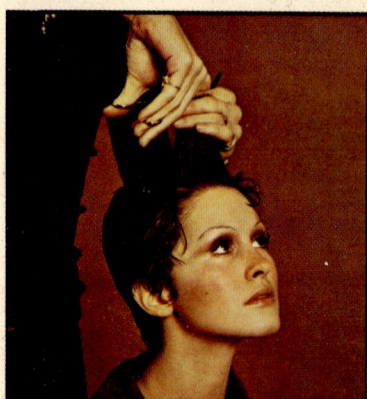 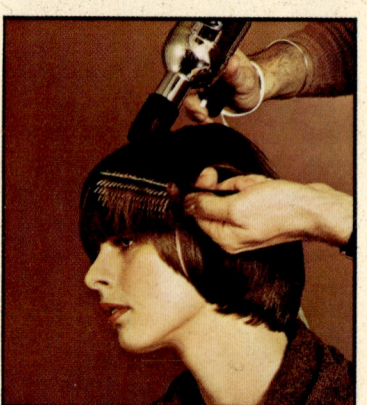
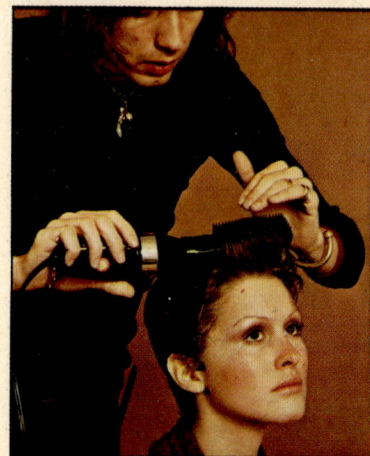 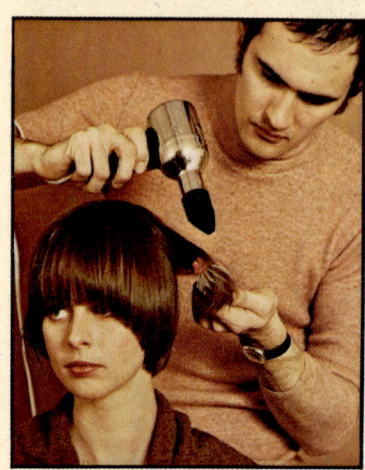

Here is a completely carefree hairdo *(opposite page, and far left)* —one that proves *very* short hair can be sweet and feminine. This hairdo suits the face, the shape of the head and hair texture — fine, very thick and with natural curl. The cutting starts at the crown and works forward and down at sides and back, with wispy softness at the back and enough length at the forehead to be feminine and to give versatility. No-care as well as no-set, the hair can be dried quickly with a drier comb; then the forehead thatch is lifted with a brush and blown dry. The forehead hair can also be set in clip curls.

The bowl cut *(left)* falls beautifully into its shape. Just run a comb through the hair, shake the head, and the style is there again. The cut is the thing: Hair is sectioned and then cleanly and precisely cut in one-inch partings in graduating lengths from the crown so that layer falls on layer to reach the bowl-shape length all around, and the hair is "beveled" all over the head. Naturally, this hair is straight and limp and very fine, with a tendency to be oily and with no lift of its own at the crown. The cut gives the lift and width needed for the face. Hand-drying the hair layer by layer adds body and bounce, but just blowing the hair dry after a shampoo and combing into place is enough "maintenance" if the hair is cut perfectly to begin with. Well-cut hair has visible style even when the hair is wet.

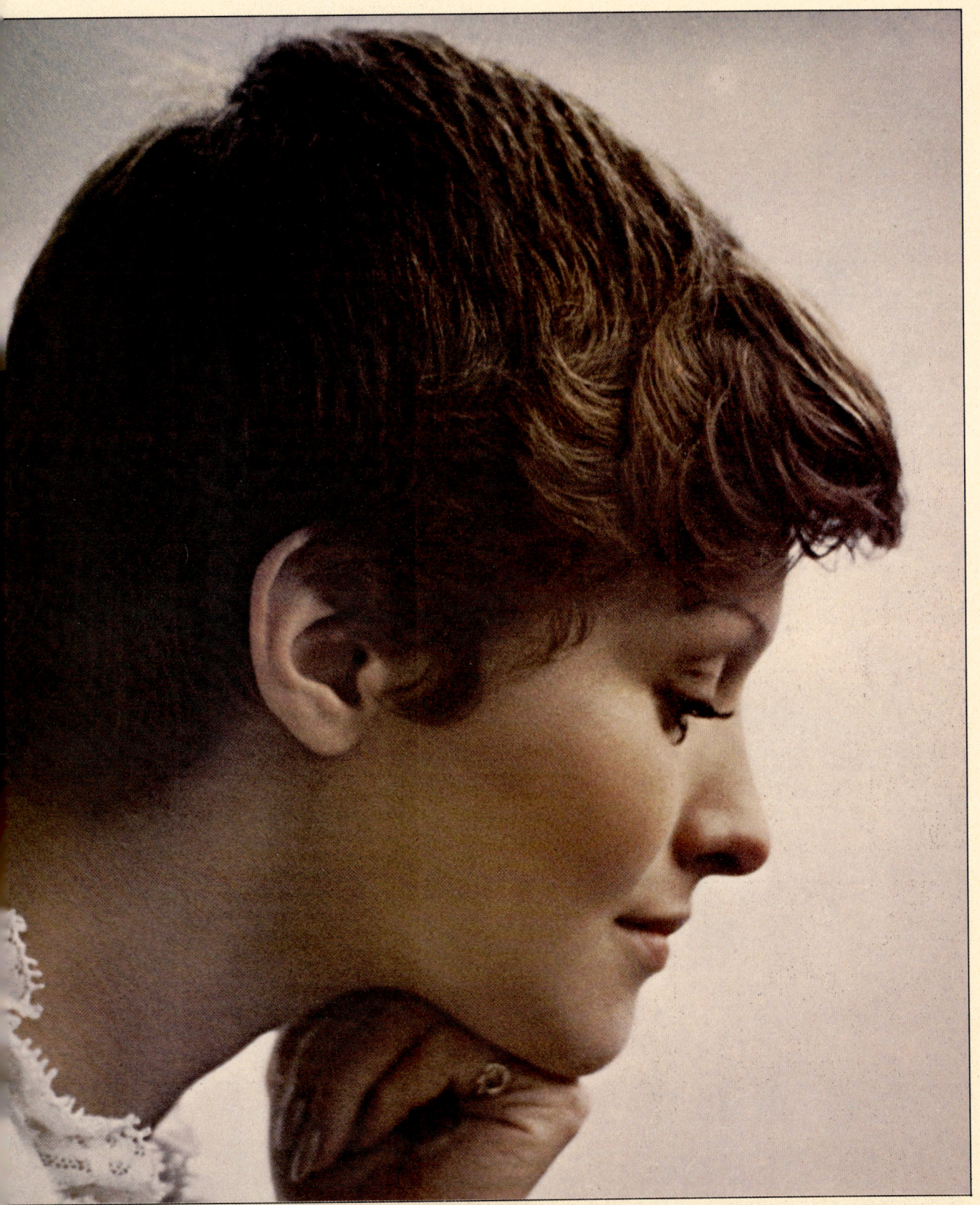

The way your hair is cut is basic to your hair style. A good haircut helps a style keep its shape and leaves the hair easy to set; the style falls naturally into place after brushing; there are no sharp points, unwanted bulk, or thin spots. Luckily, most women today can find a shop with a stylist who is a specialist in haircuts that can be washed and hand-dried and look just wonderful. Such a haircut has to be coordinated with the way the hair grows and with its texture—whether it is coarse, fine, curly, straight, has bounce or is limp is oily or dry—and also with the shape of the head, the ears, the neck, the face, even with your figure and style. Says Roger Thompson, artistic director for Vidal Sassoon International: "Hair should be easy to care for. Once cut, it should fall into place of its own accord, with very little coaxing and finishing. But to have this, the cut has to relate to hair texture—that's the secret.

"You can't just see a picture of a hairdo you like and then hope to have exactly the same thing. You may not have the kind of hair or even the face or figure for it. The cut always is individualized.

"Often the kind of no-set haircut the stylist can do for you is not one you really want. Some women are not ready for too much individuality. It's a psychological matter. Sometimes a new hairdo calls for a whole new style—and not everyone is ready to change. What suits you and your type of hair best just may not make you happy.

"When you go for a haircut, talk to the stylist first and find out what he can do for you and whether you want to go along with his suggestions. Just realize that he can do much to change your look—but you can't do much to change his ideas. So it's important to find someone who is doing the kind of haircuts you like and then to ask him what kind of a style would work for you. Then you can decide if it's all right with your idea of yourself.

"When you get a good haircut, it should need a trim only about every six weeks—and it probably won't look its best the first time till about three weeks after it's cut. If the haircut is right, it won't need a lot of finishing work. Shampoo, towel-dry and then finish drying with a hand-drier or drier-comb."

⁂ Cutting in layers helps develop a natural wave or curl; if you do not have a permanent, cutting in layers will help the setting to last longer and also will permit the hair to be puffed to give height.

⁂ Fine hair should never be thinned; it should be blunt-cut to hold its body and is best cut after it has been set on rollers, and dried.

⁂ Thick hair should be blunt-cut for the best length to mold hair to head.

⁂ Spongy, or porous, hair should be cut with a razor.

⁂ Permanented hair should be cut while wet and should be cut again as it is taken out of the rollers.

⁂ Long hair should be cut to fall all one length and then layered a little at the ends for a natural-looking line and free movement.

The layered cut. A layered cut is used for lifted hairdos, for hair that is to be permanent waved and especially for hairdos that are to be set weekly in a beauty salon. Hair is cut throughout the styling, shaped before the shampoo, and after the shampoo. While the hair is wet, it is molded to the contour of the head; after the hair has been set in rollers and dried, each lock is trimmed as it is combed so that each layer holds its place.

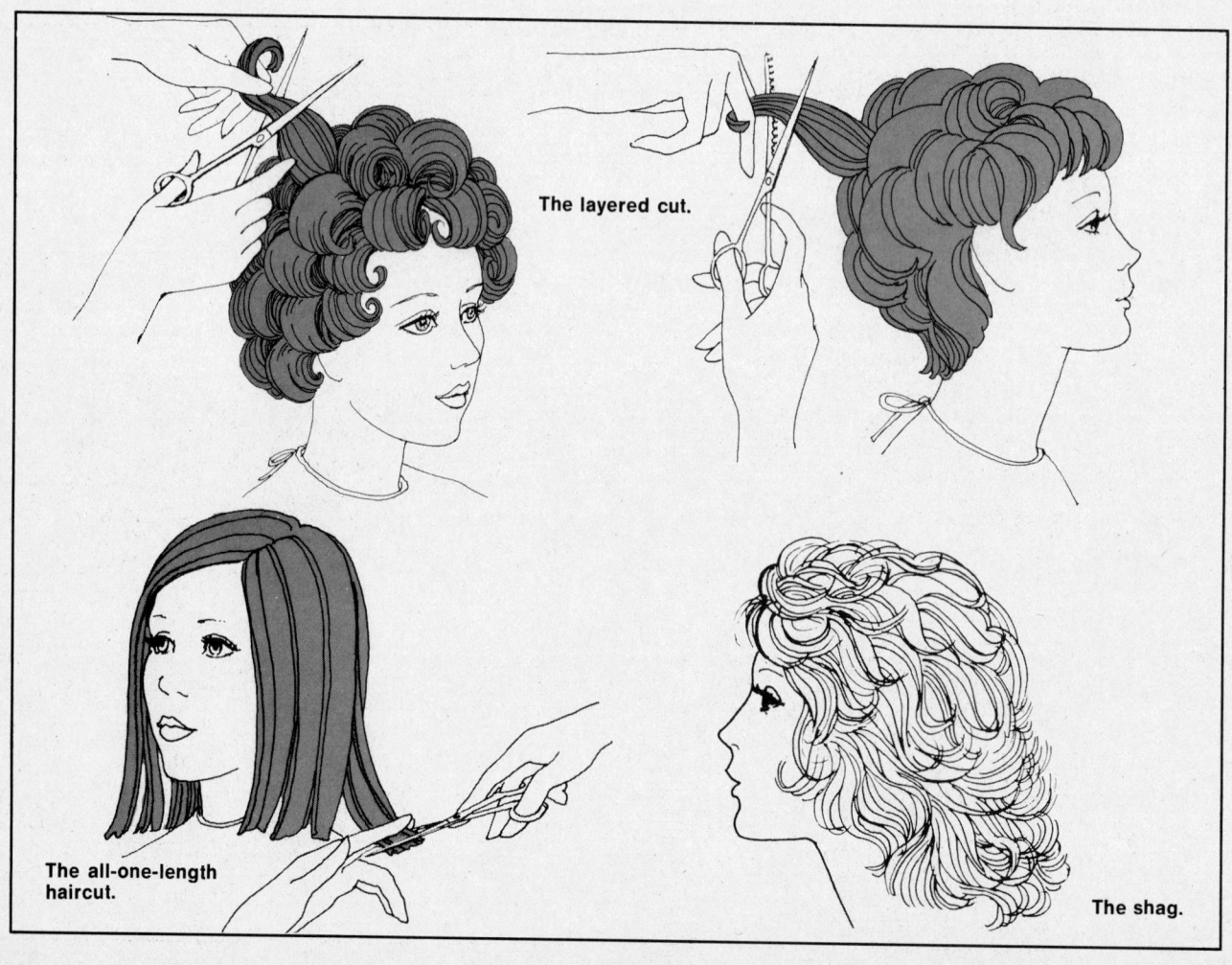

The layered cut.

The all-one-length haircut.

The shag.

✄ Rollers are removed from hair, and each curl is individually cut before brushing. Ends are first cut blunt, starting at the top and going all around the head.

✄ Each lock is measured by eye before cutting so that length will be about two and a half inches, except at the nape where hair is tapered to an inch or less.

✄ Each lock is then thinned at the ends so that it will lie in place firmly.

✄ Bangs, when cut, should reach below the eyebrows so that the hair springs back to a becoming length. Bangs are cut and thinned, as is the rest of the hair, to keep them light and slightly uneven.

✄ At the nape, hair is thinned to hug the back of head and nape. Hair is shorter here than on the rest of the head, and the shape at the back is gently rounded.

✄ Hairline is trimmed so that it looks neat, but it should still be somewhat irregular to appear easy and natural when combed.

The shag. The simplest and most beautiful form of the shag (uneven hair lengths) can be achieved with one snip of the scissors or slash of the razor—if the hair is long enough to be completely combed forward from nape to forehead and brought into one shank in front of the forehead. A rubber band is wrapped around the carefully combed shank and the hair sharply cut off just behind the band so the hair that remains falls to uneven lengths all over the head—longest at back and the bangs of proper length. The shag can also be achieved by layered blunt cutting.

The all-one-length haircut. For most down hairdos, smooth hairdos, and long loose hair, and for styling versatility, the all-one-length haircut is desirable. Hair is cut while still wet after the shampoo and then is further trimmed and shaped during the combing. The hair has shape, evenness, and graceful movement even when wet. This wet-hair look is one means of judging your finished haircut.

✄ Wet hair is combed down all around and then blocked and pinned into cutting sections. When wet, hair is docile and comes down to its longest length.

✄ Starting at the neckline, hair is blunt-cut at the ends to the desired length. After neck fringe is cut, the stylist works round the head, matching the end length in each section—four to five inches at the crown and about two inches at the neckline.

✄ Hair when trimmed falls to one length all around.

Blunt cut. A basic blunt cut—length a little below the chin, a little longer at back—can be taken care of easily and needs a trim (cheaper than a cut) only once in about six weeks. This cut also makes sense if you're letting your hair grow—it's long enough for a tieback. Add a little hairpiece or a bow—and go! (A layered cut, on the other hand, is often the costliest kind of hairdo. It needs to be reshaped and cut often and probably takes a professional setting to look its best. The layered cut is also chaos to let grow because of the uneven lengths.) Blunt-cut hair can be brush-dried into its own straight-hair style or, when you want more going-places glamour, transformed into a flip with a simple set. Have hair cut from a center part to fall to one length all around (you can change the parting as you choose) for the greatest versatility. This is the ideal cut, too, for letting your hair grow. Note that this is a scissors cut—important if hair is to be straight. The length is just about right for a tieback.

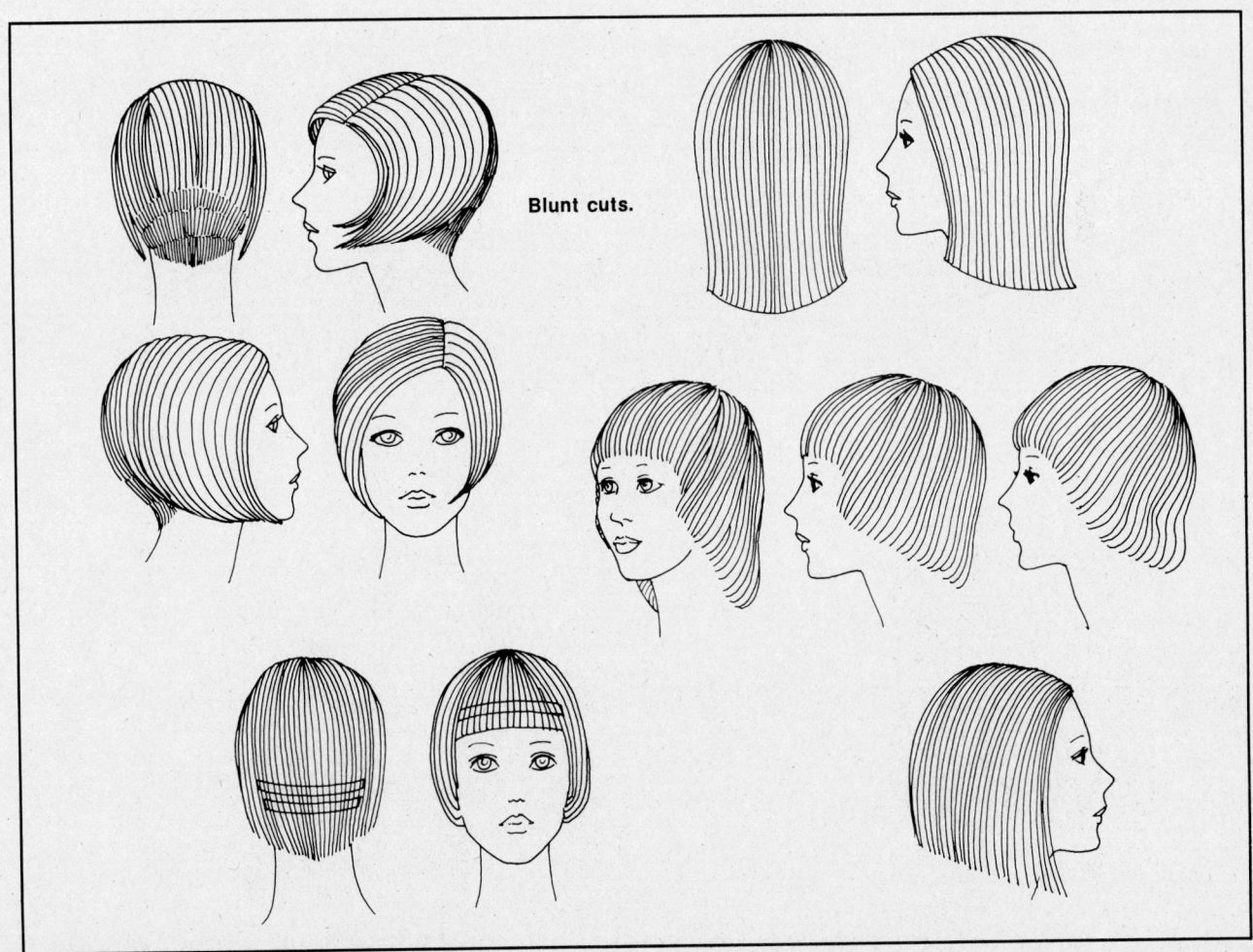

Blunt cuts.

A Hair Style That Becomes You

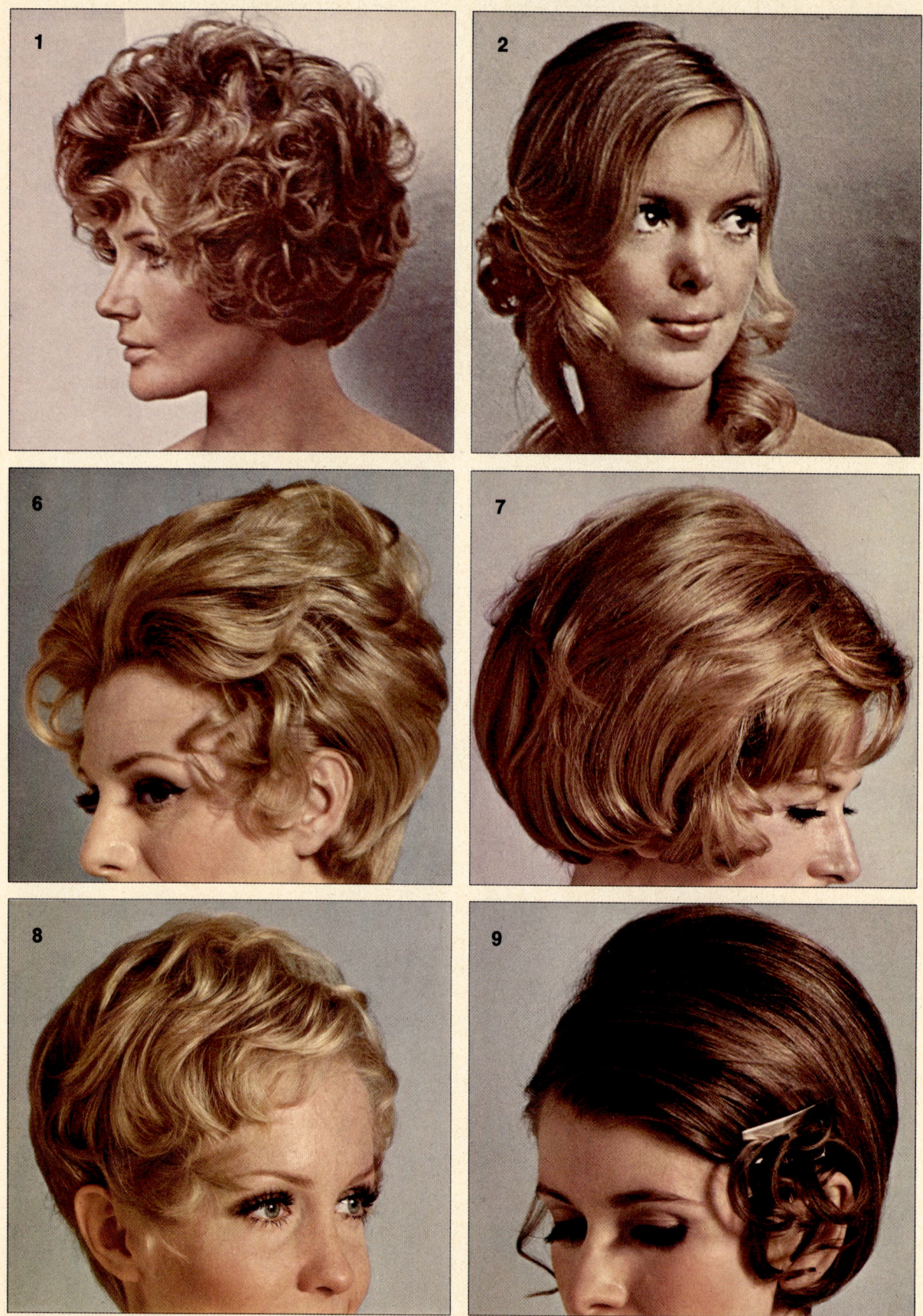

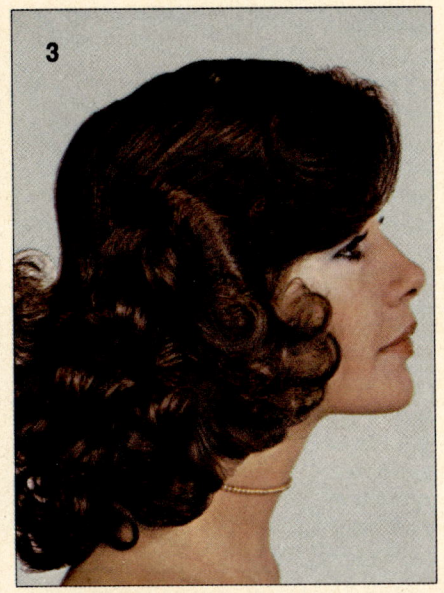
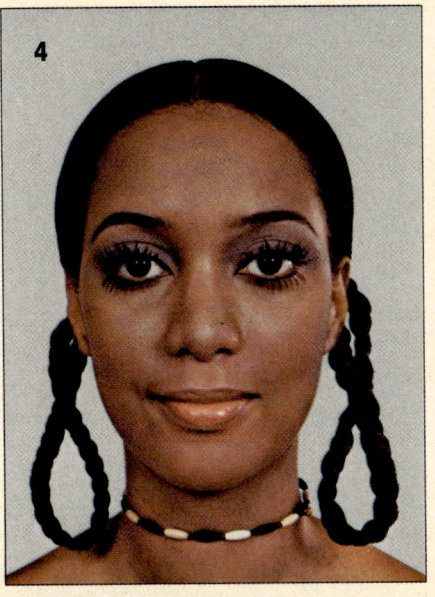
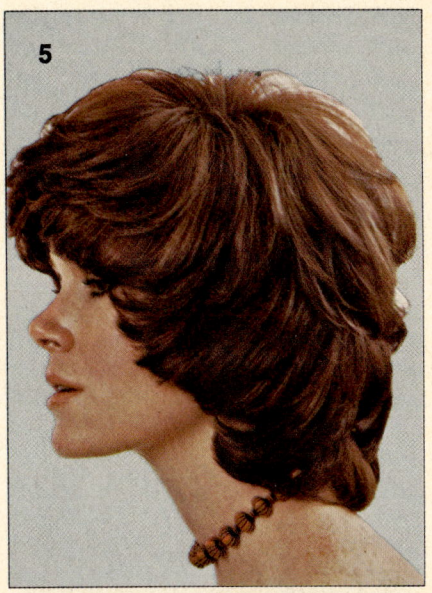
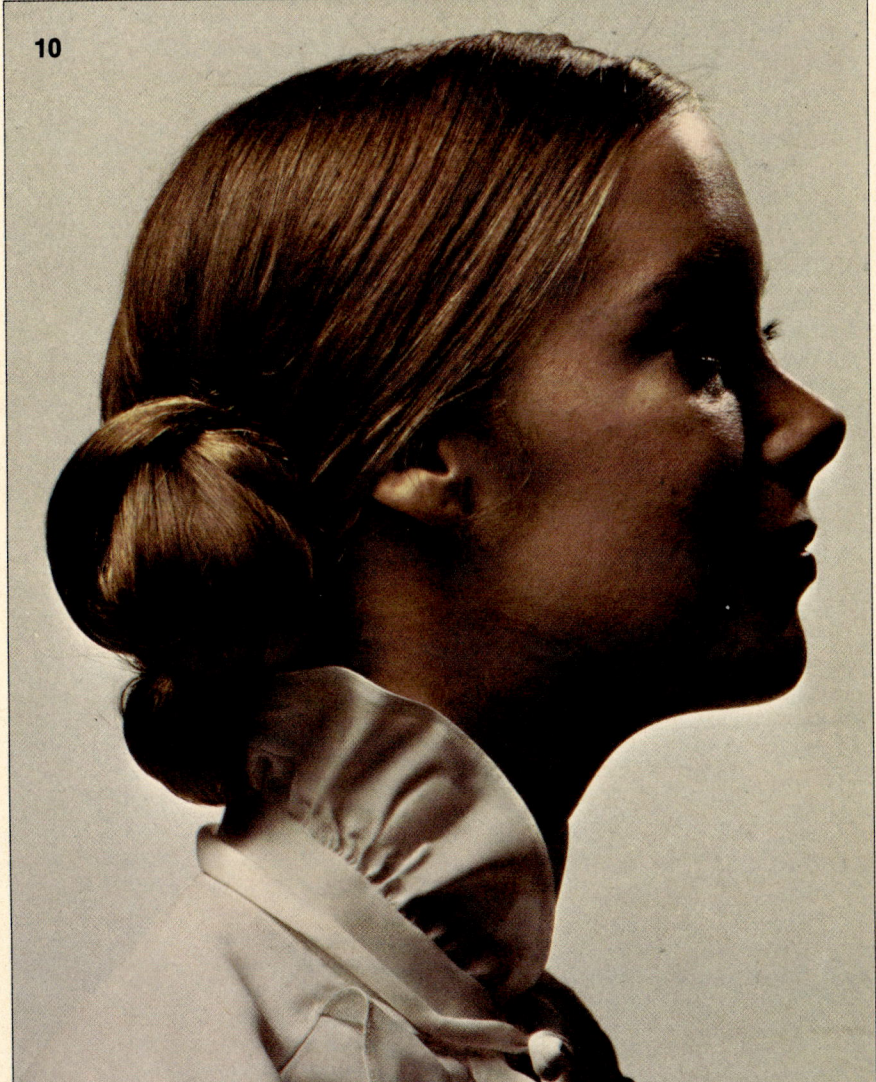
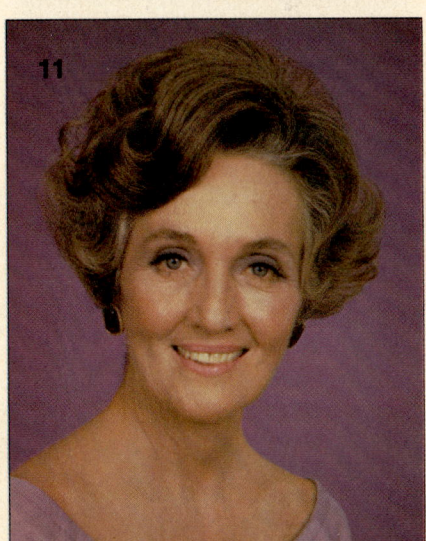
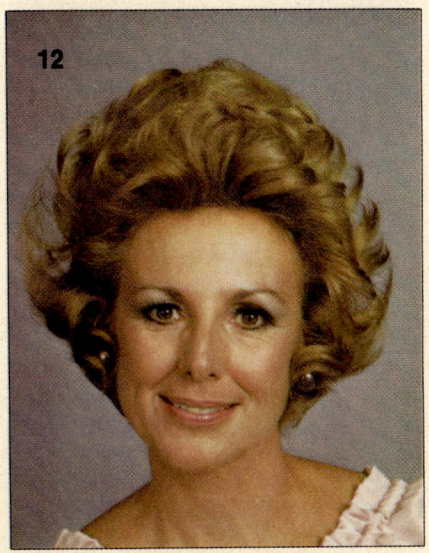

Hairdo how-tos on following pages

HOW-TOS FOR PAGES 12 & 13.

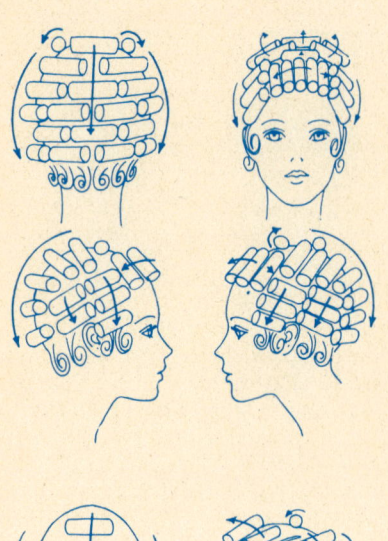

1. Tomboy or angel? You can be either or both with ringlets. Curls bounce up from a short side part and you comb your hair with your fingers when you can't find a comb. **Cut:** Hair is blunt-cut to fall about one length—4 to 5 inches at jawline, a little longer at sides and nape than at top. **Set:** Dime-size rollers are set in a stagger pattern all over the head. **Comb-out:** Brush the hair well from the side part to mesh the set into waves, and then break up with the fingers into little all-over-the-head ringlets.

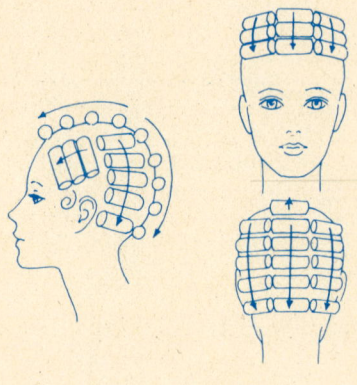

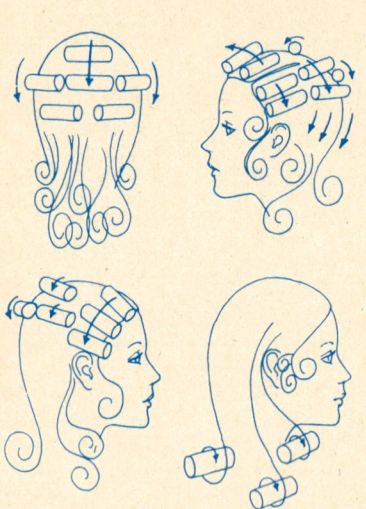

2. A romantic hairdo for hair that is growing out and is of uneven lengths. Pin-on long curls if you haven't enough hair of your own. **Cut:** Nape hair is 7 inches; sides, 5 to 6 inches; back, 6 to 8 inches. No tapering necessary. **Set:** Hand-dry (with a drier comb) and use a curling iron to form side tendrils and nape curls. If fullness is needed, set crown in small to medium curlers, tendrils and ringlets in pin curls. **Comb-out:** Brush back and side-part; tie back loosely, leaving some nape hair to shape into ringlets to fall over the shoulders. Top hair is combed down in a little bang at front and toward the ears on each side, with soft curls over the cheeks.

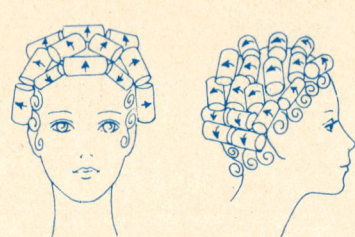

3. Young and romantic—this lots-of-curl hairdo is pretty for party-going. **Cut:** Hair is shoulder-length at back, tapered to chin length at sides. Blunt-cut with layering at the ends, side and back. **Set:** Set in medium rollers from side part. **Comb-out:** Brush all hair back to form waves at front and crown. Then brush down from side part into a forehead wave. End hair is separated into ringlets with brush and fingers.

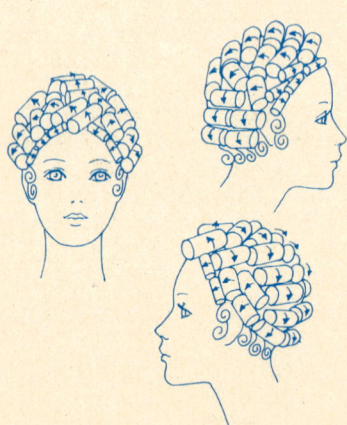

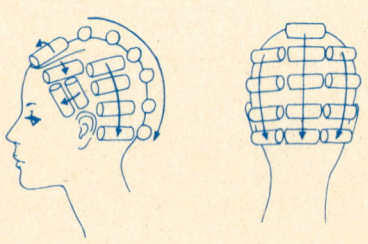

4. Skinny pigtail braids—your own or pin-ons—are neat for daytime and striking enough for evening wear. This style can be done with hair of any length. If long enough to form braids, fine. Otherwise, middle part from forehead to nape; pin ends behind ears and attach shaped figure-8 braids.

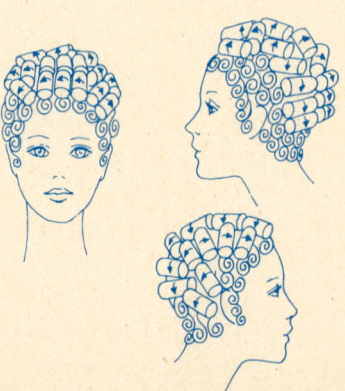

14

5. This shaggy "duster" wears well in the wind—a shake of the head brings it back into shape. **Set:** Set in medium rollers, very close together, forward and down-turning as indicated. **Comb-out:** Brush to reduce curl and then with drier brush or comb, or hand-drier and brush, brush from underneath so that underhair lies flat against face and nape and crown has lift and looseness. Bangs are split for a wispy effect.

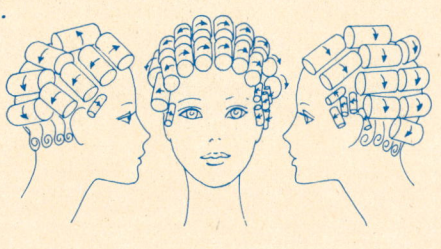

6. A short hairdo with forehead lift, casual and pretty with side curls. **Cut:** Hair is layered to be four inches at top, tapering to nothing at back. **Set:** Set in back-turning rollers, with hair around the face set on clips. **Comb-out:** Hair is brushed back strongly and then touseled by using the fingers as a comb. Side hair is turned into playful ruffles toward the face.

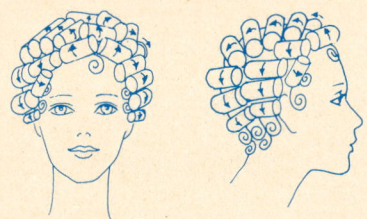

7. A go-anywhere hairdo that needs little care. Well-cut, the hair responds quickly to brush or comb. **Cut:** Blunt cut medium-short hair falls all one length except shorter at front for bangs. **Set:** This is basically a back-and-sideways set; rollers around the face are front-turned. **Comb-out:** Brush out, lifting tendrils of hair from the lines of the style to make soft cross curls. Shape front and side hair softly around the face.

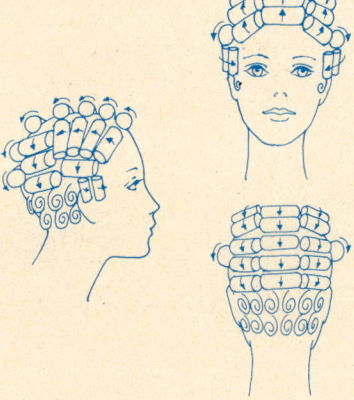

8. For baby-fine hair, a "baby-curl cut" that shows off a well-shaped head, pretty ears. **Cut:** Hair is layer-cut to be one to two inches all over head. **Set:** Short-short hair is strongly set on small-size rollers, with pin curls at the sides and at the nape to turn the hair toward the face. **Comb-out:** Brush; then comb with fingers for an undefined but head-shaping look.

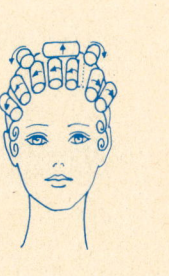 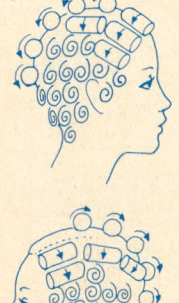

9. A smooth cap hairdo. **Cut:** Hair is medium-length, blunt cut. **Set:** Set on rollers, with the sides on small half rollers. **Comb-out:** Part low on side and comb back behind the ears. Lift side ruffles separately with brush.

10. Side-swept chignon. **Cut:** Hair that is shoulder length or longer works well. **Set:** Set in large rollers and clip curls. **Comb-out:** Part hair on the side, and comb or brush it smoothly and close to the scalp. Catch into a ponytail at back, keeping it low and slightly toward the ear on the side opposite the part. Fasten with elastic band. Separate the ponytail into three sections. Loop first section and pin above the fastening; wrap second section around the first; loop third section and pin below fastening.

11. A halo of delicate curls softens and frames the face. **Cut:** Short (four-inch) layered hair. **Set:** Medium-size rollers with dime-size rollers above the ears and pin curls at bottom back. **Comb-out:** Brush hair back; lightly back-comb top; then brush all hair away from face at top and sides, breaking the set into a halo of soft curls with the hands. Where needed, open ends of curls with fingers and lift lightly with the tip of a brush.

12. Soft lines and uplift are becoming in this side-swept hairdo with deep forehead wave and end curls. **Cut:** Hair is layered—about three inches long at the crown to an inch at the nape. **Set:** Medium-size rollers and pin curls. **Comb-out:** Brush hair back all around to reduce curl and form the setting into waves. Bring top hair slightly over the forehead in a deep wave. Comb down back hair to lie smooth against the neck; brush side hair away from the face and feather the tips.

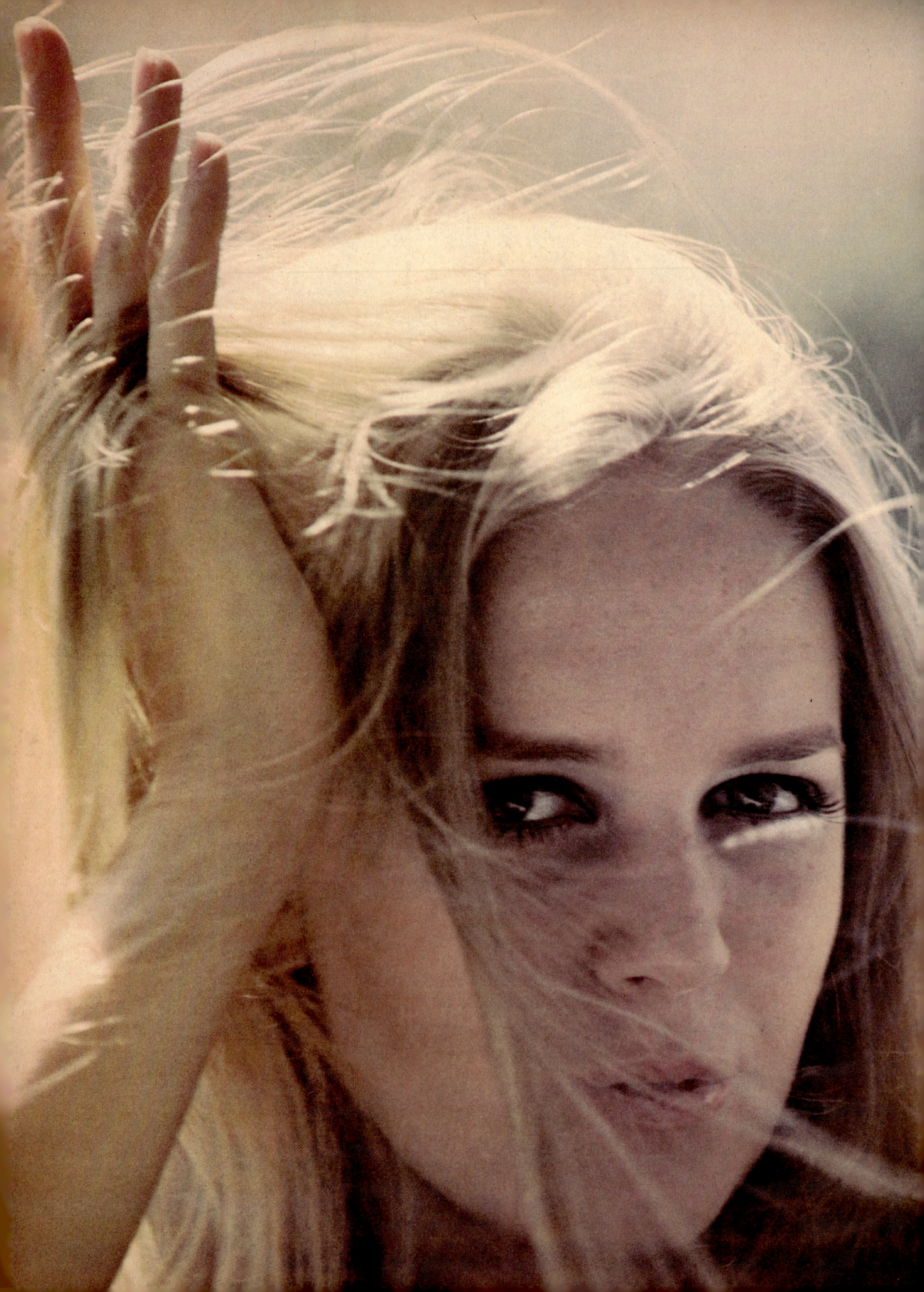

Grooming Your Hair

Brushing grooms the hair, cleans away flecks of lint, dust, and dandruff, smooths the hair into the lines of the style and meshes the strands, and distributes the natural oils. Brushing the hair after its setting is a key to a style that falls beautifully into line and holds the set well and shows no mark of the curlers. Use the brush, too, for any teasing or back-combing.

❧ The brush should have smooth bristles that will not injure the scalp or shred the hair—long bristles for long hair and shorter bristles for short and medium-length hair. When brushing, take care to keep the brush *in the hair;* do not strike the scalp with the bristles.

❧ Wash brush and comb at each shampoo but do not use a damp brush or brush the hair when it is damp.

How to brush. To stimulate the scalp, lean forward and brush against the direction of hair growth from back to front.

❧ Always brush *away* from the scalp—up and out at the back of the head, up and out at sides, and up and out at front (or from front to back).

❧ Next, brush the hair in sections, lifting a section of hair away from the scalp, brushing the strand up and out, and then repositioning it and going on to the next strand.

❧ The wrist should move with a slight twist so the brush rolls through the hair, but take care not to snarl the hair in the brush.

How to comb. Combing removes snarls and grooms the hair, is useful in arranging the hair style and keeping it in place and for parting and sectioning. Do not overcomb the hair; comb it only enough to keep it smooth and well groomed. In styling, the more you use the brush instead of the comb the softer your style will be.

❧ Use a comb with smooth rounded teeth that will not scratch the scalp or tear the hair. A rattail comb is useful in hair arrangement and setting.

❧ Start combing at the ends of the hair (this is particularly important when the hair is damp after the shampoo or has been back-combed), about two inches above the tip. When the ends are free of snarls, move backward along the strand an inch or two and comb through to the ends, repeating till the entire strand is combed. Comb the hair in sections, finishing one section before moving on to the others.

❧ Keep your comb clean—and keep it personal.

How to back-brush. Teasing—back-combing or back-brushing—should be done only at the roots, where hair is new and strong, and teased roots should not be visible in the finished style. Once scalp hair is back-combed to give a lift, ends should be smoothed over the back-combing so there is a light airy look.

❧ Take care when combing hair that has been teased. Do not place brush or comb at the roots. Instead, take the hair strand by strand, and comb out ends, working back through the length of the strand inch by inch till comb runs freely through the strand.

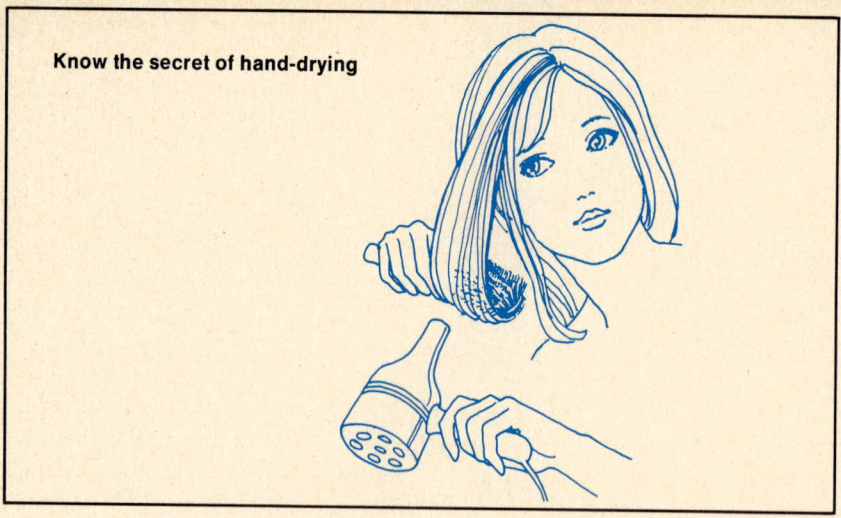

Know the secret of hand-drying. What's very great about blunt-cut hair is that you don't have to set it after you wash it; instead, shape it by drying with a hand hair drier. Just use the drier and keep putting the brush through the hair till it is completely dry. You have a straight hairdo with a very smooth look. If you want fullness and turned-under ends, shape the hair by brushing from underneath as you dry. Takes a little practice, but you soon learn.

For hand-drying, you need a drier with enough blowing power to do the job well. The more power it has, the less heat is needed. This means that the drier need not be held very close to the hair, and there will be less heating of the hair. Too much heat is not good for hair. Rolling the brush through the hair from underneath while you dry gives lift and body. Keep the brush moving so you don't overdry any one section.

Hair driers. A hair drier saves you time, in your hairsetting and, if not used for too long a time, at a very high heat, or too frequently, it won't harm your hair. You can, of course, just set your hair damp and go about your work till your hair dries at room temperature, but leaving rollers in the hair for too long a time, especially if they are tightly wound, does the hair no good either. Both driers on a stand and the cap type are effective, so let your experience dictate your choice.

Hand driers, drier combs, and drier brushes are useful for styling as well as for drying. The drier comb works well on short hair; the drier brush—or hand drier used with a hairbrush—is better on longer hair. Work from underneath, layer by layer and do not use too much heat, do not hold the drier too close to the hair, and, treat the hair gently.

SECRETS OF THE COMB-OUT

If you use a drier, dry the hair on moderate, not high heat. If you let your hair dry in air, remove the curlers as soon as ends are dry. Hair must dry evenly and thoroughly for the set to take properly. Remove curlers gently so as not to tear or to snarl the hair and test ends to be sure they are dry.

✤ Let hair set a few minutes before brushing. Then brush hair back firmly all around, turning hair under at the nape. Brush gently but firmly and do not be afraid you will take out the set. The brushing makes the set last and removes the marks of the rollers.

✤ After brushing, start with the top and place the hair into the sections that create the style. Pin sections into place and then arrange the ends.

✤ If you want ends to flip up, place a hand over bottom hair and brush the hair up over the hand; if you want hair to turn under, place a hand under bottom hair and brush the hair down over the hand.

✤ Brush top hair into place.

✤ Use the brush and fingers to lift feathery ends, to place side or forehead curls, or to make wispy bangs.

✤ Spray lightly to hold the hair style. Too much spray can straighten curl.

✤ Spray can be used to tack forehead and side curls and bangs and to control wispiness.

✤ Keep any parting in the hair indefinite unless a clean line is called for.

To revive a set. Hair spray can also be used in the comb-out or to revive a style.

✤ To give fluff to the hair, spray it lightly and lift side hair with a brush; hold the hair up and fluff hair down over ear. Spray again to hold.

✤ To build up forehead hair, spray hair lightly and then gently back-brush the hair section by section near the roots. Brush hair back and then respray to hold.

✤ To give a gentle lift all round the head, spray hair lightly and then section by section lift the hair up with the brush with a rolling motion; then roll into a side movement or back flip. Spray again to hold.

✤ To lift side hair all around, slightly ruff, or back-brush. Then smooth hair down and spray.

✤ To smooth the back, spray lightly across the nape hair. Place brush at neckline and brush ends up in choppy little strokes; do the same at sides. Then brush down and spray.

How to make a French twist. The French seam, or twist, is useful in many up hair styles.

✤ Brush hair back and up so that it is massed at the crown and then part the hair at middle back from crown to nape.

✤ Take right half of hair and fasten it with a rubber band about midway up the head.

✤ Lift ends of banded section so hair swirls upward and then to the left. Fasten at crown back.

✤ Brush left half of hair smooth and wrap it up and around the banded section, bringing ends up to crown.

✤ "Lace" left section over right section with invisible hairpins to form a seam.

✤ Brush ends of both halves together so they cover band.

✤ Brush in wisps at back and neckline and spray to hold.

NO-SET HAIRDOS

Windblow. Wind and rain can't upset this hairdo with its own natural wind-swept look. Layered (but not a shag), it lifts to frame the face and has thickness at the back, where it is needed for balance. Hair like this—coarse and straight—has to be cut in a way that gives body. The front is short enough to be lifted by hand-drying and to hold its shape. Finished, it has the roundness, softness and fullness needed to balance the features and width of the shoulders.

Cap cut. This round "cap" hairdo is short and sleek but has body and movement and can be shaken into shape. Hair is fine and very straight; cutting it to fall more or less to one length all around gives the needed body. The roundness, with hair brought over the wide cheeks and forehead, flatters a square face. The back is cut close to the nape and layered toward the crown to conform to the shape of the head. Brushed forward and then hand-dried with brush and drier layer by layer, the hair falls like a cap.

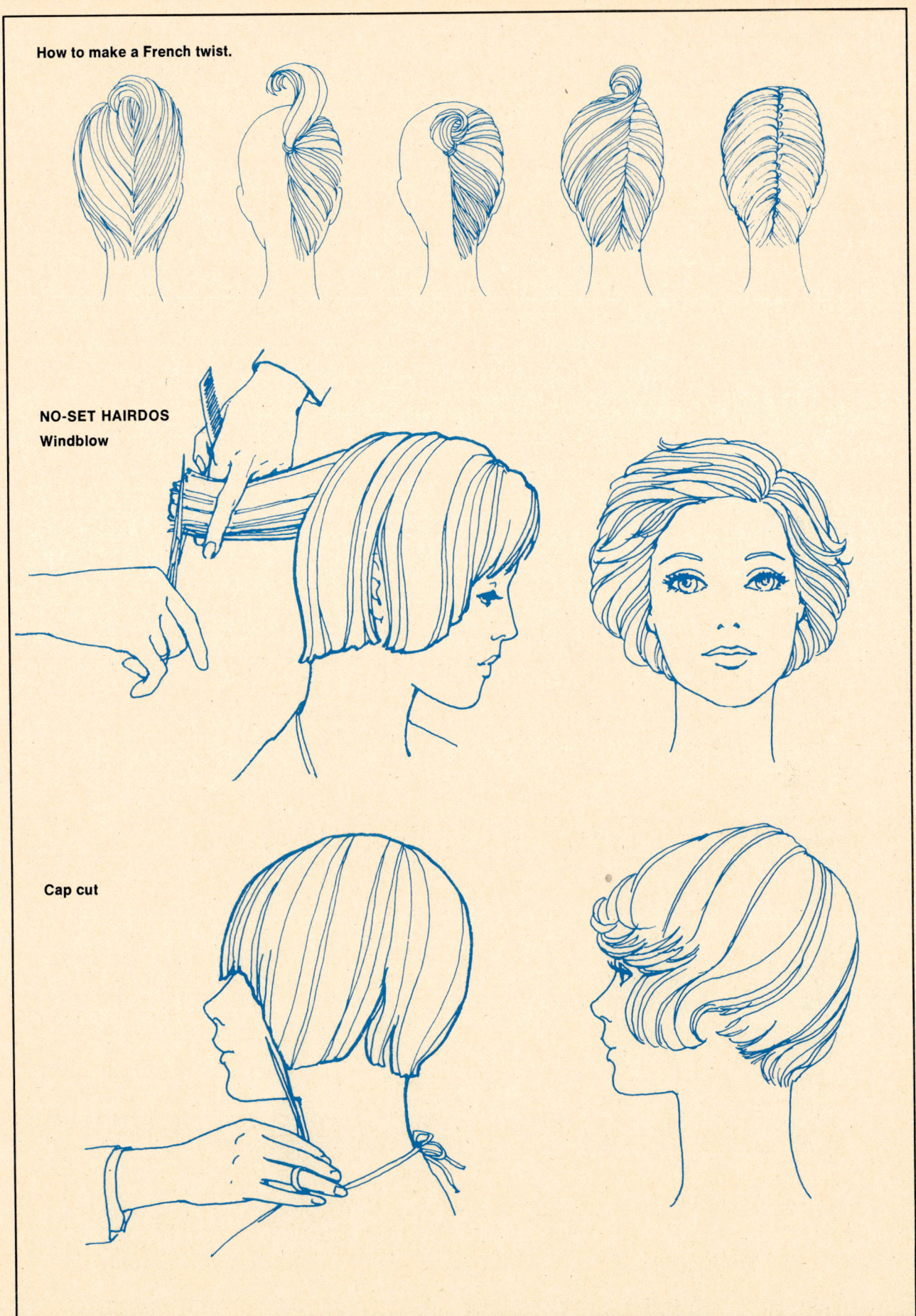

WHAT LENGTH IS YOUR HAIR?

Finding the right length for your hair for a style, for your face, and for fashion means you are sometimes letting it grow. When a short haircut is growing out, the hair often seems to be a mass of jagged awkward ends. This is because hair grows at an irregular rate—no two hairs grow at the same speed. To hide irregular lengths, the hair should be trimmed every three to six weeks to keep its shape. Here is a guide to hair length:

Short hair—This means *really* short, under four inches at the crown, two inches at sides and back, and an inch at the bottom, tapering to nothing at the neckline. This short hair should be cut to a length that will catch the natural wave of the hair and will follow the direction of the growth of the hair. Very short hair needs frequent trims—every three to four weeks.

Medium-short—This is four to five inches at the crown, tapered to about ear-tip length at the sides. Trim every four to six weeks.

Medium—Hair is cut five to seven inches all over the head (two inches at nape) and falls to a length just below the chin line. Trim every four to six weeks.

Medium-long—Hair falls to an inch or two above the shoulders. Trim in five to six weeks.

Long—Shoulder length or longer; long hair can be done up, and any length that can be pinned up can be considered *long* hair. Even long hair should be shaped and trimmed to avoid split ends and too much heaviness. Trim every six to eight weeks.

Hair grows from one-half to three-fourths inch a month—somewhat faster in summer, making summer a good time to grow a new hair style—but hair usually does not grow longer than four feet. A hair normally falls out when it reaches that length.

LONG-HAIR HAIRDOS

Long hair—even if it is only shoulder length—is versatile; it can be worn

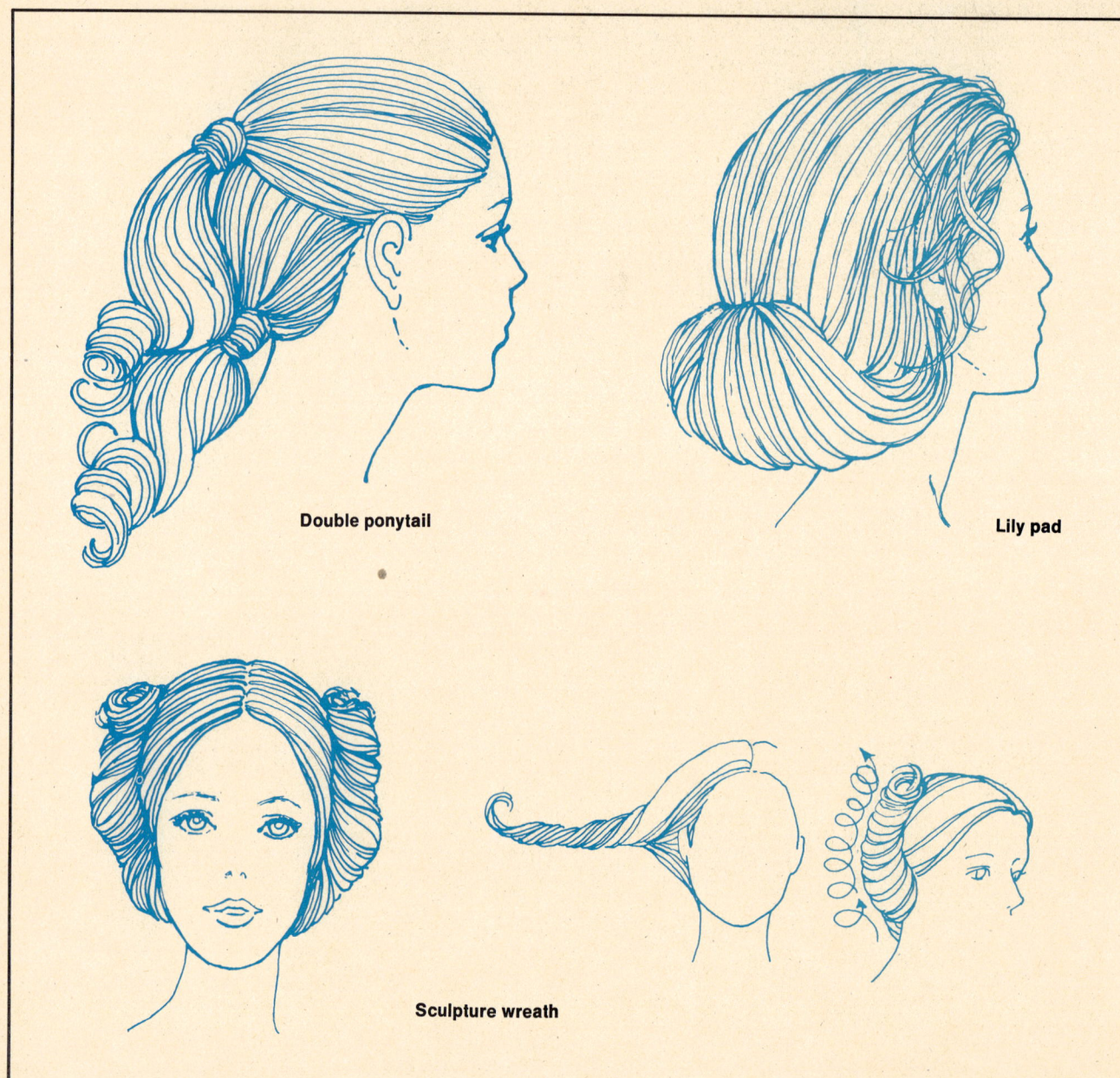

Double ponytail

Lily pad

Sculpture wreath

down, tied back, or put into a variety of becoming styles. Keep ends trimmed for movement and bounce when hair is worn down and slightly feathered to hold an updo.

Start your hairdo by setting the hair in the basic set (see page 30) to give it body and easy handling.

Double ponytail—Wraparound strands hide holder. Ends are twisted to form banana ringlets.

Lily pad—A short full look for long hair. Tie ends, lift, and then pin against the head at lower back.

Sculpture wreath—Middle-parted from forehead to nape, hair is smoothly brushed, coiled and pinned with open ringlet ends.

Oriental elegance—Loosely coiled locks are looped, tied into knots, pinned behind ears. Back hair falls in a bridal-train effect.

Updo—Brush all hair to top of head. Fasten in elastic band at crown back. Do back hair in French twist. Shape ends into large ringlets and place them forward-turning over crown and forehead. Stick-in curls can be added.

HAIRPIECES

A hairpiece is a happy attachment when you have short hair and want a long-hair look, to add to your own long hair, or for a party dress-up. Useful too in summer when you want to pull your own hair back and still look pretty.

How to use a hair piece. Work it into your own hair to give body, height, width, fullness, or to cover loose ends. Attach the woven base of the hair piece firmly to a formation of pin curls; then arrange the style, blending your own hair with the hairpiece hair.

✤ Practical and low-cost are hairpieces of precurled manmade fiber.

Barrette wiglet—Versatile is the short curly wiglet with attached barrette. This little hairpiece also comes without barrette (it can be pinned on) and lends itself to adding your own comb or bow.

Switch or ponytail—Another good addition to a hairpiece collection. This can be worn as an add-on ponytail or braided or looped for use as a chignon.

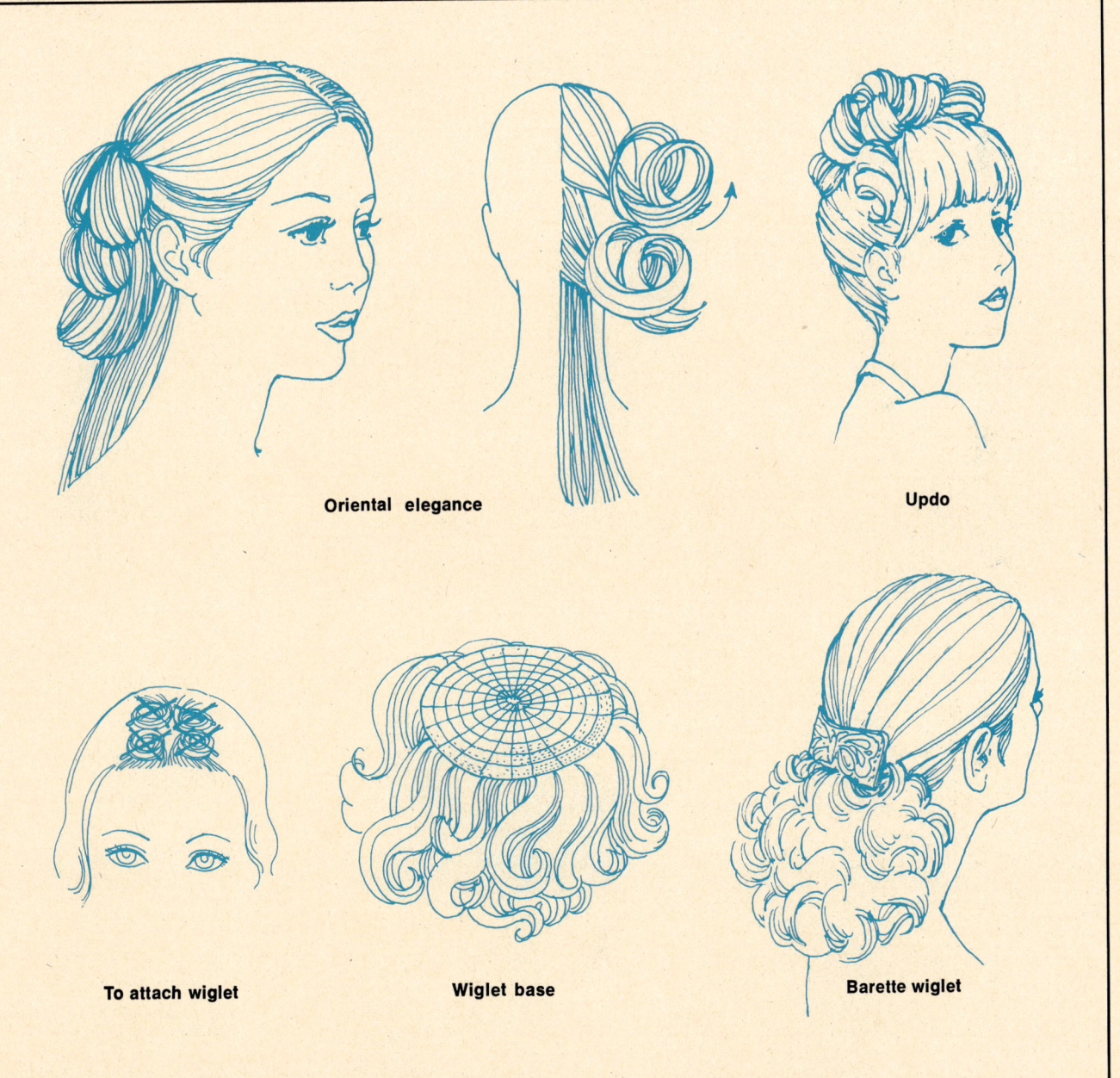

Oriental elegance

Updo

To attach wiglet

Wiglet base

Barette wiglet

21

Fall—Perhaps the all-time favorite; wear it over your own hair or underneath to fill out your hair or reverse and use as a shag.
Chignon—Comes in a variety of sizes (the switch can also be wrapped into a chignon) and can be worn at the back or the top of the head or over one ear.
Braids—These are of assorted thickness and lengths. Some in two or three tones of blond, for example, are excellent add-ons for sports or for parties (add jeweled ornaments here).
Pin-on curls—Tendrils, ringlets, guiches are all helpful hair additions.

Hairpiece hairdos. You will invent many of your own once you have a hairpiece. Here are suggestions to start you off.
Barrette wiglet—Pull all hair to the top of the head and fasten with an elastic band. Clip on hairpiece and brush into curls at the crown.

Pull hair back into a ponytail, fasten with an elastic band, and clip on the hairpiece. Smooth with a brush; the waves fall in naturally without fuss. You can brush and tease the hairpiece to give it a fuller look. It's surprising how big this little piece is when fluffed out.
Braid—Skin hair back and attach a shaped figure-8 braid at crown back.
Fall—A fall is attached at crown. Decorate with a bow or barrette where it joins your own hair.
Braid bow—Make a switch into a big chignon and attach a braid bow.
Switch—Skin hair back and pin or catch in an elastic band. Form one switch into a chignon. Below it attach a ponytail switch and let it fall down your back. Hold it with a decorative ponytail clasp.
Braided chignon—Problem with a chignon is placing it too low on the neck. Keep it high to balance the headshape.

Hairpiece ideas. Use your hairpieces to save your time, your hairdo, your looks.
Active afternoon—A pageboy fall has its own neat trick: Hair ends turn under and are tucked beneath a headband; side tips are pinned under the band.
Hair control in an open car—A chignon of false hair is pinned at back of head over tucked-in natural hair ends.
For cabana, beach, or poolside—A loosely braided switch of false hair is a fun feature and camouflages your own wet locks or lack of curl.
For sightseeing—A short-hair look is created with a round hairpiece pinned to crown back and fluffed into curls.
Daytime shopping—Your own hair in a topknot with a pin-on bun makes you quickly trim.
Cool your summer—A quick groomer that gives splash to your looks is add-on hair—a yard-long ponytail is an instant beauty maker.

WIGS

A wig saves time, money and your own looks in an emergency. Those of manmade precurled fiber are relatively inexpensive, super-easy to care for, and come in a wide choice of styles and colors—including gray and silver and fibers that simulate Black hair. Wigs can give you a change of style, color and length for times when you want to be different, or can be so like your own hair that no one will even ask if you're wearing a wig. Choose a shade slightly

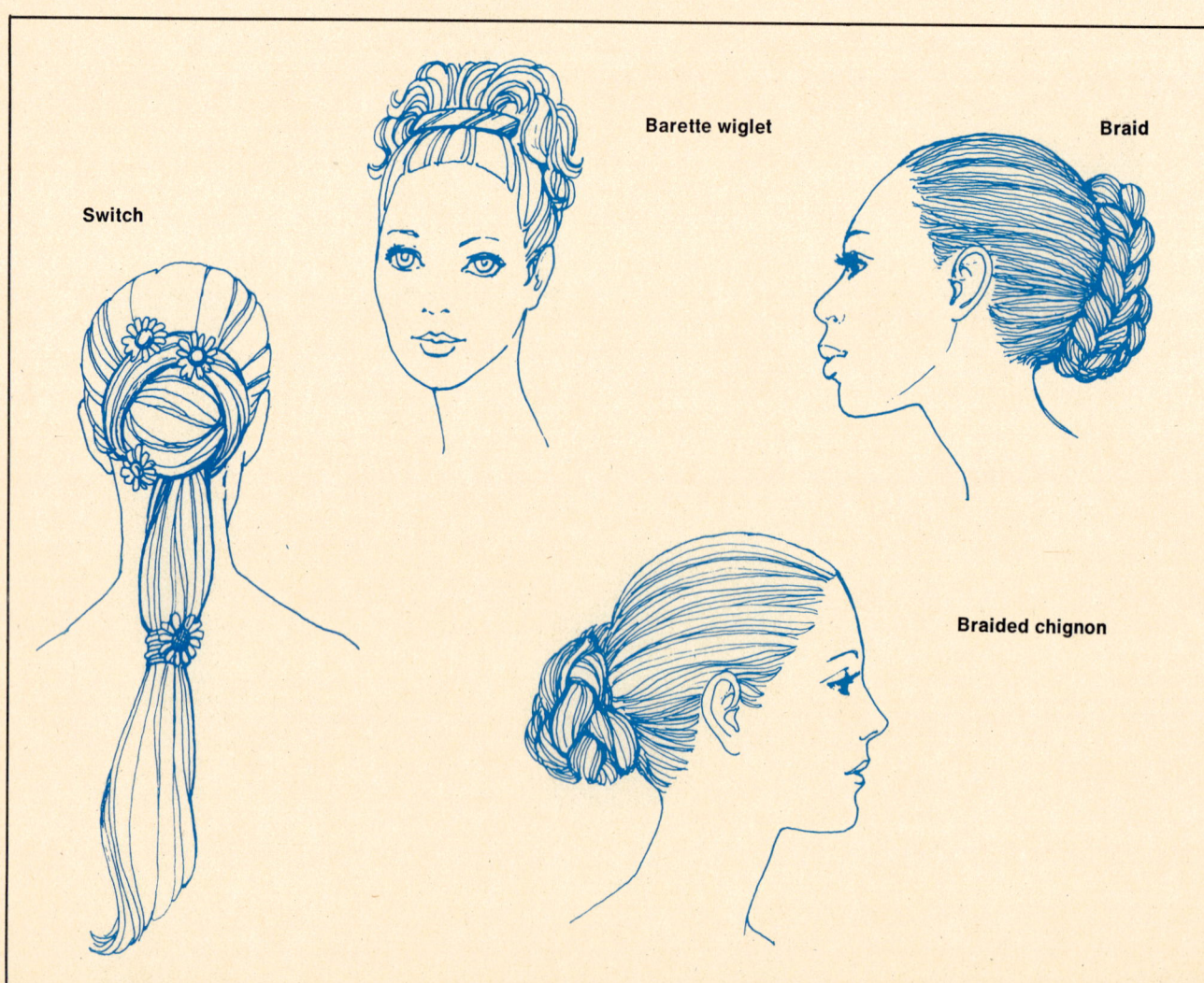

Switch

Barrette wiglet

Braid

Braided chignon

darker than your own hair color so forehead wisps give a frosted effect.

Wigs now are being made with ventilated bases so that they are more comfortable to wear in warm weather; those with the full woven cap do more to keep your head warm when the weather is cold—and so take the place of a hat.

These preset wigs need little care—you can fold them up and put them in a suitcase or a bureau drawer or in a box on your closet shelf. When you are ready to wear your wig, just shake it out, brush into the lines of the style, put it on, and rebrush. You do need a wire-tooth wig brush for grooming and brushing your wig.

Because wig fibers resist soil from the air, you need wash your wig infrequently (even if you wear it a lot). Then just swish it through cool water to which you have added a little mild detergent. Remove from water, shake out excess (do not squeeze) and hang up to dry (a doorknob will do for drying). When completely dry, rebrush. The shape, setting and curl will return. You need not reset or back-comb.

How to choose a wig. All wigs are not alike. There are different fibers that go into different brands and some have an advantage over others in one way, some in another. You will want to seek a wig in a fiber that has a natural look—the look of real hair—without too much gloss and with natural-looking color. Some fibers tend to frizz when exposed to heat (like that from the oven when the door is open); others have overcome that problem.

❧ Examine the base of the wig to see that it is well made. Some fibers are lighter than others; some wigs have more fiber and so are heavier than others. The way the base is sewn and the way fiber is attached to the base should be examined and compared. Check the base carefully to be sure there are no rips or loose or uneven stitching.

❧ Styling and color are very important. Beautiful as a wig may be on its stand, unless it looks well on you, don't buy it. The best way is to try on a variety of styles and shades—take your time to make the right choice. First, find the color and then try for style. The wig should feel comfortable and stay in place over your own hair.

❧ The variation in cost in a wig depends not only on the fiber used but also on the craftsmanship of the wig and the styling and design. Very well made wigs can sometimes be found for a relatively low price in wig-outlet stores when a style has been discontinued.

How to put on a wig. Turn the wig so the base is outside and hold it in one hand with the fingers pinching the center front. With the other hand, swirl your own hair around so that it is all on top of your head, placing the front of the wig against your own hairline and bringing it down over the back of the head (releasing the hand that is holding the hair), and then fit it properly over the ears, tucking in any hair that may be showing. You can, if you prefer, pin your hair up in large pin curls before putting the wig on. With a ventilated wig, you can bring some of your own hair through the open spaces for a varied effect.

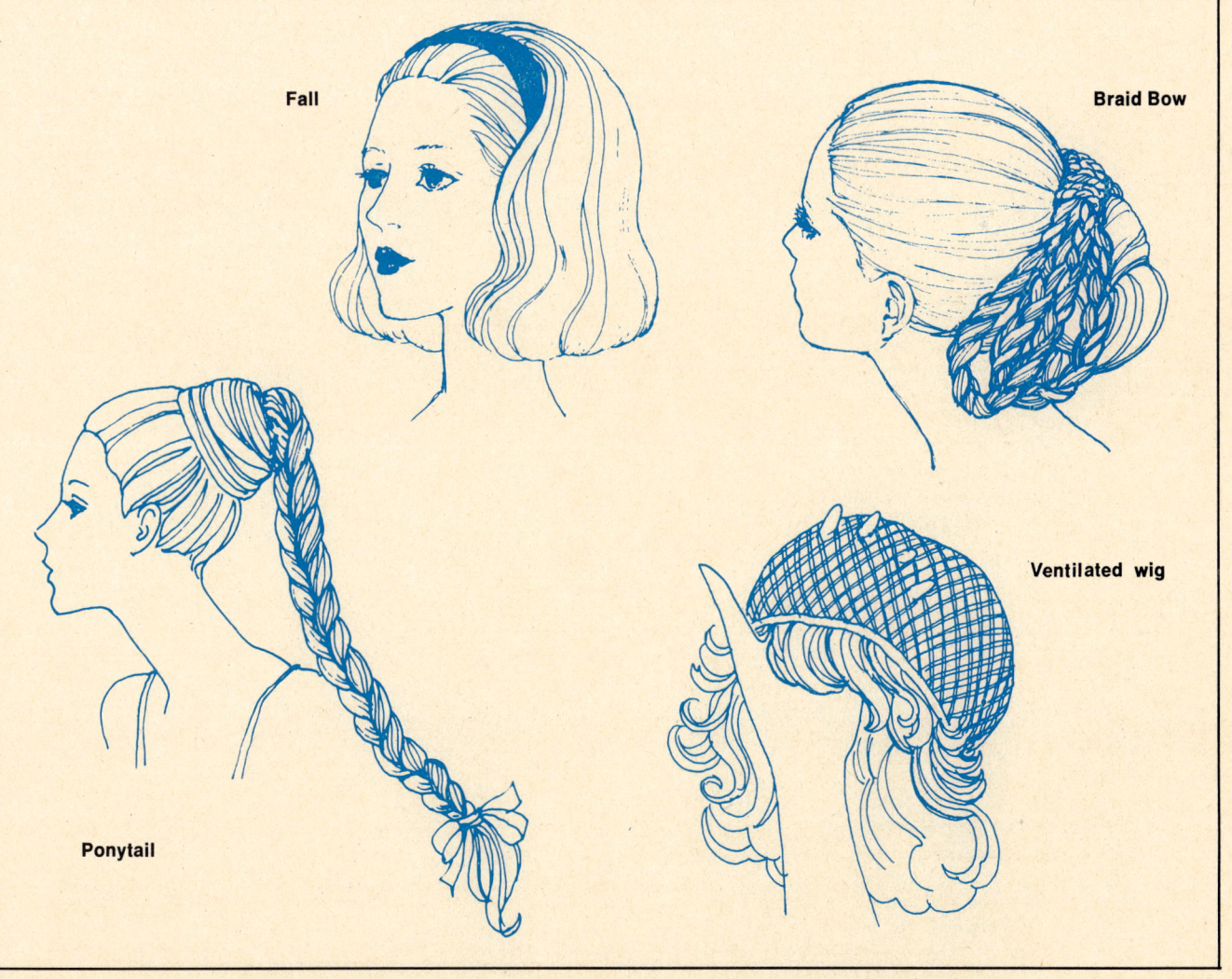

Fall

Braid Bow

Ponytail

Ventilated wig

WHAT IS YOUR FACE SHAPE?

In styling, work with the length of the hair, the direction of line (up, down, or sideways), and the degree of curl or smoothness.

Hair that looks natural and pretty can do much to improve your face shape. But, it should not do away with the distinctive features that individualize you. Some women look most beautiful when they emphasize a distinctive face shape or an irregular feature. Others of us feel happier if our hairdo (and makeup) is somewhat corrective to modify a feature or our face shape.

To analyze your face shape, start with a "naked" makeup-free face. Pull your hair back out of sight, away from your face (put on a high turtleneck to hide your throat if need be) and, looking directly into a mirror, try to visualize the outline—hairline, jaw, chin—as a circle, an oval, a square, an oblong, or a diamond. Realize that many women with an oval face don't seem to identify it; a distinctively square, diamond (wide cheekbones), round, or long face is more easily recognized.

Oval face—A side-parted layered hairdo might be hard to wear except for an oval face—which offers few problems. Form waves on both sides; lift tips of hair with a hairpin to be light and fluffy.

Round face—A middle part is often pleasing with a round face. Bring hair smoothly down and back, covering sides of forehead, cheeks, tops of ears, and pin at crown-back for height; shape ends into curls with tendrils at nape.

Long face—This is an ideal face for a romantic Victorian look—straight wispy bangs, hair puffed for fullness around head and brought down and pinned below the ears; then left loose in a cluster of curls at the neck.

Square face—A full rounded hairdo with flipped-up side sections and the suggestion of a middle part breaks up strong angles and softens a square face. Bring hair close to the head at temples and along the bottom.

Heart-shape face—Side interest in a hairdo—one with a side part, brushed into a soft wave with flip and tendrils—enhances a heart-shape face.

Wide face—A fluffy hairdo with full bangs enlivens a wide face—without being really corrective—and still gives a wholesome look. A layered cut gives the style direction and movement.

Diamond-shape face—Wide cheekbones and a narrow forehead and chin (usually pointed) can appear oval if the side hair is brought over the cheeks; have split bangs of becoming length on the forehead, and below-chin-length hair to give width to this area.

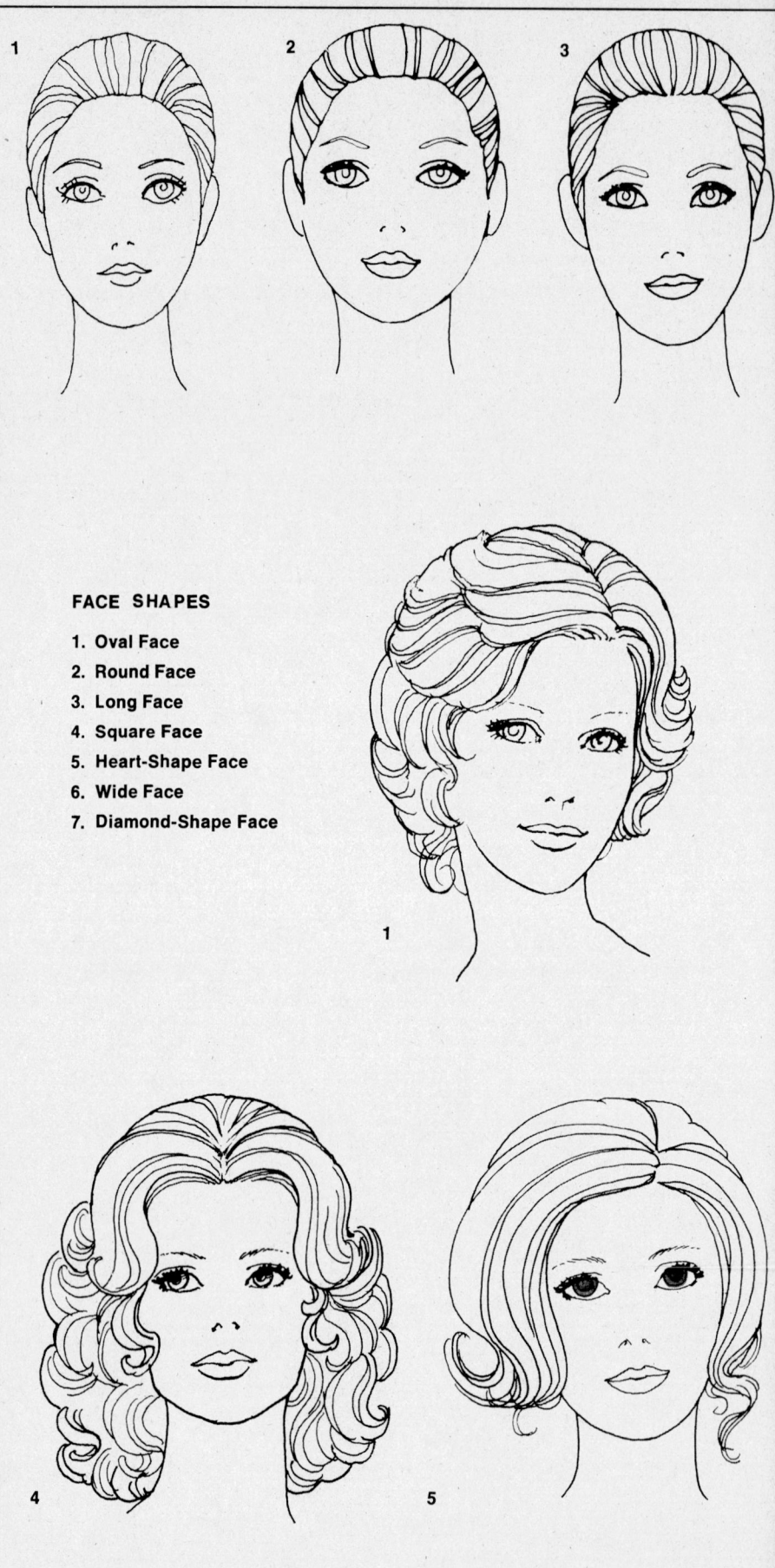

FACE SHAPES

1. Oval Face
2. Round Face
3. Long Face
4. Square Face
5. Heart-Shape Face
6. Wide Face
7. Diamond-Shape Face

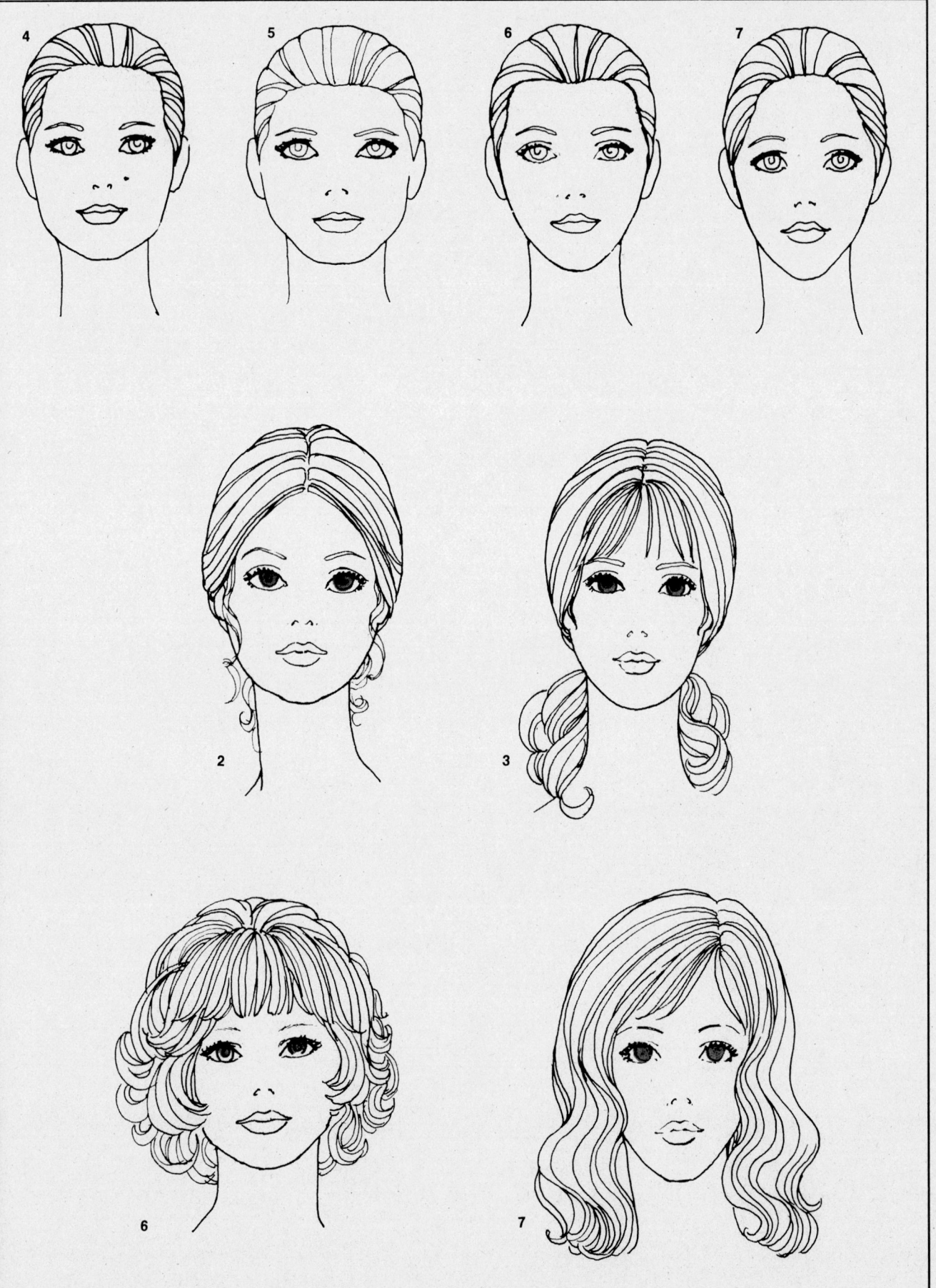

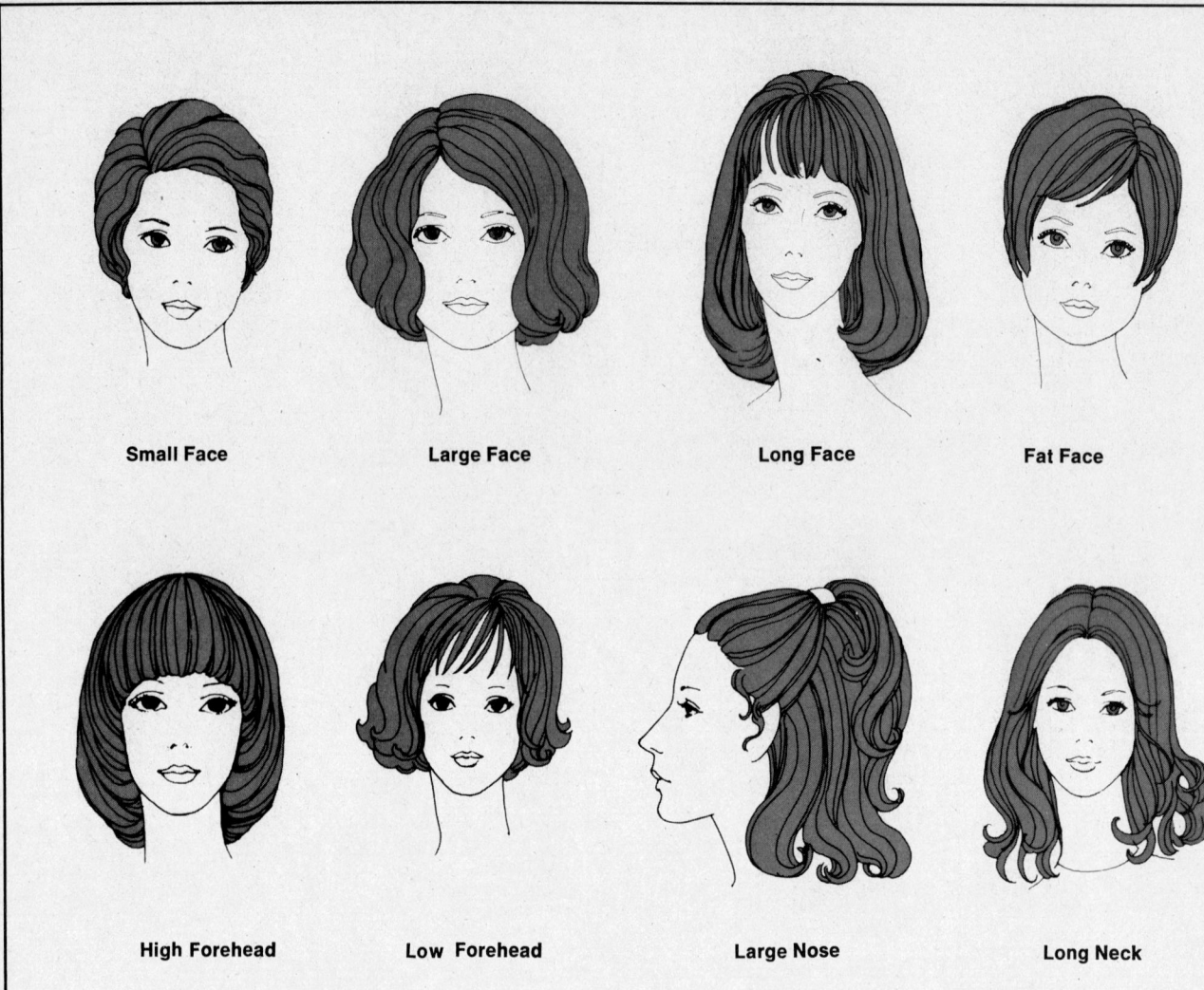

Small Face   Large Face   Long Face   Fat Face

High Forehead   Low Forehead   Large Nose   Long Neck

BALANCE YOUR FACE

A hair design can make the face appear more nearly oval and—more important—minimize any faulty feature. Analyze your face to find out how to create a more pleasing outline. Then use your hair style to create the illusion you want. Once you have made this basic change, revise the makeup of brows and mouth to complete the illusion. The neckline of your dress and your jewelry also lend themselves to feature balance. The hair design should also be in proportion to your figure.

There are few basic forms to work with in your hair style but there can be many variations for any one face.
Dimension—You add *length* to the head by sweeping the hair up to the top of the head. Add *width* by bringing the hair out in wings at forehead, cheekbones, or below the ear. But also use the *balance* between length and width.
Direction—Bringing the hair back and away from the face exposes all the forehead and chin you have, makes face appear larger. Bringing the hair down to cover forehead and cheeks makes the face appear smaller.
Balance—Changing the part helps you to balance irregularities in the face with hair mass. A low side part gives top bulk; an off-center part or a diagonal part also can give mass where you want it. Your head has side and back views, too. The profile is balanced by the bulk and positioning of the crown and nape hair.
• Massing the hair at the crown or back of the crown helps a small chin.
• Bangs of the right length solve forehead problems.
• Massing the hair low on the nape modifies a long neck.
• A cap hairdo puffed about the crown rounds the head shape.
• A full, lifted hairdo makes the head seem larger.
Changing your outline—While hair is wet from the shampoo, experiment with your hair styling. You may want to exaggerate any unusual feature—a square jaw, high forehead—rather than minimize it. But note the effect from side and back as well as from the front. From the front, the face gets the attention; from the back and sides, others first see your hair style and head shape.

HAIRDOS THAT SOLVE PROBLEMS

Small face—A close-to-the-head hairdo, with the hair worn away from the face, will make the face look larger.
• Brush all the hair away from the face and give it a slight lift all around. Hair thus serves as a frame and gives you all the face you need.
• Keep the hair slightly lifted over all the head, but rounded and shaped to the natural hairline, just above the tips of the ears in the finished hairdo. Showing a little ear will make the neck and face appear larger.
Plain face—The plainer your face, the more dramatic you can be in hairdo and makeup.
Large face—A full hairdo that brings the hair out all round the face and cuts into both the forehead and cheeks makes the face seem smaller.
Long face—If face is long and neck is

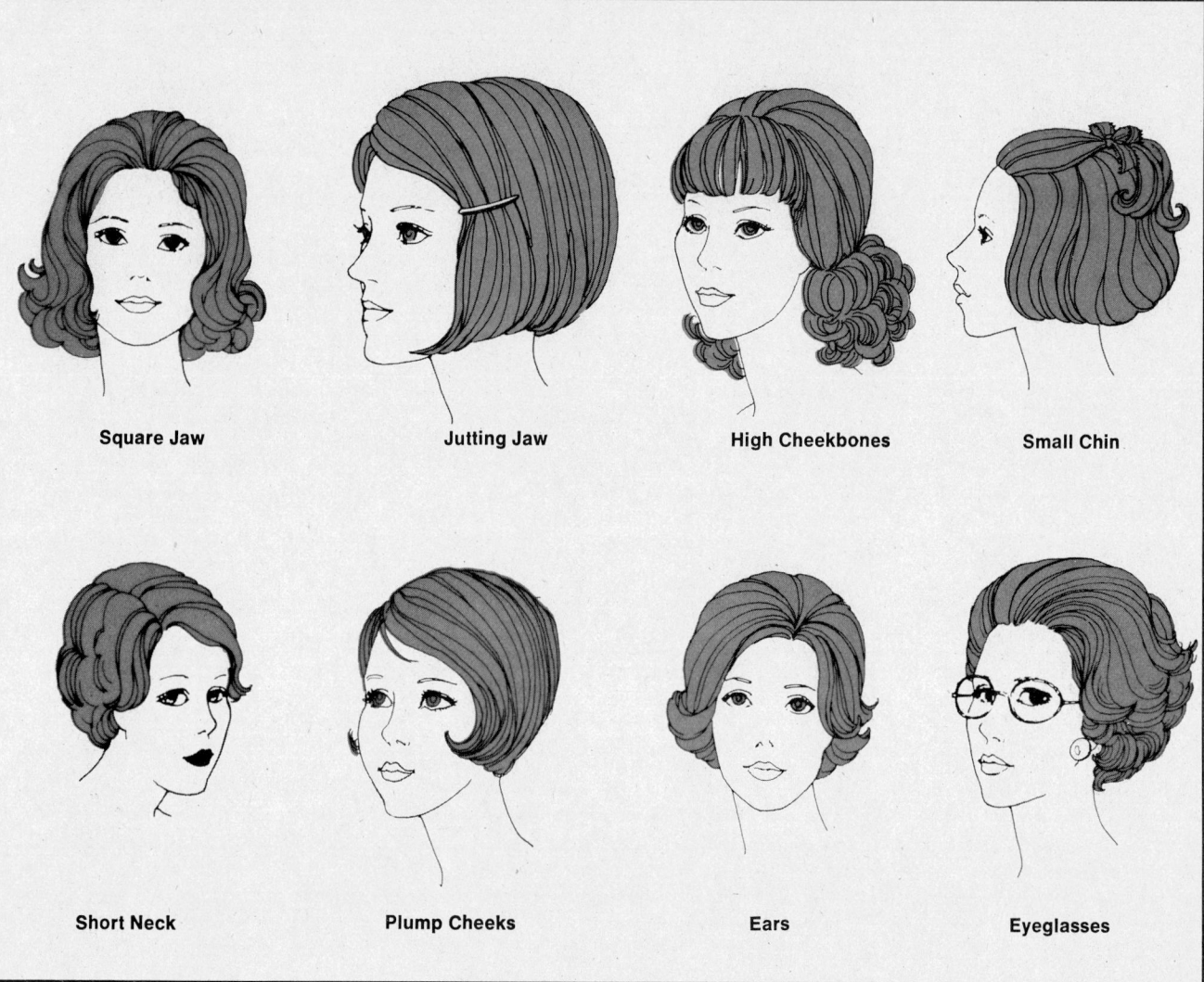

Square Jaw   Jutting Jaw   High Cheekbones   Small Chin

Short Neck   Plump Cheeks   Ears   Eyeglasses

also long, add wideness and fullness to the hair at the crown and just a little forehead height. Full bangs cut down the forehead area; let hair fall to mid-neck length in a full pageboy.

Fat face—If face is short and plump, keep the hair high above the ears and close at sides to cover the face at cheeks and temples.

Irregular features — Long layered hair that falls in a cascade of waves from a brief middle part to below the jaw line eases irregular features or prominent cheekbones.

Square jaw—For a wide jaw, add forehead width and fullness at chin line.

Strong jaw—Softening in effect are tendrils of delicate curls framing the entire face.

Jutting jaw—If jaw is square and very prominent, bring long points of hair in from below the ear to follow exactly the line of the jaw to a point just below the middle of the eye.

High cheekbones — If cheekbones are prominent, keep the hair flat to the sides of the head in this area and full above and below the cheekbones. Cut bangs so they are wider than the forehead to give an illusion of width.

Small chin—If chin is small or receding, pull hair up close to the head and into a mass at the back of crown; keep roundness at the nape.

Forehead—For a low forehead, bangs should be short and high, separated or rounded. For a high forehead, bangs should be long and wispy. A broad forehead is cut by a middle part and hair smoothed down at sides.

Nose—If nose is large, mass hair at top back of head and pin it high; then let a fall of curls, a single curl, or a smooth pony tail fall down to the hairline at the back. Length at the back of the head brings the nose into balance. Bangs, by closing in the forehead, help a small nose become important.

Long neck—A long neck is modified by breaking the line with a chignon or medium-length pageboy. The nape hair should not hug the head.

Short neck—If neck is short, get all the length you can with a lifted hairdo that fits close to the head at back and sides. Hair pulled back to create space behind the ear will also be neck-lengthening.

For a full throat—Tendrils of hair brought gracefully down along the neck on each side, with one small curl against the cheek to soften the line, break up the expanse of a full throat.

Plump cheeks—If cheeks are extra-full and plump, turn a large C-curl over the middle cheek, coming in on a curve that starts with tip of the earlobe.

Ears—Do not expose the ears, except the tip, unless they are well-formed. A hair style that is full and fluffy over the ears conceals protruding or overlarge ears.

Eyeglasses—If you wear glasses, choose an away-from-the-face hair style with a forehead lift and fullness over the ears. Hair should be neither too severe nor too fluffy. Look for a style that is softening and somewhat full to balance the emphasis glasses give to the eye area. Wear earrings when you wear glasses, and the face will appear to be better balanced.

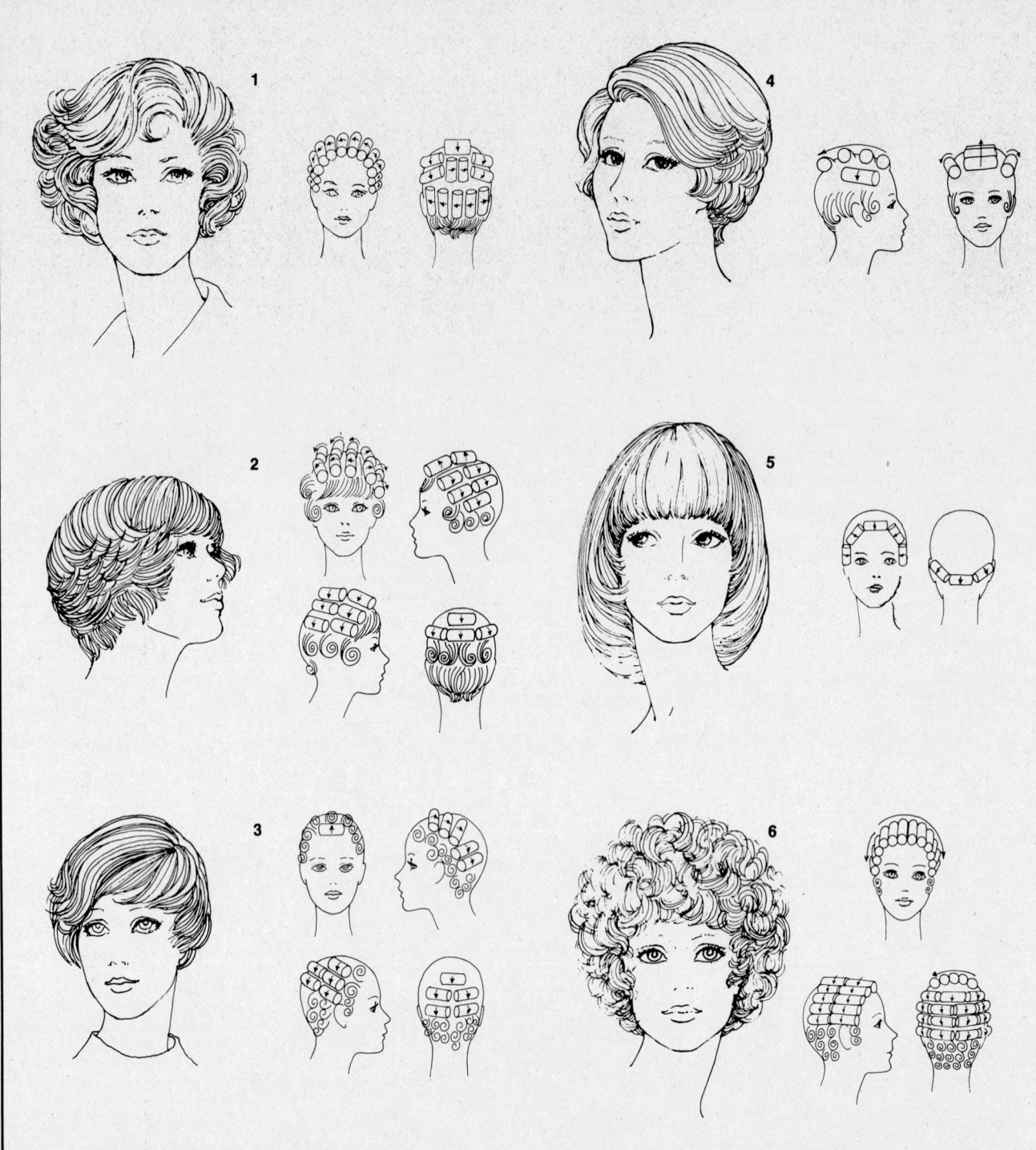

12 BEST-LIKED HAIRDO'S

1. The side sweep. Becoming, pretty, and easy to wear, this down hairdo is adjustable to your hair length and your kind of hair. Here the style is softened with forehead curls and a little duck's tail curl at the back.

2. The brush cut. A short fluffy hairdo that can be brushed into shape is the handiest for many young women and is always becoming when some fullness is needed about the face. Hair can be directed front, back, or sideways and can be worn with or without bangs to suit the face shape.

3. The wind-blown hairdo. This soft casual short cut is a favorite for the woman who wants hair that is easy to care for. Works best in hair with a hidden wave that can be brought to life with a layered cut.

4. The cap coif. Short, curly, and close to the head, the cap coif in its many variations is the stand-by hairdo for many women.

5. Full-bang bob. The full-bang bob is always with us in some form or other. Today it becomes a cheerful change for women who reluctantly give up their long-hair style.

6. The pouf. Straight or curly, severe or soft, the pouf in one version or another is always in fashion. Here the

28

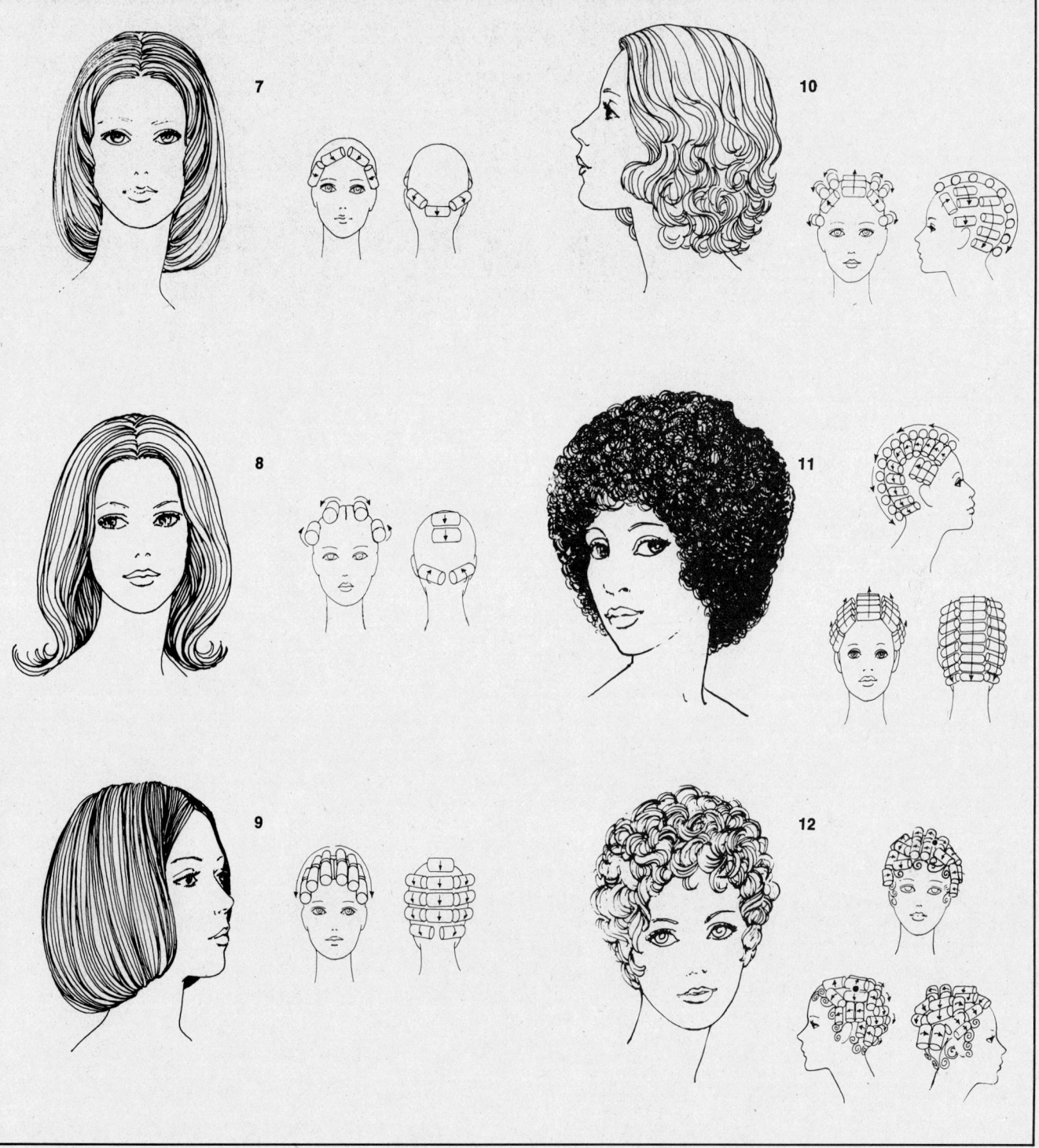

style relies on a softly layered cut and close-set rollers and pin curls to have lots of curl.

7. The pageboy. Short, long, or medium long, with or without bangs, the pageboy with soft underturned ends is often a style a woman can happily return to from time to time at any age.

8. The flip. A much-loved look for the young woman is the end-flip hair style, with or without bangs.

9. The straight-line look. A smooth seemingly simple hair style with a straight-hair look is something many women want. A body permanent may be needed for straightness with control.

10. The glamour bob. Partless, side-parted, or crossed over at the forehead, the glamour bob continues a favorite among women who want hair long enough to wear both down or up.

11. The curly Afro. Wash, condition and creme rinse hair; towel dry lightly. While hair is still very wet, brush oil into each section and set on small sponge rollers all over the head in small sections. Let dry completely on rollers. Comb with Afro pique; do not brush.

12. Angel cut. A short curly hairdo that can be finger-combed for a tumbled look. In setting, there must be a point (see dot in the setting diagram) to start with and to give direction to the design.

WHAT SETTING FOR YOUR HAIR?

The way the hair is set determines the beauty of the hair style and how long the style will hold its shape. Choose your curlers for the finished effect and follow setting patterns carefully.

Basic sets—Although different hair styles require different setting and directions of curls and size of rollers, most women find it useful to have a basic set that they can do without thinking too much. The basic roller set works well for most medium to long hair styles. The pin-curl set is good for a mass of curls in short to short-short hair.

Rollers—These are for lifted hair styles and for styles that are to have a straight-hair effect. Rollers come in a variety of length and sizes. Their diameter is often referred to in relation to the size of coins: The small ones are "dime-size;" the medium, "quarter-size;" the large, "half-dollar;" and the big ones become jumbo. Length of rollers is also important to your setting: Short (one inch), medium (two-inch) and long (two-and-a-half to three inches) will be needed in various sizes.

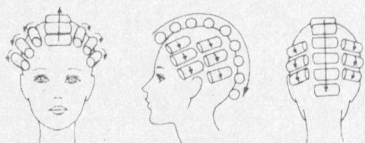

Clip or pin curls—These are good for close curl and are also used to set hard-to-curl sections—neckline, temple, or bangs—and to finish off the hair style at the bottom.

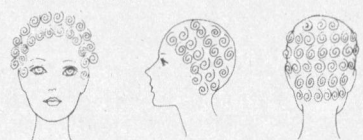

Hot curlers—These can be used for setting the entire head or for turning ends under, upward, or forward. Usually, hot curlers work best for resetting the hair between shampoos when it is not "too clean." But with the help of special setting spray for use with hot curlers, you can do simple after-shampoo settings with them after your hair is dried. If hair is easy to curl, the regular dry curlers (used with the setting spray) are fine; for porous or hard-to-curl hair, the steam curlers or steam-plus-conditioner curlers may be preferred.

Cotton—Cotton rolls are useful to give a lift to neckline hair or to set full lifted bangs or to wrap around a cheek curl—or guiche—so that it will not become overcurly.

Hairsetting tape—Wispy bangs, side curls, and cheek fringe can be combed into place while damp and held against the skin with transparent tape till dry. Use instead of clips on "pin" curls.

Wave set—Some conditioning rinses serve as a setting solution, and you then need no other wave set. Water alone can be used in setting hair. Or you can use a setting lotion; this comes in light strength for a soft curl and in firm-hold strength for hair that is overcurly, hard-to-manage, or for an emphatic curl.

Hair spray—This can be used for dry-setting the hair and can also be used as a hair-set reviver or to form the style during the comb-out.

How to set the hair. The first setting after the shampoo, especially if hair is permanented or curly or if it is hard to curl and doesn't hold a set well, is best done with hair damp, using setting lotions, rollers and/or clip curls and your hair drier. If correctly set, hair will handle well during the comb-out and hold the set well. Towel-dry the hair after the shampoo and set hair while damp.

• While hair is wet, comb each strand smooth and then comb the hair smooth against the head.

• Then section the hair into the lines of the hair style—crown, sides, back, and bangs (if any).

• Comb each section into the direction of line of the hair style. This is most important if rollers and clip curls are to be correctly placed; direction of line determines how a strand of hair will fall once it is brushed out.

Setting helps. When inserting clip or pin, take care not to disturb roller or pin curl.

• Never stretch the hair while setting; stretching causes frizz. Keep the curl firm but free of tension.

• After the set remove the rollers gently so as not to disturb the curls.

• The more curls on the head and the smaller the diameter of each curl, the firmer the set. Fine or thin hair should be set on small-diameter rollers.

Winding—Each roller or pin curl should be directed in the line of the section of which it is a part.

• Start each curl by separating a strand from the rest of the hair and combing the strand away from the scalp.

• On the crown, hold the strand up and away from the scalp to create a lift in this section: at the sides and back pull the strand straight *out* from the scalp; at the forehead pull the strand forward from the scalp. Then wind each curl all the way to the scalp.

• The size of the roller or pin curl depends upon the length of the hair and style you want. The larger the curl, the softer and smoother the set. For each curl, part off a section slightly shorter than the length of the roller and one inch deep.

Strength of curl—For both pin curls and rollers, the firmness of the curl depends on how it is wound in relation to its base. The base is the section of scalp from which the strand arises.

• For the firmest curl, comb the strand back from the base at a 45° angle before you start to roll and roll from this angle, firmly attaching the roller or pin curl *directly over* its base.

• If you pull the hair directly away from the scalp at a 90° angle and fasten the curl half on and half off its base, the curl will have more softness and flexibility in the comb-out.

• If you pull the hair 45° toward the direction in which you are going to wind and fasten the curl ahead of its base, the curl will give direction to the hair style but the shape of the curl will brush out.

Roller setting—Comb the strand smooth and, holding the hair firmly, place a folded end paper over the middle of the strand. Slide the end paper down to the ends of the strand and then place the covered ends directly against the roller before you begin to wind.

• Roll the curler in the direction of the line of the style and roll evenly so the hair will be smooth.

• Clip the roller in front if you rolled it forward; at the back, if you rolled it backward.

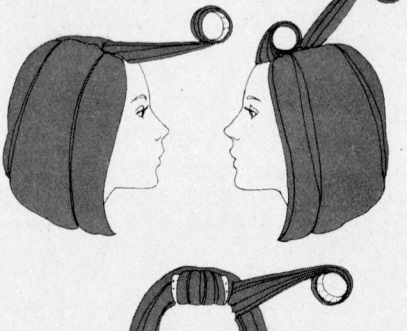

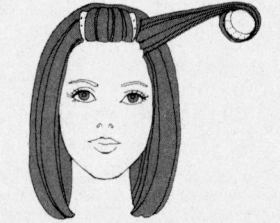

How to make pin curls. You can make many kinds of pin curls for various effects. Again, the larger the strand, the looser the curl. The direction of the curl and its placement on or off its base will also determine the firmness of the curl. Comb the curl into wet hair just as you want it to lie when it is dry. All stems—the section of the strand as it comes away from the scalp is "the stem"—for each section should move in the same direction. Neckline curls may, however, be turned toward ears on each side. Do not draw a sideburn curl back before turning it forward.

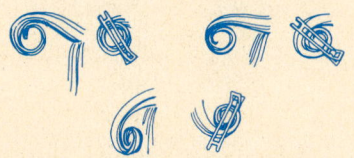

Sculptured curl—Part off as much hair as you want for the curl and hold the strand up and out. Comb it smooth and do not twist.

❧ Press a finger of left hand firmly against the scalp to create a hollow at the base of the curl. With the comb in the right hand, draw the strand forward stretching it to a point.

❧ Now, using both hands and starting at the tip of the strand, roll the curl carefully in a small series of rings to the base of the pin curl. The inner ring should be smallest and the outside ring the largest.

❧ The finished curl should fit neatly against the scalp.

❧ Pin or clip through the curl, not through the stem—the unwound part of the strand closest to the scalp.

No-stem curls—These clip curls are firm and long-lasting. Start the curl by pulling the hair back from the direction of winding at a 45° angle and form the circle directly over the base. Clip through the base to hold.

Full stem—This curl is pulled forward in direction of line at a 45° angle, and the circle is fastened ahead of the base; this curl gives direction only.

Half-stem curl—This curl is started with the strand pulled out at a 90° angle and lies half on and half off its base.

Stand-up curl—Pull the strand straight up from the scalp and then comb back at a 45° angle from the base; wind in a series of rings to the scalp so that the curl stands up from the head. Pin or clip at the base.

WHAT CARE FOR YOUR HAIR?

Hair has uses other than adornment. Hair acts as a sunshade, keeps the head warm, and serves as a buffer to protect against bumps. Once hair is visible, it is "waste tissue," as are the tips of the fingernails. Just the same, hair beauty depends upon good health. Illness, a change of diet, anxiety, overexposure, or simple neglect can quickly show up in dryness and lack of luster, reflecting changes in the scalp condition. Hair beauty comes with balanced diet, exercise, and other simple ways of well-being. Hair beauty can be protected by careful handling, too. Here are ways to care for your hair—by proper cleaning and scalp massage. Here, too, are suggestions on what to look for in a permanent and in hair coloring.

Your hair. A human hair looks to the naked eye like a smooth strand of silk—but under the microscope it shows a layered outer coat made up of overlapping tooth-edged cells. This layer is translucent and colorless and is called the *cuticle*.

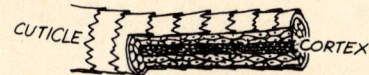

In healthy hair—and untreated hair—these outer cells lie flat and are closely interlocked. When you comb or brush the hair away from the scalp, the layers are not disturbed. Much back-combing and back-brushing can loosen the layers —and this makes for rough, "damaged" hair.

How can you avoid becoming a "hair cripple"? If your hair is damaged, a short cut may be the answer for you. Hair closest to the scalp is younger and consequently stronger (unless it has been carelessly bleached) than the ends.

❧ If top hair is overexposed to sun and hair spray and therefore drier than the rest, can be helpful to change the direction of your hair style from time to time to expose another section of hair.

❧ Don't overbrush, overtease, or overspray your hair. Handle it gently when you comb it, brush it, roll it up, and take it out of curlers. Avoid the highest heat on your drier; don't make use of a curling iron or other heated curling device a daily habit.

❧ Use a water softener—or hardwater-use hair preparations—if you live or vacation in a hard-water area.

❧ Always rinse your hair thoroughly; a hand spray helps when rinsing out shampoo or hair conditioner.

❧ If hair is long, keep the ends trimmed and shaped. A six-inch strand is about a year old at the end and has been through about 52 washings and sets and perhaps a thousand combings. If ends split, they should be trimmed at once; otherwise, the splitting will gradually continue up the hair shaft. Sacrificing a quarter inch or so of length will help to keep long hair healthy.

How to massage. Massaging for five minutes a day keeps the scalp exercised and fresh. Massage before brushing so that any particles of shed skin will be removed by the brush.

❧ Starting at the back of the head, place both hands against the scalp and gently rotate the scalp skin; repeat at sides, crown, and forehead till skin feels loosened.

❧ Then, starting again at the back of the head, place fingertips (not nails) of both hands against the scalp and move the fingers in small vibratory circles. "Walk" the fingertips all over the scalp, making small circles with the fingers at each location, till the whole scalp has been covered.

❧ A dandruff-remover preparation or warm oil can be applied with the massage; hair should then be brushed and shampooed.

Washing and rinsing. Choose a shampoo for your hair type, for the condition of the water (hard or soft), and for the dryness or humidity of the air in your area. Cream, liquid, or lotion shampoos are easy to apply. Bar soap tends to tangle the hair and often leaves soap deposit. Most liquid shampoos should be diluted one-quarter or one-half with water before using. Use as little shampoo as possible so it will all be rinsed out.

Soap shampoos—Wonderful in soft water, soap shampoos may form scum or fail to lather in hard water.

Detergent shampoos—These shampoos lather well in soft or hard water.

Dry shampoos—For emergency use, dry shampoos are available, but these are not recommended for regular hair cleaning or for frequent use.

❧ Apply the shampoo section by section with a cotton square so as not to disturb the set and follow directions carefully. Brush out thoroughly.

What shampoo for your hair type? The test of a shampoo is how well it lathers and in what condition it leaves your hair. After shampooing, hair should feel clean, the scalp should be comfortable (not dry or itchy), and hair should have luster or gloss.

❧ For oily hair, herbal shampoos and detergent shampoos are excellent and leave the hair oil-free and really clean.

❧ For dry hair, use a shampoo designed to remove soil but not natural oils—a shampoo incorporating lanolin or other fats. Shampoos of pure castile soap have a high oil content and little alkali and also are good for dry hair.

❧ Shampoos for normal hair should be used by those who have no unusual scalp condition and who need no special water softener.

❧ If you have dandruff, shampoos that help this condition are at hand.

❧ For color-treated hair, use a neutral shampoo intended for hair that has been lightened or tinted. Other shampoos may affect the hair coloring.

How to shampoo. Before the shampoo, massage the scalp and then brush the hair to remove tangles.

✤ Rinse hair in warm water to remove loose dust and skin particles.

✤ Pour or dip up a small amount of shampoo into one hand, and apply the shampoo to the scalp with the fingertips.

✤ Work the shampoo over the scalp with massage movement to get the scalp really clean and then work the lather down through the hair section by section. The first application of shampoo will lather only slightly.

✤ Rinse hair thoroughly to remove shampoo, loosened dirt, and dandruff.

✤ Reapply shampoo to the scalp with the fingertips and again work the lather down the hair by sections.

✤ Rinse thoroughly—and when the hair feels well rinsed, rinse again. Any shampoo left in the hair will dull its gloss.

✤ Towel-dry the hair, blotting not rubbing, and comb—do not brush—while wet.

What rinse for your hair? Hair, like all skin and skin products, is normally slightly acid. Cleansers such as soap and detergent are slightly alkali. An acid rinse—vinegar or lemon juice—restores the acid state of the hair; do not use an acid rinse if a conditioning rinse or color rinse or other treatment is to be applied.

✤ Creme rinse or spray leaves the hair easy to comb. Creme rinse is applied to the hair in the final rinse water—or is sprayed onto towel-dried hair. These rinses control static electricity and make the hair less flyaway. They also restore lost oils and give the hair gloss and manageability. Some serve as setting lotions; no other setting lotion need then be used. If you use a color rinse or conditioner-setting lotion, apply it to towel-dried hair.

Egg shampoo. Egg shampoo cleans the hair but also acts as a conditioning treatment. Some of the components of egg yolk are believed to have value for both skin and hair and make this an excellent softener for dry, brittle, and damaged hair and a glorifier for any head of hair.

✤ Separate two or three eggs and whip up the whites to a froth; add a tablespoon of water to the yolks and stir to a creamy consistency. Recombine whites and yolks.

✤ Rinse the hair to remove superficial dirt and towel-dry.

✤ Apply the egg froth to the scalp with the fingertips in a massage motion and then work the egg well through the damp hair. Add cool water if needed.

✤ Rinse hair in cool water (so as not to cook the egg) and then repeat the application till all the egg mixture is used up.

✤ Rinse again till all egg is removed.

✤ You need not reshampoo the hair. Simply dry as usual after rinsing.

HAIR CONDITIONERS

Don't wait for hair damage before you look into today's hair beautifiers. Conditioners are based on proteins and oils similar to those the hair loses from weathering and overtreatment. These preparations usually are applied to towel-dried hair after the shampoo and rinse. Some are left on only for a minute; some, for five minutes; others for half an hour. Some require use of heat or the wearing of a cap during treatment. Some also serve as a setting lotion.

✤ After the shampoo and rinse, setting-lotion conditioner is worked for a minute into towel-dried hair and is not rinsed out. The conditioning action goes on as the hair responds to the warmth of the drier.

This conditioner gives body to thin fine hair and makes any type easier to handle. It can be used on dry or oily hair; for best results, use regularly after each shampoo.

✤ Rinse-out conditioner in the form of a thick lotion is applied to freshly shampooed, rinsed, and towel-dried hair. Work it through for a minute (or leave it on for two to five minutes according to directions) and then thoroughly rinse it out. This conditioner improves gloss and manageability and keeps the hair strong. Use it after each shampoo to build hair strength.

✤ For dry, brittle, damaged, weathered hair, cream-conditioning treatment is advisable once a month or oftener. The treatment should also be given before permanenting and can be combined with lightening, toning, and tinting touch-ups. Conditioner acts as a filler to the hair and builds hair body with continued treatment. Cream conditioner is applied generously to the hair and scalp. To apply, lift the damp hair strand by strand and apply upward, away from the scalp, with a gentle pulling motion. Work in well, and then leave on for 20 to 30 minutes. Afterward the hair is rinsed thoroughly.

✤ While new growth near the scalp is being tinted or toned, cream conditioner can be applied to the rest of the hair. Once the color has developed in the roots area, the color can be combed down over the hair ends without the conditioner's interfering with the color process. The hair is then rinsed and shampooed. If lightener is being used, it should be applied first to the roots; then the cream conditioner is applied to the rest of the hair. The conditioner is rinsed out with the lightener.

✤ If you color your hair, you will find that the coloring preparation has a built in conditioner. After color treatment your hair will probably look and feel better than usual, have more gloss and body. Hair that has been lightened may not react this way; to prevent drying and breaking, a conditioner should be applied with the lightener and after each shampoo.

✤ For hair that lacks gloss, a cream dressing that is rubbed in sparingly but well before the comb-out—or one that is sprayed on after the comb-out—adds light and brilliance.

How do conditioners act on your hair? Basically, a conditioner detangles snarls and reduces frizz and has antistatic-electricity ingredients to make hair less flyaway when brushed or combed. It also gives gloss to the hair and adds body.

✤ Some conditioners help smooth down the platelets on the outer skin of the hair and fill in lost body and also seal split ends. Protein conditioners are needed on fine limp hair, on color-treated hair, and long hair that has aged through frequent shampoos and other treatments. These body-building conditioners coat the hair and each strand actually becomes thicker—as well as more springy.

✤ Instant conditioners (setting conditioners) help hair hold the set and also deposit protein to fill out the hair strands.

✤ Corrective conditioners help the hair hold moisture, soften dry and brittle hair, and make the hair more supple and resistant to breaking.

✤ Balsam gives sheen to the hair. Protein helps restore natural body.

Hot-oil treatment. As a preshampoo conditioner for sun-dried, brittle, and over-dry hair, hot-oil treatment is helpful. Hair oil, creme conditioner or a lanolin preparation can be used.

✤ Heat the oil to comfortable temperature and, with a cotton ball or square, apply the oil to the scalp, sectioning the hair with a comb to be sure the entire scalp is covered. Massage the oil into the scalp till skin feels warm and tingling.

✤ With a comb, bring the oil down through the strands of the hair.

✤ To complete the treatment, dip a bath towel in hot water and wring the towel dry; wrap the hot towel round the head and leave on till warmth is gone; apply another hot towel; continue treatment for 20 minutes.

🌿 Your hood hair drier turned to very warm can be used instead of a hot towel; or if you have an infrared lamp (not ultraviolet), comb the hair under its warmth and light for 10 minutes.

🌿 Hair should be shampooed after treatment.

Dandruff treatment. Dandruff is often simply normal scurf—dead skin particles that drift off the scalp as they do from the rest of the body skin. The particles are caught by the hair oils or sift down upon the shoulders. Severe dandruff sometimes accompanies excessive oiliness of scalp and facial skin and then may appear as scales and crusts; frequent shampooing will be helpful. Dandruff may also come with excessive dryness and there may be itchiness and inflammation; then dandruff is considered a form of dermatitits. Dandruff can also be a germ disease and in this case should have the attention of a dermatologist.

🌿 Shampoos, rinses, and preshampoo treatments for dandruff make the scalp clean and comfortable and keep the dandruff down, but frequent shampoos are often needed.

🌿 Daily massage and brushing will also help keep the hair dandruff free.

Are you alarmed about hair loss? There is a normal hair loss daily—between 50 and 100 hairs—but hair tends to drop more rapidly in spring and autumn when most creatures have a "molting season." Often a new hair is growing in when the old one falls, but sometimes follicles become dormant and rest for a few years; other follicles are meanwhile reawakening, so in normal circumstances the number of hairs on the head will remain about the same.

Heavy hair fall is usual after pregnancy and sometimes occurs during the menopause. At this time there may be a great deal of thinning but rarely does it reach the state of baldness.

Many young women today have alarming hair loss that cannot be completely explained. If the loss is excessive, certain precautions are recommended:

🌿 Keep hair clean; excess oil may act as a depilatory.

🌿 Avoid tight headbands, hats, and styles that skin the hair back from the face.

🌿 Do not use brush curlers in the hair; do not roll any curlers very tightly.

🌿 Avoid overfrequent use of permanents and hair colorings.

🌿 Brush and comb the hair moderately or use scalp massage as a substitute for brushing. This improves circulation.

🌿 Do not rub the hair after shampooing; blot hair dry and then use a drier set at moderate heat.

🌿 Keep fit—eat a balanced diet and get enough sleep and exercise.

🌿 See a dermatologist if the condition becomes alarming.

PROTECT YOUR HAIR

When hair is damp or newly treated with coloring or waving lotions, handle it gently. After shampooing, blot hair dry with a towel; use a comb, not a brush, to prepare the hair for setting.

🌿 In setting, do not roll the curlers overtightly; go easy with snarls so hair is not broken in combing. Dry the hair under moderate heat. Remove curlers gently.

🌿 Do not overtreat the hair. Shampoo as often as you like, but have coloring jobs and permanents only when you really need them.

🌿 Sun and wind can dry and bleach the hair and split the ends; so will overly dry indoor air.

🌿 Avoid tight hats and headbands and hair styles that tug at the hair; too much tightness can destroy hair roots.

🌿 Back-comb the hair as little as possible and then only close to the scalp where the hair is new and strong.

🌿 Do not *over*brush. Long hair needs brushing to keep it unsnarled and well-groomed, but short hair needs little brushing except after the setting. Instead, exercise the scalp with regular massage.

🌿 Give your hair an occasional rest. Try not to roll up the hair every day; instead, find a style that holds a set for five to seven days or needs only a few clips to revive it.

🌿 Sleeping on rollers is unwise. If at bedtime hair is turned into a few large curls and these are pinned into place under a net, hair will be soft and well-groomed the next day.

HAIR-CARE HELPS

🌿 Have your hair shaped and trimmed often. Hair grows somewhat faster in summer, so spring is a good time to get rid of ends that from overexposure or overtreatment are likely to become dry and to split. Short or long, hair needs trimming to avoid wispiness and signs of uneven growth.

🌿 Change your part often. Top hair often becomes sunburned and dry. With a change of part that exposes healthier underneath hair, your whole head can look silkier and better groomed.

🌿 Shampoo frequently. In winter, a hairdo usually lasts only about five days even with good care. Holding a set for a full week is even harder in summer, when the scalp perspires a lot and warmth stimulates oil secretion. Wash your hair whenever it needs it for a soft, fresh look. Frequent washing won't dry it out if you use a shampoo that is right for your hair condition—color-treated, dry, oily, or normal.

🌿 Rinse after a swim. If your hair gets wet with salt water or treated pool water, rinse it right away to get rid of salts and chemicals. This is most important if hair is color-treated, particularly if it has been prelightened.

🌿 Dry hair carefully. Treat wet hair gently. Blot it dry with a towel—or dry it with a blower set at low or medium temperature. So the hair will dry quickly, towel-dry it before setting it in curlers. When using a hood drier, keep it at low or medium heat.

🌿 Use a hair conditioner regularly. A conditioning treatment every three or four weeks keeps healthy hair looking well. For dry, damaged, or lightened hair, use a conditioner once a week—or with every shampoo.

🌿 Don't overtreat the hair. If the hair is sun-damaged, dry, and strawlike, don't expect a permanent wave to solve your problem. It may make it worse. Instead, cut away damaged hair before having a new permanent. If you lighten your hair, keep touch-ups about four weeks apart. And allow a week between any coloring job and a new permanent.

🌿 Avoid oversunning. A hat, a scarf, keeping to the shade—these limit exposure to sun and protect the hair against streaking and overdrying. Hair dressings, rinses that coat the hair shaft—these give protection while sunning.

🌿 Wear a swim cap. You protect both your hairdo and your hair color if you wear a close-fitting cap when you swim. Some water may still seep under the cap, and the hair at the temples, nape, and sides may get a little damp. After you swim, carefully rinse out these damp sections of hair. You need reset only these parts. Such little attentions protect your hair coloring and your set.

🌿 Avoid wind-whipping. In windy places or while you ride in an open car or in a fast boat, keep your hair tied up in a scarf or tucked under a cap. Wind-whipping can split hair ends and create tangles that may result in breakage when you comb your hair out.

🌿 Don't overcomb or overbrush. Unnecessary handling puts a strain on the hair. Comb only enough to keep your hair neat; brush only enough to keep hair polished and well-meshed. Set your hair as little as possible and do not wind tightly on rollers. A firmhold setting lotion, spray, or gel will fix your curl better than will tight winding. Remove curlers as soon as hair is dry.

🌿 Avoid hair-setting emergencies. A home hair drier will prove a good friend—so will a scarf or hat. A wig or a hair piece that fills out or covers your own hair and looks natural—or a fun hairpiece, such as an extra long braid or flounce—will help you through emergencies. If your hairpiece is of man-made fibers, it will be sun-resistant.

🌿 Take advantage of hair coloring. Hair colorings add body to the hair and can improve texture. Many of today's hair colorings contain conditioners, so the hair feels better and looks better and is more manageable after color treatment. Hair that is lightened and toned should be treated as delicate hair; exposure to summer sun and to chlorinated water should be avoided.

MONEY SAVERS

You do your hair yourself at home, and that saves money—right? But do you pinch all the possible pennies? Do you . . .

🌿 Carefully measure shampoo, conditioner, creme rinse, whatever, so that you use enough but not that extravagant too much. More important than extra detergent to a shiny, clean-hair look is lots of rinse water; rinse at least once again after the water runs clear.

🌿 Use hair color wisely. Most practical is semipermanent color in your own shade—a six-week color job. Money-saving in the long run, even if they're a bit of work at the start, are frosting and streaking. Great on light browns and ash blondes—and you can go three months without restreaking. As you add streaks, the sunshine effect just gets prettier. If you use one-process or two-step permanent hair color, don't over-color your hair. A partless hairdo hides the color line. But don't let the new growth go too far; the difference in texture between treated and untreated hair can lead to breakage—and you would hate that!

🌿 Spray lightly. The soft look in hair-doing requires little spray. Complaints about "how quickly that container empties" are mostly a result of over-spraying. Try spraying your hairbrush and then running it over the hair to smarten your do.

🌿 Follow directions. Permanents, hair colorings, conditioners, shampoos—they all have that useful fine print. If you do what it says, you get good results. For example, if the conditioner is to be put on towel-dried hair and left on for five minutes—that's the way to do it.

🌿 Shop for beauty-shop bargains. We all want a beauty-shop do sometime. And somewhere in your town there's bound to be a special—or a discount day. Do take advantage.

WHAT YOU WANT IN A PERMANENT

A permanent, whether it's a salon or home wave, can give as little or as much curl as you want. A body wave gives very little curve to the hair—just enough to give it body and to help it hold the set. A shadow wave gives slight wave only, in the pattern in which the curlers were set. A permanent can also produce a tight and springy curl, and this will allow you to have the curlier hair styles.

To get what you want in a permanent, choose the waving strength for the kind of hair you have; choose the rods for the kind of wave you want—small or medium rods for a tight and springy curl; large rods for a loose and casual body wave. Then follow all the directions in the package exactly.

Hard to wave—This is hair that refuses to hold a set for even three days or is baby-fine, limp, or droops easily, or is very straight. Children's hair is always resistant.

Easy to wave—This may be coarse hair, hair with natural curl, hair that is porous from color treatment, or hair that has recently been permanented.

Damaged hair—This is hair that is bleached, broken, or overdry; damaged hair should not be waved till it is in good condition.

Normal hair—If you have not used a permanent-wave kit before or if you have no outstanding hair problem or if your hair has not been color-treated, choose the regular-strength solution for normal hair.

What kind of wave? The size of the wave pattern—loose and casual or tight and springy—and the lasting power of the wave are controlled by the size of the rod and not by the processing time.

Wound on the usual home-permanent rods—large, medium, and small—the wave will be permanent. It will last till the ends are cut off. Set on large-diameter plastic rods, the wave cannot really be called a "permanent." It will last only two to three months, but the wave will be loose and casual and easy to handle. With a salon wave wound on large-diameter rods, you will also need a new wave in two to three months. Again, the soft effect is often worth the extra time and money.

Rods should be chosen according to the texture of hair and the place on the head where the rods are to be used.

🌿 *Coarse hair* should be set on large rods because this hair curls easily.

🌿 *Limp baby-fine hair* should be set in small strands on medium rods. Fine hair needs this smaller rod to get the same style that can be had with thicker rods on coarse hair.

🌿 *For short hair,* use short rods; for long hair, use long rods.

🌿 Large rods should be used at the crown for a soft effect; medium rods at the sides, and small rods at the neckline.

🌿 Always use small-diameter rods on neckline hair but never use these small rods on the rest of the head.

🌿 The size of the rod controls the size of the curl at the ends; the form of the rest of the wave depends also upon the amount of hair sectioned off for the strand and on the length of the strand that is wound.

How to get a good permanent. Home-wave kits come in a variety of styles.

🌿 Trim the hair before the wave to get rid of the old ends that may frizz if rewaved. Taper but do not thin medium or coarse hair; fine hair should be blunt-cut after a shallow tapering.

🌿 Condition the hair before shampooing and after the permanent but do not use conditioner *after* the pre-permanent shampoo. Shampoo before the permanent so the hair will be clean and free of oils and will take the softening lotions well. Do not condition the hair after this shampoo; oils will interfere with the wave process. And do not brush the hair immediately before the permanent.

🌿 After the shampoo and before winding, gently towel-blot the hair; don't rub, for this creates tangles and may cause scalp sensitivity.

🌿 Wait 10 days to two weeks after your last color treatment before having your permanent.

🌿 Do not have a permanent if hair is out of condition, if scalp is irritated, or if hair is badly damaged; instead, have hair-conditioning treatments weekly for three or four weeks before waving.

🌿 Assemble everything you need—timer, plastic comb, cotton, towels, glass or china dish for waving lotion, and your wave kit before you begin your wave. Allow plenty of time—this is no occasion to rush.

🌿 Take a swatch test—a sample curl—before you begin your permanent to see how your hair reacts to the wave. This means that a swatch of hair is treated to the waving lotion, wound, timed, neutralized, dried and combed out as a preview of what kind of curl the kit will give you in your hair.

Winding. Have the hair slightly damp when you start your wave; if hair is too wet, the waving solutions become diluted and are less effective.

✄ Block the hair as instructed and wind sections in the order suggested, starting with the neckline hair, going on to sides and back and then to the crown hair (wound last because the wave here should be soft).

✄ Apply lotion one inch from scalp and to the end of the strand and then comb the lotion through the strand. The longer the hair, the wetter the ends should be in wrapping.

✄ The strand should be as wide as the curler—one-fourth inch deep at the neckline; one-fourth inch to three-fourths at the crown.

✄ End papers make winding easier and avoid bunching of hair ends and prevent hooking of ends. Use only one end paper on each strand. Fold end paper and place it over the middle of the strand and then slide the paper down to cover the ends.

✄ In winding, hold the strand out from the scalp and perpendicular to it. Do not overstretch the hair, but wind evenly and firmly so the rod is close to the scalp and stays put; the curl should be firmly wound but without tension—loose enough so that it can be rocked back and forth when in position, but not drooping.

✄ Use the right amount of hair on each curler. The more hair on the rod, the looser the curl, but the curl should not be wound so thick that lotions cannot penetrate. If this happens, ends will be straight. Too tight winding also prevents penetration of lotions.

✄ Make all curls in each section the same size and wind the curls under so the wave will hug the head. Use enough curlers—36 to 48—depending on the amount of hair.

✄ Be sure to start the curl with the very tips of the strand against the roller.

✄ If you wish smoothness near the scalp; wind curls only one inch higher than you want the curl to be. To have lift near the scalp, hold the rod up and wind all the way to the scalp—one turn above where the lotion was applied. Neckline curls should be wound all the way to the scalp.

Processing. Waving lotion softens the hair so that it takes on the shape of the rod; neutralizer fixes the hair in this new pattern and thus makes the curl permanent.

✄ Be sure each curl is saturated and rewet each curl thoroughly at the second application. Use all the lotion provided with the kit.

✄ Time carefully for the kind of hair you have and for the kind of wave you want. Easy-to-wave hair takes about 20 minutes to wave; resistant hair 30 minutes. In addition to this time, you will have waiting time after the rinsing of 30 minutes.

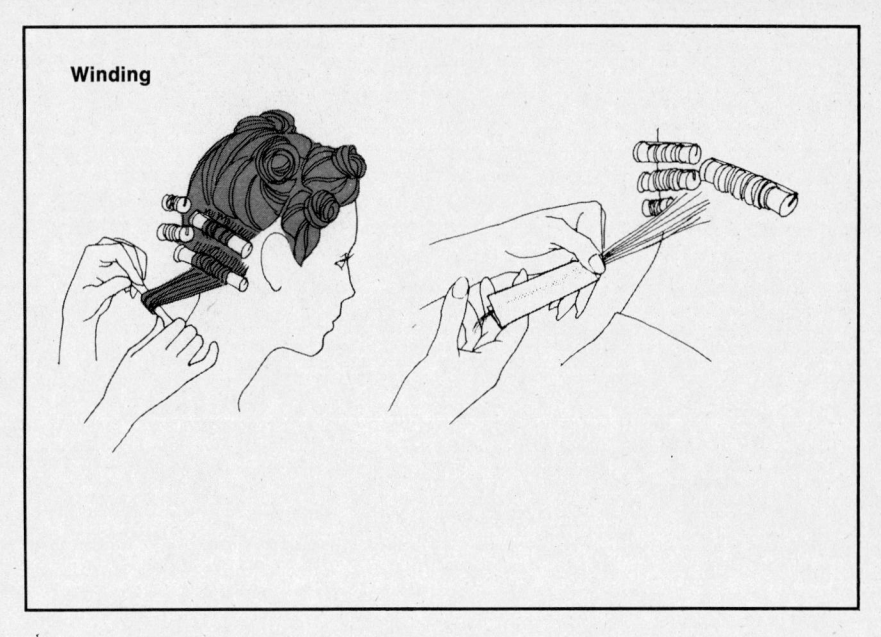

✄ Make a test curl as soon as hair is wound. And make a test curl each time you have a permanent because hair condition varies. Blot the curl. Then release the rod and unwind the curl one and a half turns. Relax the hair across the hand to see how the wave has developed. Take care not to stretch the curl. If wave is developing, rewind carefully and continue with the processing. If not, rewind, wait a few minutes and test the curl again.

✄ Be sure to neutralize according to directions and neutralize thoroughly; this makes the wave permanent. Rinse out neutralizer in tepid water.

✄ If you have had a loose wave, you can hand dry it with a drier brush or hand drier. Otherwise, set it in rollers or pin curls and dry.

After permanent hair care. Do not reshampoo the hair for at least five days after a permanent.

✄ Delay any color treatment for at least one week—preferably two—after your permanent.

✄ Set the hair on jumbo rollers to have a smooth set. If hair seems straight after the permanent, look at it while it is wet. If it is curly when wet, your permanent has taken; if it is nevertheless straight when dry, it may not have been set to pick up the wave properly.

✄ Hair "dryness" after a permanent is usually frizziness from faulty winding, not lack of oil. Care must be taken that hair ends and each section of the hair are properly wound.

✄ If hair is limp after a permanent, the cause may be one of many. If you used a home wave, write to the manufacturer with your query. If you had a salon wave, tell your troubles to your hairdresser; in some cases the limpness can be corrected.

HAIR STRAIGHTENING

Hair straightening is the opposite of permanent waving—the same process of softening the hair so that it relaxes and takes on the shape that is applied to it, and then neutralizing to fix the new shape. If hair is coarse and in good condition and not too curly to begin with, the process usually works well. Fine hair is harder to straighten than coarse hair.

✄ The softening solution is applied to the hair, starting at the nape and is combed through the hair till the hair becomes straight. This is repeated over the entire head—or in whatever parts are to be straightened. Then the hair is neutralized and rinsed and shampooed.

✄ Straightened hair always has a little bend left in it. In humid weather it may become curlier or even a little frizzy. A hard-hold setting lotion will help avoid this.

✄ As new hair grows in, straightened hair becomes curly at the crown and the new hair has to be straightened as soon as this becomes a problem. Although the straightening effect on the hair that is straightened is as lasting as permanent waving, the problem of new growth is harder to deal with. A growing-out and even trimmed permanent stays curly at the ends, where curl is wanted. The straightened head of hair becomes curly near the scalp where curl is wanted least.

35

HAIR-COLORING GUIDE

Should you color your hair? Sooner or later, you may say "Yes." Big questions: "What shall I use?" "What shade do I choose?" "If I don't like it, can I change back?" "Will it cost a fortune?" "How much time does it take?"

Before you consider hair color—or a change—you need to be aware that some home-use preparations are designed only for previously untreated hair—for example, sunlighteners, frosting and streak kits, some blonders and six-week, or semipermanent, colorings. If you use a preparation such as the froster or streaker, you should not lighten your hair by another process until your streaks have entirely grown out—or are ready to be cut off. With other products, like the six-week semipermanent colors, you can switch to one-process permanent hair coloring—or even double-process blonding. Before you switch from one type of coloring to another, ask yourself: "What have I done to my hair?" And if you've treated it a lot, or it's out of condition, get a professional's advice on how to change.

Two big items are extremely important in successful home hair coloring—the *patch test* and the *strand test*.

🌿 The *patch test for sensitivity* consists of mixing the color with its developer and applying a few drops behind an ear, where you leave it undisturbed for 24 hours before you use the color on your hair. If irritation develops, don't use the preparation. This test protects you against certain allergic reactions you may have—or may later develop—to the hair coloring.

🌿 The *strand test* is done on a single strand of hair to determine how long the preparation should be left on your particular type of hair and to guide you in timing the process. Proceed according to directions—and remember, the time it takes to do a strand test must be added to the time it takes to color the rest of the hair and, of course, to shampoo and set and dry it.

Protect your hands with rubber or plastic gloves when you do your hair coloring.

Keep in mind that—except for two-process blonding, where the hair is first lightened to a pale shade and then colored to a particular blond or light-red shade—the hair coloring reacts *with your natural hair color* to form the new shade. Temporary and semipermanent hair colorings should be chosen in a shade near your natural color. If you use one-process permanent color and have some gray in your hair, the gray takes the color differently from the hair that still has natural color. But this light and shading gives a pleasing, natural effect. If hair is very dark and resistant, it may take as long as two hours—and maybe several applications of lightener—to prepare it for a light shade of coloring.

🌿 The natural coloring matter, or pigments, in the hair—what makes it brown, black, red, gold—lie in an underlayer of hair called the *cortex*. Any hair coloring or lightener that is permanent—that will not wash out and will last till the hair grows out—has to penetrate to this pigmented layer. There the natural pigments will be removed by the processing (lightening) or new color will be deposited (tinting). In order for the cortex (pigmented layer) to be reached, the outer layer of flat tooth-edged cells, the cuticle, has to be softened enough for the bleach or dye to penetrate.

To get a decided change in your hair color or to lighten your natural hair color, you have to use a pentrating hair coloring or a bleach that acts on the pigmented layer of the hair.

🌿 The pigments that give hair its natural color are (1) of the brown variety—combined with proteins and fairly easy to remove; (2) of the yellow and red variety, containing iron and more difficult to remove.

Once you have bleached or dyed your hair, the natural color will not come back into the treated hair. But new growth at the roots will come in with the natural pigmentation and will have to be bleached or dyed to match the previously treated hair.

Hair grows at the rate of about a quarter-inch to half-an-inch a month (faster in summer than in winter) so a touch-up of the new growth in three to four weeks is necessary. The hair at the back of the head is usually darker than the rest of the hair and, in lightening the hair, this part is done first. Because scalp heat accelerates lightening action, when the hair is bleached for the first time, hair closest the scalp is done last.

🌿 Blond hair has little pigment and this hair will often fade or darken in early youth. To remain blond, such hair will need lightening.

🌿 Red hair also often loses its redness, fading or darkening to brown; then some kind of color reviver is helpful.

🌿 Brown appears in a variety of hair shades—some with reddish casts, some with golden casts, some so dark as to appear black. Brown hair may turn dull and may need warmth (adding of red tones) or brightness.

🌿 Black hair is truly black. But most hair that is considered black is really dark brown. Dark brown or black hair shows any gray readily because of the contrast in color. Covering or blending in early gray is often desirable.

🌿 Hair becomes gray and then white by losing its natural pigments. No one is quite sure just why hair grays—and natural color cannot be restored. Early graying is probably a hereditary trait. Except for color, gray hair is often normal; but if the skin generally is dry, the hair will also be dry. Gray and white hair may turn yellowish in sunlight and from certain wave solutions; special rinses liven the gray color or add silver, blue, or lavender tones. Scattered gray hairs can be blended or made less noticeable with rinses or covered with tint, toner, or very dark semipermanent color.

WHAT HAIR COLORINGS DO

When choosing a hair color, remember that *temporary colors* and *semipermanent colors* do *not* lighten the hair—they enhance the natural color, give highlights and blend in gray. The lightening shades of *one-process permanent color* (lotion tints) lighten only up to nine shades (on very dark hair). The shampoo-in tints lighten only up to four or five shades. When hair is lightened, it goes in *stages* (depending on its original color) from black to brown to red to red-gold to gold to yellow to pale yellow. These are the *stages* in lightening—and are *not* what is meant by *shades* of lightening. The shades are much slighter changes, being the points at which a visible difference in the hair color is apparent. Light brown hair, lightened nine shades, will become a light blond; dark brown in nine stages lightens to a red-brown (auburn shade). One-process permanent color acts with the natural hair color to produce the new shade. To lighten and tone the hair, it must be lightened to the stage indicated on the toner package to produce the same shade.

Some preparations are designed for previously untreated hair—these are the sunlighteners, and frost and streak kits. Frosting kits and sunlighteners work best on medium brown to blond hair; streaking kits are recommended for brown hair or darker.

Temporary color is color that can be shampooed out; hair that has been exposed only to temporary color is *not* considered to have been previously treated. Use of any other hair coloring or lightener or blonder means that your hair has been color-treated—observe precautions.

In permanent hair coloring it is usually suggested that a woman (particularly if she is over 30) go to a shade that is lighter, rather than darker, than

36

her own coloring. If you are now gray, it is also suggested that you go to a lighter shade than your original coloring. If you darken your hair and don't like it, don't change it yourself, consult a professional hair colorist.

Except for temporary color, a patch test for sensitivity is required before using a hair coloring.

When your hair is color-treated, it needs special handling—use a shampoo for color-treated hair; use a conditioner after each shampoo. Do not subject color-treated hair to too much sun or other hazards (such as swimming-pool chemicals). Do *not* have a permanent at the same time as you have a hair-coloring treatment. Wait a week after the permanent before you color your hair, or a week to 10 days after your hair treatment for a permanent. Use only a *gentle* permanent on color-treated hair; time carefully.

Change your makeup colors when you change your hair color—a new lipstick and foundation will help your new hair color *go*.

HAIR-COLORING PREPARATIONS

Hair-coloring preparations include the temporary colorings—color rinses, metallic powders, color crayons—that can be removed by shampooing; the semipermanent colorings — longer-lasting color that fades with three to five shampoos; permanent hair colorings—tints and toners that cannot be shampooed out and that permanently change the color of the hair; lighteners—which bleach or permanently remove natural pigments from the hair; and preparations to create special effects—streaks—in otherwise untreated hair. Except for the temporary colorings, a patch test for sensitivity is required. A strand test may also be necessary to time your processing correctly. Rubber or plastic gloves (sometimes included in the hair-coloring kit) must be used to protect the fingernails (they take color similarly to the way hair takes color) when you work with most coloring preparations.

Temporary hair colorings. Color can be shampooed out. Temporary hair coloring can be used on human hair wigs and hairpieces as well as on your own hair. They cannot produce a decided color change. They color-coat the outside of the hair shaft only, and do not penetrate to lighten or change the natural color.

Color rinse—Highlights, tones and enriches natural color, reduces brassiness on lightened and toned hair between touch-ups, evens the color in gray and white hair. Washes out with each shampoo.

Highlight shampoo—This incorporates a temporary coloring in a shampoo. Do not confuse with shampoo-in permanent hair coloring or semipermanent foam-in color. Highlights, tones, and enriches natural color; evens gray or white.

Spray-on powder—To accent or highlight; or to streak or tip; also to cover new growth at scalp between touch-ups.

Color crayon—For temporary retouch on roots when new growth begins to show. Apply to untreated areas only where new growth is visible.

Semipermanent colors. Do not rub off or shampoo out, but do fade with three to five shampoos. The coloring affects only the outer layer of the hair shaft and does not lighten the hair or make a decided change in the natural color. Choose a shade near your own hair color or darker. Blends in gray and enhances natural hair color; most products incorporate conditioners that give luster and body.

Color rinse—In applicator bottle; conditioner incorporated in product or included in kit. Apply to dry hair before shampooing. Product lathers and cleans while it colors.

Foam-in—In applicator can; conditioner incorporated in coloring product. Plastic gloves included in kit. Can keep leftover for touch-up. Apply to clean, dry hair.

3-week-rinse—Powder (in capsule). Incorporates conditioner. Mix with water before applying to clean towel-dried hair (after shampoo).

Sunlighteners. Gentle oil bleaches slightly lighten hair—but do not tone (add color) as they lighten. Lightening action takes place only while hair is damp. The warmth of the sun or the heat of your hair drier is needed to activate lightener. Can lighten whole head or be used to streak hair (apply only to individual strands) for a sunlit look. Best for natural blondes, medium to light brownettes, with previously untreated hair. Can also be used for retouching roots later.

One-process permanent hair colors. These are the lotion tints and shampoo-in tints that penetrate to the inner shaft (cortex) of the hair *(see diagram, page 31)* to change the natural color—either by lightening and toning (the lightening shades) or by infusing color (the darkening shades). The coloring acts with the natural hair color to produce the new hair color. The change is permanent in the treated hair—the color will not shampoo out. Protect tinted hair from overexposure to sun—as it continues to oxidize and set the color for the first 24 hours.

Lotion tint—One-process tints can give you a decided change in hair color, covering 100% of gray, lightening your natural color up to nine shades (in dark hair) or darkening your own natural color, producing reds, browns, black, or blond hair color depending on the combination of your natural hair color and the shade of tint chosen. Except for "two-process permanent hair color," which can give the delicate pale shades of blond or red, one-process lotion tints produce the most decided color change.

Shampoo-in tint—Will lighten hair about half as many shades as the same color in a lotion tint. Shampoo-in tints change color depth and tone, lighten up to four shades, or deepen hair color, and cover up to 35% of gray.

One-process blonders—Blonders—for the woman who wants to lighten blond hair, keep it light, or to add gold or red highlights to darker hair. One-process blonders act on the cortex (pigmented layer of the hair) to remove natural color—and thus to lighten the hair. May also be used to streak and tip. Available in kit with fast-acting lightener, accelerator, or as one-process lotion, which lightens and tones in one process. Conditioner incorporated in product.

Two-process permanent coloring. This "double blonding" is needed for delicate light-blond and pale-red hair colors. The first process—lightening—removes the natural color from the pigmented layer of the hair shaft (but does not add color). Any degree of lightness can be achieved, but the lightener may have to be reapplied several times to bring very dark hair to a pale shade. Black hair goes from black to brown to red to red-gold to gold to yellow to pale-yellow as it lightens. It is necessary to check the toning product (see "Toner") to learn what stage of lightening is required for a particular shade. Even gray or white hair needs to be pretreated for 45 minutes to make it porous enough to take a toner. Lightener with developer and accelerator and toner with developer can be bought as individual kits or individual items; complete two-process-color kits are available.

Toner—A toner penetrates the hair shaft to give the new delicate color to previously lightened hair. It doesn't lighten the hair itself. On first treatment, hair must be treated by lightener for at least 45 minutes to make it porous enough to accept toner. The toner package will tell you what degree of lightening is required for a particular toner shade. Lotion or shampoo toners are available.

Toner may be in kit with developer and plastic gloves, or toner and developer can be bought separately.

SPECIAL EFFECTS

Coloring for special effects—frosting, tipping, streaking—is really two-process color (lightener plus color rinse). The at-home preparations are for use on previously untreated hair, and should not be used on previously lightened hair, nor should another lightening process be used on the frosted, tipped, or streaked hair till treated sections have grown out.

Frosting—Consists of lightening and color-rinsing strands all over the head for a sunlit look. Tipping involves lightening and color-rinsing wider strands of hair chiefly around the face. Streaking is the lightening and color rinsing of wider (one-half-inch) strands of hair (one to six strands) around the face. The same effects can be produced on previously treated hair by two-process color or even by one-process blonders, depending on the hair shade, but this is a job for a professional colorist. Sunlighteners and powders are other preparations that can be used for streaking hair that has not been otherwise lightened.

Frosting and tipping—Hair is lightened to the desired shade and then toned with a color rinse. Kit includes lightener and developer, color rinse, perforated cap (through which individual strands of hair are drawn), hooked "needle," mixing spoon and bowl, plastic gloves, and heat cap.

Streaking—This process is for lightening and color-rinsing sections of hair one-quarter to one-half inch thick; use only on untreated hair; not recommended for blondes. Kit includes lightener and developer, color rinse, mixing spoon and bowl, plastic gloves, foil wraps. You must provide your own conditioner (for use in application) and cotton strips and bobby pins.

CHEMISTRY OF HAIR COLORING

Certified color—These are the "acid" colorings used in temporary rinses and do not require a patch test before using.

Developer—20-volume peroxide usually in a cream formula. The 20-volume peroxide is used to "develop" the action of permanent tints and bleaches and most toners. Usually the developer is bought in a 6-ounce bottle for home use (unless developer is included in the kit), and this is enough for three treatments. It is unwise to buy in larger quantities for home use as "freshness" is important in the action.

Lightener—This is usually bleach in either cream or powder form. The cream is mixed with an accelerator (to speed the lightening action) and with a developer—20-volume hydrogen peroxide—to make the action take place. The powder bleach is usually mixed with 20-volume hydrogen peroxide, which serves as the developer.

Semipermanent colors—These contain aniline (organic) derivatives (as do tints, see below), but are not mixed with peroxide. The color penetrates only the outer layer of the hair. A heat cap is usually worn, as scalp warmth accelerates the action. With foam-ins, air is the oxidizing agent, and the heat cap is not needed.

Tint—These permanent colorings are aniline-derivative (organic) dyes that act on the cortex (inner layer) of the hair shaft and require a patch test for sensitivity. The tint is mixed with developer (20-volume peroxide), which helps it penetrate the outer layer. Never store any *mixed* tint and developer. Unused tint (unmixed) can be stored if kept tightly closed.

Toner—Usually a dilute tint (aniline derivative) mixed with developer and applied to previously lightened and softened hair. Some toners, like semipermanent colors, need no developer, but do require a heat cap to develop the action.

Vegetable and metallic dyes—These are "permanent" dyes but do not require a patch test. Henna is the only vegetable coloring now used as a hair dye. The metallic dyes coat the hair shaft and give a less natural appearing coloring than tints but can be used if one is sensitive to the compounds in tints.

Drabbing drops—These drops are used sparingly as an additive to tint or bleach. They cut down reddish or gold notes to avoid brassiness in the new hair color. As we pointed out earlier, the red and yellow pigments are difficult to remove from the hair. When you use a drab tint or toner, you may still get a reddish or brassy (yellowish) effect because red-gold pigments still in your hair show up. Drabbing drops are used sparingly in the tint-developer mix to help knock out these pigments.

PRECAUTIONS

Do not use a hair-coloring preparation if your scalp skin is scratched or for any reason irritated. Postpone the hair treatment till the problem is relieved. Take care, in the several days before your hair-coloring treatment, not to strike the scalp sharply with brush or comb or to scratch your head too much or otherwise to irritate the scalp.

If your skin is tender (or even moderately so), you may feel a burning sensation on the scalp if you use a bleach. This may not be abnormal, and probably will be relieved as soon as the bleach is removed. But because the discomfort may be disturbing, it is often wise to have the first bleach job done by a professional who can evaluate your reaction. Many women are very good at doing their own lightening and toning, but many women aren't—and it is our recommendation that for the first time—and even for touch-ups—this is a job for the beauty salon.

BEFORE YOU USE A COLOR PREPARATION

Before you buy, decide upon what type of coloring you want and be sure that you are buying the kind of preparation you want. For example, do not confuse foam-in semipermanent coloring with shampoo-in tint or highlight shampoo. Do not use home streaking or frosting kits on previously treated hair.

❧ Read the label carefully to be sure you are getting the kind of coloring you want for your kind of hair and to learn what is included in the kit.

❧ Be sure you know *everything* you will need to complete the treatment—plastic or rubber gloves (if not included in the kit), shampoo for color-treated hair, conditioner (if not included in the preparation or in the kit), developer (for tint or bleach) if not included in the kit.

❧ Read the directions in the package carefully and follow instructions.

❧ Do a patch-test 24 hours before using a hair-coloring preparation.

❧ Do a strand test for timing, if suggested, before you start.

❧ Assemble your supplies and be sure the package has all the items necessary to do the job or that you have assembled them individually.

SPECIAL THINGS TO DO

❧ Be sure to use rubber or plastic gloves during your hair coloring.

❧ When used, hair coloring and developer should be at room temperature; store any unused tint or developer where it will not get too warm or too cold.

❧ Discard any mixture of tint or bleach and developer. Do not store *mixed* hair-coloring preparations at any time.

❧ Unmixed leftover hair-coloring preparations may be stored, but the bottles should be tightly closed.

❧ Use plastic, glass or china bowls for your mixing and a plastic applicator. Metal should not come in contact with hair-coloring preparations.

❧ To avoid stains, protect your clothes and your surroundings from splashes of your hair-coloring preparation. If these happen, rinse away quickly.

❧ Do not let your hair-coloring preparation get near your eyes. Keep eyes tightly closed during rinsing.

❧ If hair coloring gets into the eye, wash eye thoroughly with clear cool water (15 minutes). See doctor.

❧ Keep hair-coloring preparations out of the reach of children.

❧ Know how the shade you buy will react with your own hair color—do you want a lighter or darker shade than your own in a tint? Will you want a drab or warm color in a shade near your own?

❧ Semipermanent color should be chosen in the shade nearest your own hair color.

❧ Shampoo-in tints should be chosen in a shade *near* your own color.

CHOOSING A HAIR COLOR

In a permanent hair coloring, it is usually suggested that a woman (particularly if she is over 30) go to a shade that is lighter rather than darker, than her own coloring. If you are now gray, it is also suggested that you go to a lighter shade than your original coloring. The reasoning behind this is that skin tones also change as hair grays—and lighter hair becomes more flattering. The question: How light is light?

A good rule to follow in selecting one-process color is this: If hair has little gray, choose a hair coloring two to four shades lighter than your present hair color. If 50 percent gray, choose a coloring two shades lighter than your present hair color. If hair is all gray, choose a coloring one shade lighter than your natural color. To match natural color of the hair and to cover gray, choose a shade close to your natural color.

Skin tones relate to the choice of hair coloring:

❧ If your skin is clear and fair and pinky fresh, you can be very flexible in your hair coloring—pale blond, soft brown, red, auburn, and if you are very young, dark brown, even black.

❧ If you have a very light skin, light warm tones will be becoming—but you can also be flattered by warm browns.

❧ If your skin is neutral—beigy—avoid the extremely dark tones. You need warmth and brightness.

❧ If your skin is very ruddy, stay away from harsh reds, but warm reddish brown or warm tones of blond can be becoming.

❧ If skin is olive (brunette) and you have naturally dark hair, stick with auburns, warm or dark browns, and avoid too much light and brightness in color. Blond hair is great with tanned skin.

❧ If skin is brown or dark brown and accompanied by natural black hair, hair can be colored to a richer black or blue black or lightened to a warm dark brown. Often the red notes that appear with lightening are not becoming.

Important in choosing a hair color is the distinction between the warm colors—those with red or red-gold cast—and the drabs, or ash, shades—those without the red or red-gold notes.

Because of the red and yellow pigments in the natural hair, the red and gold notes often appear in hair that is lightened, even with a drab shade of hair coloring.

If hair is white or all gray, these natural pigments are reduced and the ashy shades of hair coloring will come out drab. This may produce too dull an effect if skin is also beigy. In this case, you should choose a warmer shade of hair coloring.

A warm color on hair that has strong red and yellow pigments still in the hair can come out too red or goldy. If your present hair is dark ash blond or darker, the ashy (drab) hair colorings will still produce a warm effect.

The very best way to find the right color for you is to have your first hair coloring done for you by a professional colorist in a salon. This is particularly important if you are going to take a big step—go to a decidedly different hair color.

Apart from that, the general rules are these:

❧ In temporary color (rinse), choose a shade near your own or in a shade to produce a special effect—silvery, gold, reddish, or even pastel pink, blue, yellow.

❧ In semipermanent color, a shade that matches your own hair color.

❧ In one-step permanent color, a shade one to two shades lighter than your own (lightening shades) or near your own (darkening shades).

❧ For two-process blonding, get professional advice.

❧ If you darken your hair and don't like it, don't change it yourself, consult a professional hair colorist about making a change.

❧ Think of hair color in terms of the *drabs*—colors without red tones—and the *warm* colors—those with a reddish cast—and the golds.

❧ The more contrast between natural and artificial color, the more noticeable will be new growth. Style your hair so you can keep your touch-ups as far apart as possible—preferably four weeks apart, no closer than three.

❧ Do not use durable color for two weeks before a permanent wave or for one week after.

❧ Keep a record of your color formula and of your timing as a guide to the next treatment—and consider that a formula must be changed from time to time, particularly if you are graying.

❧ Before you color your hair, snip a small strand of your own hair color and keep this for a guide in case you want to recolor your hair in your own shade.

❧ Do not overexpose color-treated hair to the sun; most colors oxidize and change in sunlight, as does natural hair, and hair may become brassy or reddish.

❧ Use a neutral shampoo or a shampoo for color-treated hair.

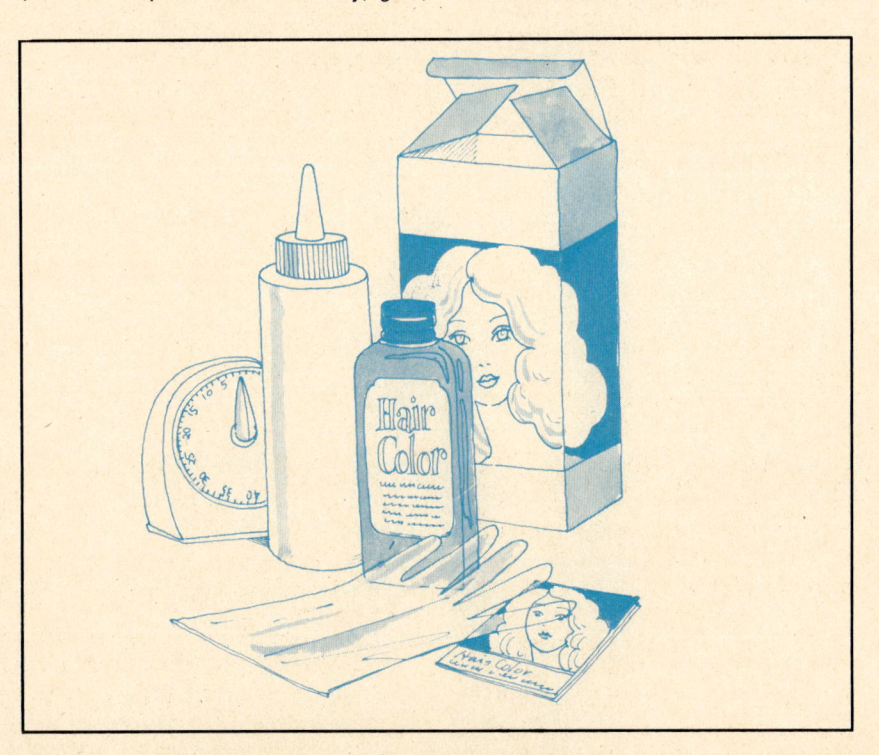

GIVE YOUR MAKEUP A MAGIC TOUCH

Makeup is the art of illusion. Once you know what to do to create this illusion of beauty, you can get the effect with surprising ease. Selecting colors and harmonizing colors is a key. Part of the makeup—foundation and powder—must be chosen to bring out and enhance the lively tones of the skin; other elements—eye shadow and lipstick—bring eye and clothes color into harmony.

Are you omitting the important "first step"? You should start with a clean face; if skin is dry, two cleansings with cream; if skin is oily, use a liquid cleanser. But when skin is fresh and clean, there is still the need for a "normalizer" before makeup is applied. This is the first step in a makeup that stays fresh. Apply a moisturizer if skin is dry, a toning liquid if skin is oily; or, if you have dry and oily areas, a moisturizer where that is needed and a toner where oil appears (usually the center of the face, from forehead to chin). The moisturizer prevents flaking, helps makeup last. A toner helps keep oily areas dry; excess oil can cause makeup colors to change, and your illusion of beauty will be lost.

Have you found your best foundation color? Some women have a perfect complexion, and for these women it is true that matching the skin tone will give the right foundation color. But most women have problem skin, and the right color choice can improve it.

Many women have a florid skin and should choose beige tones to subdue the pinks, but care should be taken that all the natural color is not toned out. Enough should show through to give a lively look to the complexion. Other women have a pale or sallow complexion and need color in their foundation, pinkish tones to bring out the highlights and make the skin look alive. Great care should be taken to choose a foundation that will not change color on the skin.

Do you remove the excess foundation? To apply foundation, put little dabs over the skin of the face and throat and then spread the foundation gently over the skin with the cushions of the fingers in upward strokes till the skin is smoothly covered. Don't rub; smooth on gently. Then the excess should be removed. Wrap tissue around fingers, and, starting at the chin, work upward gently. A foundation so applied and so removed will minimize tiny skin imperfections, highlight the complexion, and never make the face look hard and old.

Do you ignore lights and shades? To highlight, use a lightener in all expression lines, in the curve around the nostrils, in the dark shadows about the eyes and also in the hollows of the cheeks if they are pronounced. This not only softens the shadows but rounds the contour of the face; used around the eyes, lightener makes deep-set eyes brighter and seems to bring them

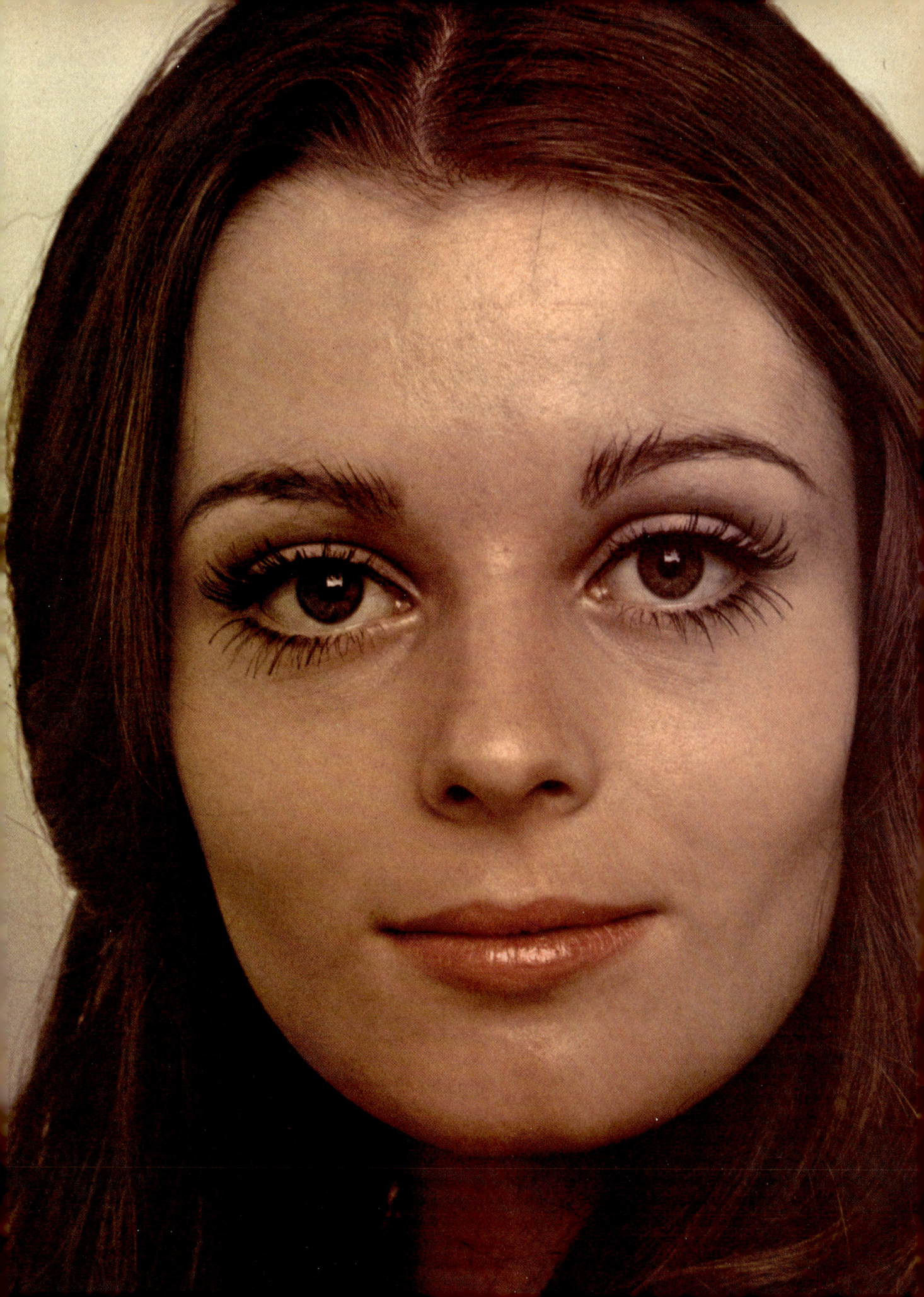

forward. Use also on any pigment spots and birthmarks. Press the lightener into the lines; remove excess with tissue. For shading, use brown contour cream, or brown shadow, which is soft and spreads easily. Smooth onto the fatty area below the brow, and around the eye; use around the eyes if sunglasses or regular eyeglasses' rims have left white areas; use too, on the pale V-shape area below the chin. If lights and shades are applied where needed and blended in well, they can make the whole face beautifully modeled. Apply lightener under foundation, shading over foundation.

Do you neglect neck and throat? If the throat is smooth and pretty, you needn't use makeup on it. Just blend in the foundation at the jawline. But many women need to do something about the neck and throat, particularly when the throat skin is dry. Cover the entire skin of throat and neck with brown shader and tone it in well. This will shape and firm the jaw line, minimize a double chin, make the entire throat appear smooth and beautiful, and help to concentrate attention on the face.

Are you afraid of rouge? Rouge should harmonize with the lip color and should be applied to give a natural blush, a healthy look. Start with a single dot on the cheek under the center of the eye and blend carefully toward the outside of the face in a half-moon shape on the part of the cheek that lifts when you smile. Never bring the rouge below the lower tip of the nostril and keep the color high and to the outside of the face, not bringing the color close to the nose. If face is full, blend the dot of rouge in a V-shape to below the lower tip of the nostril but stop above the line of the upper lip. Use a tissue folded over the fingers to tone rouge and work in upward rotary strokes. Teenagers should apply rouge lower on the face than does the mature woman.

Have you forgotten about loose powder? Loose powder should always be used in the first makeup of the day. Loose powder gives the skin a fine texture and adds a delicate touch to the complexion and also helps the makeup stay fresh-looking. Pressed powder can be used for touch-ups during the day, but these will not often be needed if the first makeup is done well. Lightly pat on translucent loose powder with a puff till you look as if your face had been in a flour barrel; then, using outward strokes, brush off the excess with a powder brush till only a fine mist remains.

Does your eye makeup become too theatrical? Shadow, liner, and mascara can be used to enhance the eyes without creating an exaggerated look. Eyeliner is becoming if skillfully applied; it goes on easiest if you use a liquid liner and a sable brush. Start at the inner tip of the upper lid and swing the line delicately across the lid at the roots of the lashes; stop at the outer tip. Shadow is then applied to soften this line. Use cream, stick, or cake eye shadow and, again, apply with a sable brush just above the lashes, increasing slightly upward at the outer tip of the eye to give a soft line and up as far as the crease in the upper lid. Shadow is keyed to the wardrobe color—and you will need a variety of shades. Frosted shadow is pretty for evening, and a little frosted topaz in tiny, scarcely visible strokes on the fatty area just below the brow gives a nice open look.

Can you avoid a hard line in the brow? If you have trouble penciling brows, darken them with brow powder. After powder is applied, rough up brows, combing then from the outer tip toward the nose; then comb the brow hairs upward to leave a wide space between brow and eyes. Shape into a natural arch with the comb. Now, using a brown or black pencil (use the side of the pencil, not the tip), fill in the brow line as needed with light lines, as if you were drawing delicate hairs. If hair has golden lights, touch up with a gold pencil; if hair is black with silver lights, use a silver pencil.

Do you "tip-off" your mascara? Using

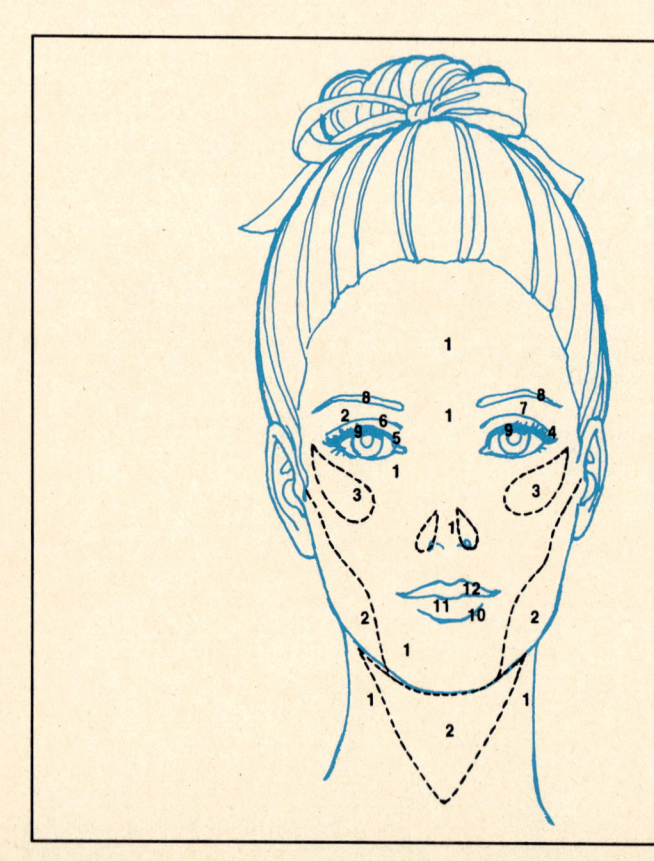

Basic makeup plan—Apply undertone to face and throat to give a soft glow. Lightener **(1)** is pressed into forehead and throat lines, around eyes, and in a thin line down tip of nose. Foundation is smoothed gently over the skin, and excess is removed. Shader **(2)** is blended under chin, below eyebrow, and in hollows of the cheeks. Cream rouge **(3)** is toned over fattest part of cheek in half-moon shape. Loose powder is then applied generously, and excess is removed with powder brush. Upper lid is lined **(4)** with a brush and liner; shadow **(5)** is applied to the lower half of upper lid, with darker shader **(6)** in crease and lighter **(7)** above. Brows are first darkened with powder **(8)** and then filled in with pencil. Lashes are darkened with brown or black mascara **(9)** and tipped with colored mascara. Lips are outlined with lip-liner pencil **(10)** and then filled with lipstick **(11)** and glossed **(12)**.

a mascara wand, apply the color with a rolling motion, under and up, to the undersides of the lashes; to make a definite upsweep, hold the wand upward against the lashes till they dry. Apply two coats, combing the lashes after each application to prevent sticking or beading. Then use colored mascara on the tips; it will not be obvious but will be very lovely.

Have you learned about lip liners? You need at least two lipsticks—a bright color and a muted transparent gloss. The lip should first be lined (use pencil or brush) to give the mouth a definite shape. The liner prevents smudging and seeping of the color into the fine lines around the lips. Apply lipstick generously within the lip line. Apply a second coat of lip gloss with a sweeping stroke that gives fullness to the lips. You can use a lighter shade in the middle of the mouth.

How can you judge your makeup? Applied with taste and knowledge, your makeup will give the illusion of beauty. But how can you really be sure that your makeup is exactly right? The best way to evaluate is to use a magnifying mirror. If, in this mirror, the effect is slightly more vivid than you would like it to be, you can be sure that it will be just about right as other persons see you—even in sunlight.

HOW TO CHOOSE AND USE THE NEW MAKEUPS

Gels, translucents, cover-ups — which should you choose? Makeup super-simplified—that's the *sheer gels*. If you have a clear complexion that needs color but not cover-up—if you want a healthy no-makeup look—these gels are for you. Shiny, reflecting, glowy—*translucent makeup* is for you if you want a little covering (to hide freckles or blotches, maybe?) and still let your own healthy skin show through. You need a good complexion underneath—and it helps to have a bit of natural blush. *Cover-up makeup* isn't only for the girl who has something to hide—it's also for anyone who wants a completely finished look to her complexion. Take your time with it. This makeup should be flawlessly done to be just that—flawless.

Sheer gel tints. These offer the simplest of makeups and give a wonderful just-you look. Color choice is by skin and hair tones—golden shades for brunettes, peach for blondes, pink for brownettes, coral for redheads—with the undertint in a shade that brings out your best. Use green (yes, green!) to tone down an overblush and produce beige skin tones; pink if skin is sallow; peach or coral to add glow. To apply, squeeze some of the gel into one palm and pat over the face with the fingertips of the other hand. Use sparingly; pat thinly over wide areas; before you put on the next tint, give the skin time to react to the earlier one. Don't be too quick to put on the next tint or take the next step.

🍃 Start with a thin coating of a face-tint gel. Pat thinly over entire face and throat and let dry.

🍃 Cheek gel is thinly patted over a generous portion of the sides of face and on cheeks, with just a touch on the chin. Blend edges well.

🍃 With the little finger, spread shadow gel over the upper lid very close to the lashes and up to the fold, blending outward toward the temple. A tiny touch of a brighter but harmonizing shadow gel in the middle of the upper lid emphasizes color.

🍃 Use a transparent liner to line lightly the roots of the lashes on the lower lid and to line upper lid. Mascara lightly.

Translucent makeup. This makeup takes time and a lot of skillful brushwork to add up to a wholesome mini-makeup effect.

🍃 Your complexion is pretty but not perfect. So start with a pearlized undertint to give basic glow. If skin is yellowish and could look healthier, use pink; if you want to add glow, use peach or coral. Spread the undertint all over face and throat gently with the fingertips. Let it set before putting on foundation.

🍃 Translucent cream foundation in a neutral tone is spread evenly with the fingertips over face—cheekbones, nose, chin, forehead, throat—and let set.

🍃 Now for your brushwork: Start with a pearlized highlight cream. Under the eyes, brush it from the lash line into a downward V that tips out on the upper cheek right below the middle of the eye. This blocks out any under-eye shadows, gives the eye a new shape and dimension, and creates a very flattering highlight on the upper cheek.

🍃 Apply the highlight above the eye, too, close to the brow and just under the bone, lifting at the middle to emphasize this area and to give the eye up-and-down dimension.

🍃 Use the highlight, as well, to contour the cheeks. Starting from one ear, brush on highlighter in an elongated V-shape from ear to cheekbone but not overlapping or even quite touching the highlight. Use blusher one shade lighter above the highlight, again in a V-shape, along the top of the cheekbone from ear to tip of cheekbone. The edge of the line should be softened but not blended with the highlight.

🍃 Brush the entire face—chin, under chin, throat, eyes—with translucent powder.

🍃 Slightly above the natural crease of the eye, brush in hollow shader, lifting and emphasizing the color slightly at the middle of the brow line. If either corner becomes too heavy, lighten it with a cotton-tip stick.

🍃 Apply brush-on shadow in color in a dome shape on the upper lid to the crease, slightly elongating the lid at both corners. Blend the colored shadow lightly into the contour color at the fold so as to leave no definite line.

🍃 Draw a thin line of liner on the colored shadow, close to the base of the upper-lid lashes. This line should be right next to the lashes.

🍃 Above this line draw a very thin line of black, using an extra-fine brush.

🍃 Use a bright see-through-lipstick with translucent makeup.

Cover-up makeup. The total cover-up is the makeup for the woman who wants an absolutely flawless finish on her face. Choose a base to bring up your skin tone or match it.

🍃 Light cover makeup is spread evenly over the face and throat with the fingertips. It must be smoothly blended, and after it is applied, it is helpful to go over the entire face with a damp sponge to blot and smooth.

🍃 With a puff, press loose powder into the foundation over the entire face and throat so makeup will be long-lasting.

🍃 Brush contour makeup gently over the entire lower jaw—from the middle of the ear inward to the edge of the cheekbone and down close to the jawbone—so as not to have a definite edge (though the contoured area is square).

🍃 Brush cream rouge over the sides of the face to the temples, coming up the side of the face past the brow line and over the highest part of the cheekbones, and also touching the chin, the tip of the nose, under the brows, and the forehead at the hairline.

🍃 Shadow the upper lid in colored shadow from the lashes to the crease of the lid, lightly blurring the shadow for an indefinite shape and rounding it over the outer tip of the eye to the lower corner between the lash lines. Darken the base of the lashes with eye liner, slightly heavier toward the outer corner but not circling the eye.

🍃 Brows are brushed with powder brow makeup.

🍃 Use opaque lipstick in a bright color, filling out the lip lines, plus a lip gloss to mute the shade.

How The Famous Salons Do The New Makeups

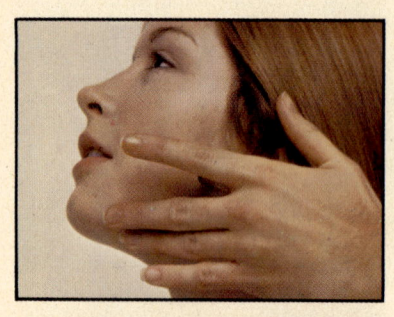

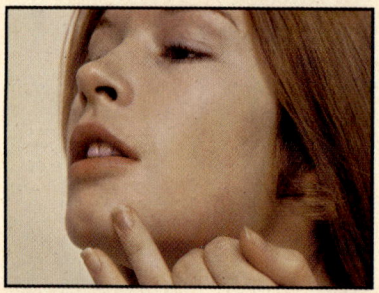

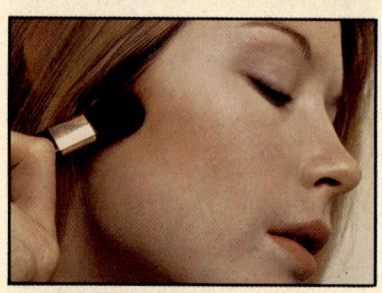

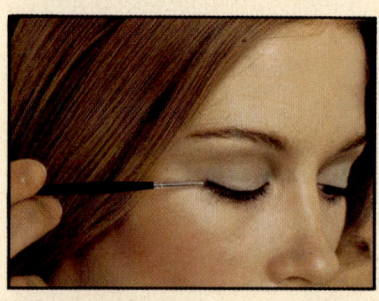

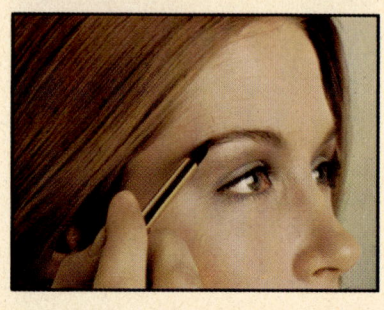

A good makeup shouldn't be hurried. Beauty salon makeups take from 30 minutes to an hour. This includes cleaning the face, moisturizing, and contouring. Use their little tricks—such as letting your moisturizer set for five minutes before putting on the makeup base and letting mascara dry between applications, and using brushes for artistry. Not rushing!

❧ Makeup starts with a good face cleaning (makeup should be an enhancement of your naked face).

❧ Use moisturizer (unless skin is oily), and use a faintly pink concealer under eyes to diminish shadows.

❧ Translucent foundation clarifies the skin and gives it an even color, but base should not be a visible covering. Your middle and ring fingers are your makeup fingers; use them to blend in foundation, stopping at the chin line. The throat usually looks better if not made up. Stop foundation at the chin line, blending it well so there is no line of demarcation.

❧ Fine, dry skin takes a minimum of makeup base; touch eyelids only lightly.

❧ To cover blemishes pat on a little extra foundation— one with more cover power than the base used all over.

❧ Shading is used almost as a straight line beneath high cheekbones to give depth and shape. Put on in a flying-V shape and blend along the cheek to the ears to give length to the face.

❧ Translucent powder is puffed on. Translucent powder helps hold the makeup and prevents caking. After 10 minutes, the powdery look disappears and only a natural glow remains.

❧ Use powder blusher as a shading in cheek hollows (below cheekbones). Creme rouge (shiny) as a highlighter on fatty part of cheek to bring out fullness, and up to the side of the eye (but not above the brow).

❧ Contour the eye socket in taupe shadow for depth and shape; the shadowing here shouldn't be at all obvious.

❧ Use pearlized color shadow on upper lid to the fold—a shiny highlight below the brow. Frosted shadow—under the brow on the upper lid and below the lower lashes, extending outward —makes eyes look larger by catching light.

❧ Line upper lid from tip to tip right in the lash line to shape the eye but so finely that the line itself isn't seen—very light on lower lid, darker on upper lid.

❧ Pencil the brows for emphasis and then brush to give a natural look to brows that need filling in and definition.

❧ To make silky or thin brows interestingly shaggy, put a little lash adhesive on a mascara brush and brush up.

❧ Mascara the tops of upper lashes to make false lashes adhere and create a single lash line. Use mascara on lower lashes, plus individual false

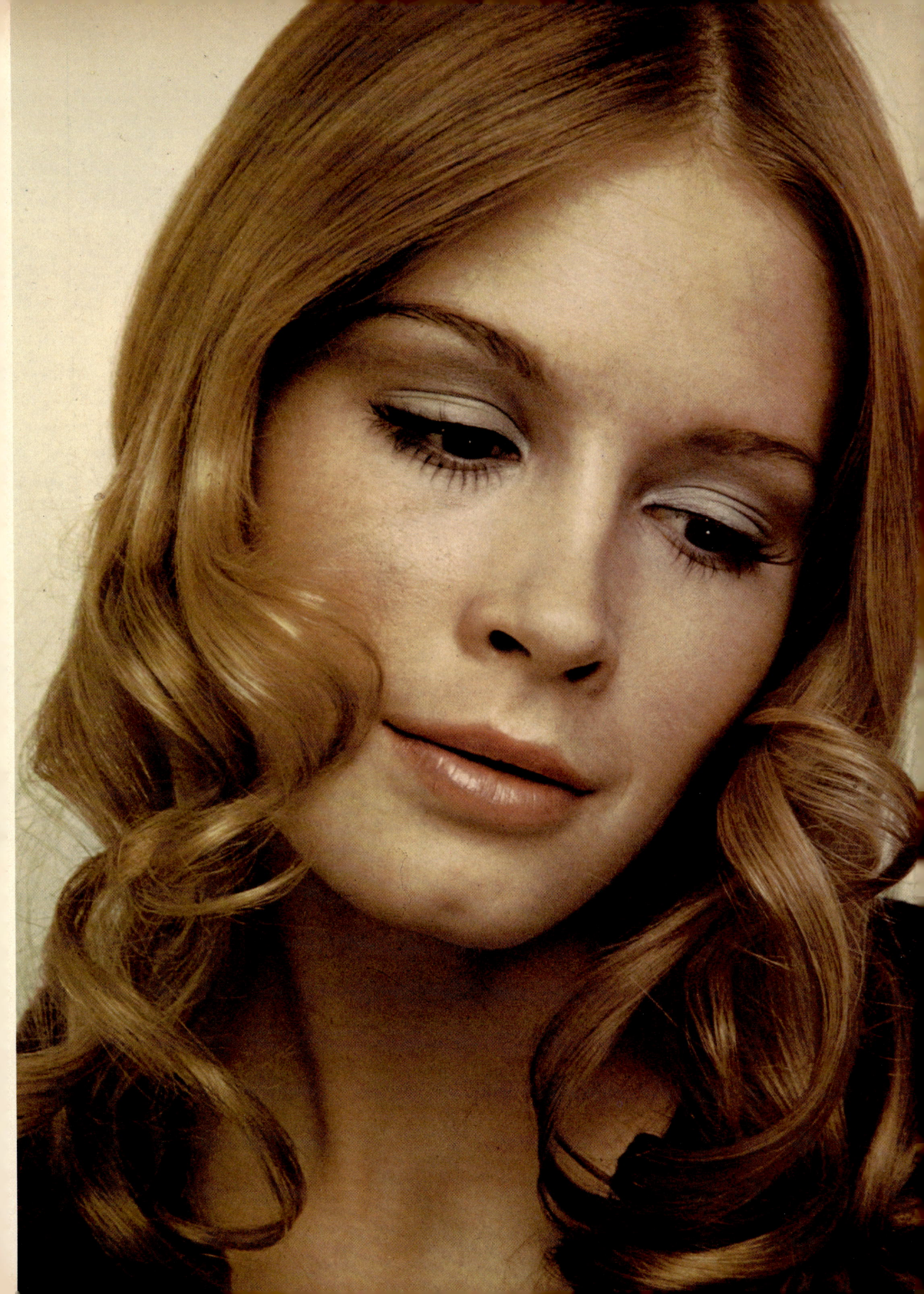

lashes, if you choose, but use no line here.

➤ False lashes are carefully cut to size. If too long, they can irritate the eye. They should begin at the inside corner where the eyelashes start and stop at the end where the natural lashes stop.

➤ To apply false lashes, grasp lashes between thumb and index finger. Apply adhesive to the base and leave for half a minute, till it gets tacky. Then hold head up and look down into a mirror so you can see your own lashes. Bring false lashes down onto your own lashes. Push lashes gently into place with a toothpick. Beginners have better luck if the lashes are on before eye makeup.

➤ Keep your mouth open slightly when you apply lip color. Use a lip brush to outline the mouth, following the natural lip line; then fill in the lip color with mouth open. A liner brush is needed with bright lip colors. Hold the brush like a pencil and rest your elbow on a tabletop till you get confidence. Do each lip from corner to middle on each side. Then fill.

WHAT COSMETICS FOR YOUR COMPLEXION?

Cosmetics today come in many different forms—and each has its own uses. What is right for you depends on your skin type and the effect you want to create. In creating your skin tones, it's the combination of foundation and powder that gives color to the complexion and evens the skin tones. The foundation gives the color and texture; the powder acts as a fixative. You should look for a clean light-texture foundation that will appear natural, will not cake on the skin, and will let the natural glow and beauty of the skin shine through.

Foundations. Your foundation can be almost anything from an invisible film to an opaque cover-up.

Tinted gel—This gives color and some tightening to the skin but almost no cover-up for blemishes, large pores and so on. Wonderful for a healthy outdoor look, letting a summer tan show through, and for anyone with a fine beautiful skin who wants only a glow. These gels are also available as leg and body make-up for instant tan. Pat on a gel with fingertips for smooth coverage. Let dry before patting on gel blusher and eye shadows. No powder needed.

Translucent liquid—Usually a powder suspended in liquid, this type of base must be mixed by shaking before you put it on your face. It gives color and minimum of cover-up. Fine for healthy young skin; great too for older skin with fine lines because it does not emphasize them. Shake bottle, apply base in dots on face and smooth with fingertips. This makeup gives a smooth clear look to the skin, and lets color show through. Best in beige tones where little added color is wanted.

Tinted lotion—This is the best all-round base for the woman with dry or normal skin who wants some color and some covering. Oils in the base give a natural dewy look. Apply lightly, remove excess and use loose transparent powder as a fixative.

Tinted cream—Heavier than lotion foundation, this gives good coverage and somewhat better protection from dryness. Use sparingly—apply with sponge and tissue off excess. Use with loose transparent powder for a lasting effect.

Cake makeup—This has good covering power and gives a matte finish to the oily or blemished skin. Apply with a damp sponge and roll makeup onto the skin so that it has a soft smooth look.

Contouring makeups—These are foundations—stick or creams—for use as lights or shades. Apply with brush, not from the stick or with fingertips, for most delicate effect. Choose one shade lighter or darker than the foundation so the contouring is subtle.

Blemish covers—These are cream foundations with greater covering power than the usual makeup bases. Closely match your foundation color and apply with a brush blending carefully into the surrounding area. Can also be used for reducing under-eye shadows.

Medicated makeup—The skin has a natural "flora"—the bacterial coating of the skin. If you have blemishes, you can help your skin (more by drying the oil than by the antibacterial effects) by wearing medicated makeup.

Hypoallergenic makeups—Most cosmetics have as few allergens as possible; perfume allergy is, however, common; hypoallergenic makeup is low in common allergens and may be worn by many (but not necessarily all) women who are allergic to other cosmetics.

Waterproof makeup—Makeup that goes swimming and stands up to storms is available. So are waterproof false lashes (attached with waterproof glue) and waterproofing liquid to coat your eye makeup.

Powder. You create your complexion color with makeup base. Powder should be neutral so that, when applied, it does not change the color of the foundation.

Loose powder—Powder sets the makeup and has the added advantage of reflecting light so that tiny lines become less visible. Powder generously all over the face; include eyelids, but powder lightly there. Then brush off excess powder with a powder brush in a downward direction. This removes excess and avoids a matte look. Then, go over the face with a damp sponge to give a natural luminous look. Pat the sponge lightly over the eyelids, nostrils and the entire face and forehead so the color, though softened, comes through. Natural skin oils also help to give a becoming dewy look. Wait 10 minutes and the dusty look of the powder disappears.

➤ Tinted powder, in the color of the foundation, adds to the tone of the makeup and is sometimes needed for a matte look.

➤ Translucent powder, or no-color powder, is preferable with most light-texture and translucent makeups.

Pressed powder—Some pressed powders combine a makeup base with the powder. This powder-plus-foundation is all the makeup you then need for everyday use; teenagers need not use a heavier base except for occasional dress-up parties. Other compact powders are face powder in pressed form (no base); these have little clinging power of their own but can be used for touch-ups over liquid or cream foundation. Do not use foundation-plus-powder compact makeup for touch-ups if you have already applied a base; the combined effect is likely to be heavy.

Blushers. Your foundation creates the skin tones; rouge adds a healthy glow. It also can be used to shape the face as rouge and blusher are really the same thing. All blushers except powder blushers are applied over foundation and before powdering. Powder blusher is put on after powdering.

Gel rouge—This transparent face color gives glow and color and should be put over large areas. Pat it on—don't rub, or it will streak.

Liquid rouge—This is usually a clear color that is applied to the face with fingertips and blended in over the foundation. It gives a clear lively glow.

Creme rouge—It has more body and is more opaque than either gel or liquid, and can be used for shading as well as for color.

Cheek gloss—It comes in a stick and can be used directly from the stick on cheeks, forehead, chin, and eyelids for glow and color.

Powder blusher—Can be used for color or shading. For color use over the high points of the face—cheeks, chin, tip of nose, forehead. For shading use under the chin, on the forehead, in hollows of cheeks and along the jaw line. Apply with large brush over the powder and re-apply frequently as it tends to shed.

Eye shadow. Shadow comes in cream, liquid or powder forms. In any case, you get the best effect if you apply it with a brush.
Cream shadow—This is soft and long lasting and gives a moist look. Apply lightly with brush so that the color is even and clear and will not crease. To prevent creasing, fill in with powder shadow.
Powder shadow—This can be applied dry over foundation (with brush) or mixed with water and applied with brush. Mixing with water makes the shadow longer-lasting.
Liquid shadow—A lighter form of cream shadow—can be transparent and luminous. Long lasting.
Gel shadow—Apply with fingertip or brush. Transparent—it gives color, no cover-up.

Eye liner. Your choices are pencil, liquid, or cake (mixed with water and applied with brush).
Pencil liner—Soft crayon pencil may give a heavier line than is wanted in most makeups today. Good for making soft dots between lashes and for a soft smudged line. Takes skill to apply correctly.
Liquid or cake liner—Liquid gives a fine line, but the same effect can be achieved with cake liner mixed with water. The cake is available in kits with your eye shadow in harmonizing shades.

Mascara. Cake, liquid or wand? You will probably want either cake or liquid for the first application and a wand for touch-ups.
Cake mascara—This is preferred by many models and actresses but it takes time to apply it beautifully. This means wetting the brush, lightly stroking it in the cake and then stroking the mascara evenly on each lash from root to tip, brushing the lashes so there is no caking. Repeat till each lash is coated.
Liquid mascara—Though less likely to cake on the lashes this also gives a heavy covering and should be used delicately.
Wand mascara—Certainly the most convenient form and is great as a carry-along. Gives today's popular light-lash look.
Lash-lengthener—If you don't wear false lashes, or if your own lashes are not long and swooping, this is for you. Fibers in lash-lengthener tend to build up. Be sure to brush the lashes well after using.

Brow color. A crayon pencil in the color of your own brows gives the most beautiful and soft line. Also useful, are the brow powders or creams—especially good for lightening, but powders tend to make the brows look a little dull and dusty. Brush with a light lash oil.

Lip makeup. Your choices are lipsticks, creams in a pot, glosses in stick or jar, lip-liner pencil and automatic lip-liner.
Lipsticks — These may be creamy opaques, translucents, and transparents. They may be pearlized (frosted) or clear. If you use pale lip color, put the paler shade underneath and use gloss or a darker shade in the middle of the mouth. If you like a dark lip color, line the lips with the deeper color and use the brighter color to fill and gloss in the middle of the mouth to mute the brightness. If you like a bright mouth, fill the lip outline with the brighter color and coat with gloss to soften the brightness. Lipstick is best applied with a brush—at least to line the mouth; or you can line with a brush, fill with stick.
❧ Opaques give a matte effect. Apply lipstick, blot to set color, and apply gloss or pearlized lip color to shine up your mouth. Most lasting form of lip makeup.
❧ Translucents should not be blotted. Again, use deeper shade to give mouth color; gloss for added brightness.
❧ Transparents give the clearest color with gleam. Great for a young mouth.
Glosses—Can be applied with brush or directly with the stick or even with your fingers (the cream kind). Keep gloss to the middle of the mouth so it will not smear the mouth outline.
Lip liner—Best results come with using a brush and your darker shade of lipstick as a liner. If you have trouble doing this, a lip-liner pencil or an automatic lip-liner brush may be helpful.

HARMONIZE YOUR MAKEUP COLORS

Skin tones change with the season and with age; let the basic complexion tone, hair and costume color guide you.
Fair—Light neutral skin that often needs enlivening. Choose pink (natural) or light beige (ivory) in the foundation.
Pink and white—This skin has delicate pink undertones on forehead and throat. Choose natural or blush-pink foundation if skin is just slightly rosy; ivory if pink notes need toning down.
Peaches and cream—This skin is slightly golden. Foundation can be neutral—beige or ivory—or light rose-beige if skin tends to sallowness.
Medium—This is the neutral medium-dark skin; often it lacks color and needs brightening. Choose light rachel or light rose-beige foundation.
Ruddy—Rosy cheeks and general high color in this skin may need to be toned down by beige-tone foundation. Choose rachel or light brunette.
Brunette—This is the neutral brunette skin. Dark rachel or rose-beige foundation can be used.
Rose brunette—The high color of this complexion often is due to thin translucent skin. Brunette foundation with no pink notes is flattering.
Olive—This brunette skin may have golden undertones. If at all sallow, use dark rose-beige foundations; otherwise dark brunette.
Brown—If your skin looks grayish because of dryness, warm it with a gold or bronze note in your makeup. This is always flattering to a brown skin. Some warmth may be needed to avoid sallowness, and this comes with a deep-rose or rose-brown note in the foundation. If skin is smooth and clear, match the skin with makeup base.
Black—Usually you will not need a makeup base—except for a moisturizer to keep the skin fresh-looking. Dark powder keeps away grayishness in the black skin. Foundation highlights with gold flecks are becoming for evening.

Eye shadow. This can harmonize with costume color, eye color, or with the natural shadows in the eye skin. These natural eye-skin shadows may be faintly blue, green, lavender, or brown.
❧ Use a shadow in harmony with your costume color as a color note just above lash line.
❧ When wearing neutral colors—beige, brown, black, gray, white—or navy blue, pick the color note that matches your eye color. Blue, turquoise, or gray-blue eyes; green or gold-green for green, hazel, brown, or golden eyes.
❧ Lavender and pink shadows are pretty on pinkish skins. Yellow on a brunette skin. Black skin needs a bright shadow—blue or green or turquoise.

Lip and cheek color. Rouge should be in harmony with the complexion color and with the lip color. The lipstick should harmonize with the costume color or the accessory colors.
Copper, orange-red, pale coral—Use orange tone lipsticks with orange, melon, yellows, yellow-brown, taupe, and all browns—and with black, white, and gray if in harmony with accessories.
Clear reds—With red costume colors, the lipstick should be a near match. Clear red is also useful with neutrals, such as gray, black, white, and beige, and often with browns when there is no conflict in accessory colors.
Pink to rose—Pinks are pretty with all pastels and with lavender and with light shades of gray and beige; also with many shades of brown and with black.

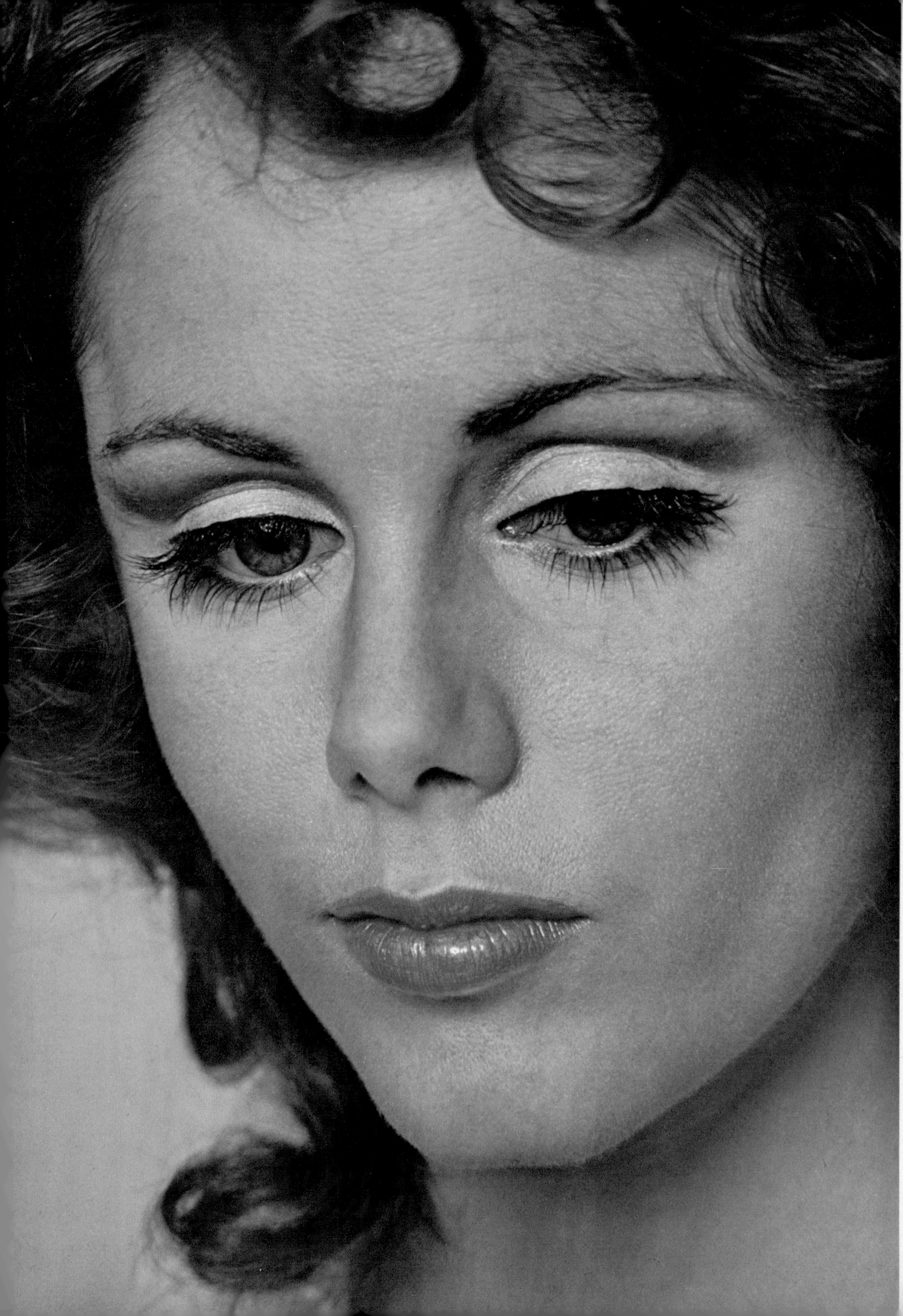

Look Your Best In Nightlight

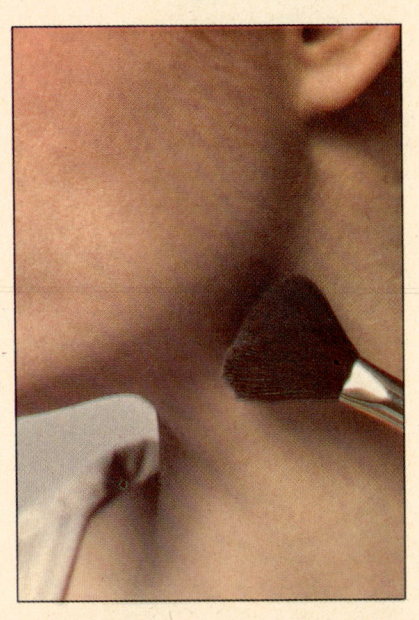

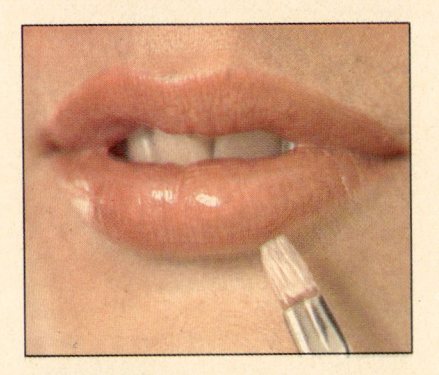

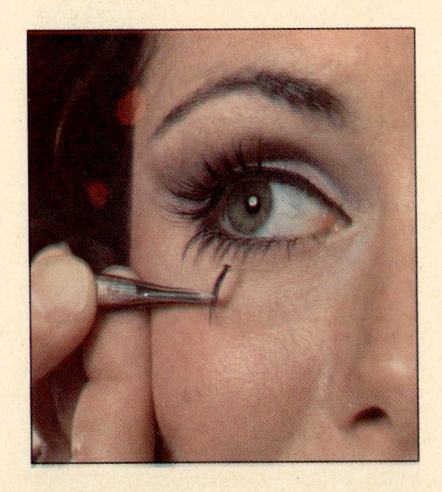

Daylight—and often the indoor light we work under—is strong and revealing. You need to make up for daylight in a very natural way. Your base must match your skin perfectly. Eye makeup and contouring (lights and shades) cannot be obvious. Lip color is clear and bright. With evening, everything changes. Lighting is soft and subdued. Lamplight is warmer (has more yellow) than outdoor light. Rooms—restaurants and theatres—are often dim. In night light, highlights and shadowing become less distinct; pale colors almost disappear; contouring fades. Makeup for evening must be done in a different way. For gala goings-on special luminous makeup can be used—pearled rouge, pearled or gilded powder, frosted eye shadow, and iridescent lipsticks. A clean light brow is part of evening beauty. Start your makeup with a freshly cleaned skin—and an eyebrow shaping. Pluck stray hairs between the brows and below the arch and any stragglers above the arch. Be sure that all daytime mascara is cleaned away. Even when the lashes seem clean, there is always some fallout of mascara onto the lower lid, and this can create an unbecoming shadow if it isn't completely cleared. Repeated action with a cotton ball moistened with freshener or cleanser may be needed. Nighttime makeup base should be no darker than the skin (test the base on the side of your throat, not on the wrist or back of the hand), but it is most becoming if it has a rose tone. If your daytime neutral beige base is used for evening, an allover brushing with light pink blusher can be flattering.

✺ For a smooth skin surface, use a skin freshener before applying makeup base. Makeup base should be spread evenly over the entire face, including eyelids and lips, and then brought down over the throat to blend away at the neckline of your dress.

✺ Contouring—highlighting and shading—must be emphasized for night. Highlights go below the brows (use lightener here even if you later apply blusher in this area; the lightener improves the effect), below the eyes (toward the temples), above the cheekbones under the lower lid, on the middle of the chin, and down the middle of the nose.

✺ Shading goes in the crease of the eyelid, along the sides of the nose, and on the sides of the face below the cheekbone and along the jaw.

✺ Blend creamy pearled rouge along the cheekbone over the highest part of the cheek, and fan it out toward the temple.

✺ Brush blusher across the forehead at the hairline, over the highest part of the cheeks, and on the chin.

✺ The eyes should have a rounded open look. Iridescent eye shadow catches the light beautifully and adds a color note. When false lashes are used, they can be heavier than your daytime lashes—but should not be overlong. Too lengthy, they cast unbecoming shadows.

✺ Apply colored iridescent shadow on the upper lid from the lash line to the crease in the lid. Powdered shadow mixed with water and applied with a brush goes on easily—and stays. If the eye is not contoured, the colored shadow can be blended upward toward the outer corner of the brow.

✺ The contour line (brown or taupe shadow) starts at the crease in the upper lid and is blended upward and outward the length of the lid. If you have trouble contouring with cream or powder eye shadow, try this trick: Mix brown cake eye liner with a good amount of water till you get a light brown wash. Do the contouring with this "water color," using a sable brush to apply it. This same watery mix can be used with the same brush to touch up and fill in the brows; the effect is much more delicate than with pencil or powder.

✺ If you are brunette, use brown eye liner—light brown if you are a blonde or redhead; charcoal if you are silver-haired. Cake liner applied with a wet brush works well. Start with a fine line along the lashes across the inner half of the upper lid. At the middle of the lid begin to widen the line a little, fanning it out into a wedge shape at the eye's outer tip. Line the eye along the lashes of the upper lid, and lightly under the lashes of the lower lid.

✺ Black mascara is usually becoming for night, but blondes may prefer dark brown. Apply mascara to upper lashes above and below. Lower lashes can be lightly touched with a mascara wand.

What finishing touches make an evening makeup glow?

✺ Use pearlized or gilded powder for a wonderfully luminous effect.

✺ Blusher (this, too, may be pearlized) should be brushed on the forehead along the hairline to the temples, below the brows, on the highest part of the cheeks, and on the chin. Touch it, too, if you like, to the tip of your ears.

✺ The first application of lipstick should be a fairly bright color; cover the whole lip area. The second lipstick should be a pale pearlescent to lighten the mouth and give it sheen. The pearlescent is applied to the middle of the mouth and blended lightly over the rest of the lips.

✺ Your evening hair style should be designed to pick up the light. Spraying with hair gloss helps pick up highlights.

✺ You can add to your nighttime beauty by putting yourself, when possible, in the best available light, standing or sitting where the light is diffused, keeping your neck long in back and your chin high so that your face catches the best light.

✺ Light coming from below chin level casts unattractive shadows on the face. At a restaurant table choose a seat that keeps candles or a low lamp at least an arm's length away. In a living room avoid a seat close to a chair-side lamp.

✺ And most important, keep an inner glow. An evening out works a special magic; let it transfigure you.

PARTY FACE FRESHENERS

Give your skin a dewy look. Even if your face is already clean from washing, or whatever, give it a quick fresh-up by running an eye-makeup-remover pad over the skin; then go over the face with a wet sponge; blot dry. Follow with a pearly moisturizer—a real party pickup.

Add some glow. Touch up the middle part of the face—forehead, nose, chin, inner cheek—with gold frost; it gives a warm gilty glow. Then you're ready for foundation. Best for party freshness (at any age) is liquid tinted "young skin" base. With its fine texture, reflecting quality, and color, you'll need little powder.

Create a natural blush. Blend cream rouge low on the cheek and to the outside of the face. There it looks true. High and on the fattest part of the cheek, it only calls attention to any facial lines or under-eye circles.

Highlight your eyes. To hide under-eye shadows, smooth a lightweight corrective cream—only a few shades paler than the skin tone—below the eyes. White should not be used here. Use white or pearl to illuminate the prominence below the brows. To shape the eye, the same beige shadow with which you contour the jaw line can be applied with a smaller brush in the crease of the upper eyelid. Brush the upper lid to the crease with transparent pearlized highlighter to keep the lid dewy.

Use little face powder. The drier the skin, the less powder you need. The youthful look is gleamy, so powder only moist or oily areas and then simply "blot" the face with the powder puff instead of patting powder on and then blotting the excess. Powder the neck, and brush off excess to prevent makeup's rubbing off on clothes.

Lift your brows. Thin pale lifted brows with a well-defined line give an open, wide-awake look to the eyes. Cleaning out the hairs below the arch and shaping the brows are instant face fresheners. Use brush-on brow powder to fill in the line (this is more natural than penciling); or use "no color" brow makeup to lighten dark brows.

Try an easy "face-lift." Starting back of the earlobe, brush tawny shadow along the underside of jaw and chin and below the chin to the Adam's apple in a believable V-shape shadow. This gives the illusion of a firm jaw line, minimizes a double chin. Use the same brush and shadow to contour the outside of the face—in the hollow of the cheeks—and to slim the nose: Squeeze the contour brush into a narrow wedge to make a strip down the sides of the nose, stopping where the nostrils broaden.

Wear added lashes. If you prefer individual lashes to a strip, take an inexpensive pair of strip lashes and clip them apart in clumps of three or four hairs (no more). Pick up a clump with tweezers, dip the end into a small amount of surgical adhesive that you have squeezed out onto a piece of freezer paper, and then place each clump on the lash line to fill in the spaces between your own lashes. Do the upper lash line from side to side; on the lower lash line, add three or four little clumps to the outer tip between natural lashes as needed to balance the weight of the lashes above.

Keep lips shiny. For the softest, prettiest mouth, coat the lips with lip balm, let set for a minute, and then clean off; this wipes away any flaky skin. Next, outline the mouth with a lip brush and a pale lip color; it is around the rim of the lips that a highlight naturally appears, and you can make the lips slightly fuller if you outline with pale lip color. Finish with a brighter transparent color in the middle of the mouth (carry this lipstick along to refresh with during the party) and a generous shimmer of frosted lip gloss.

QUICK PREPARTY PICKUPS

Bone-tired? *Don't slump!* Try instead this quick body perk-up: Stand in good alignment, feet together, arms at sides. Then jump a few inches into the air, bringing feet apart to the sides and landing softly. At the same time clap hands overhead. Jump again, bringing feet back together, arms down. Repeat rapidly four or five times. You'll find it a backbone stiffener, face freshener, and emotional energizer all in one.

Pale face? Take advantage of skin-toning facial masks. A pickup mask—gel or paste—makes the skin tingle, leaves it looking glowy. Skin freshener or astringent (if there's no time for a mask) helps, too. Pat it on with a cotton ball or square after a cream face-cleaning. If skin is oily, go for a brisk soap-and-water wash with a rough "scrub cloth."

Need to relax? A shower bath will do it. Instead of lolling in a tub bath (fine at bedtime), adjust the shower till it is hot and steamy. Scrub yourself briskly with a rough washcloth (unless skin is dry); then use a soft fluffy one). Finish with a full two minutes of water as chill as you can stand. Before drying yourself, smooth on after-shower oil as an allover skin soother.

Aching feet and legs? For about five minutes, using shower or spray, alternate (30 seconds each) hot and cold water over feet and legs from the knees down. Dry skin briskly. Follow with a body-lotion rub.

Under-eye puffiness? Sometimes it's due to poor circulation. Smooth it away and pick up your energy by lying down for five minutes, feet raised and eyelids covered with cotton balls or squares moistened with witch hazel. The five-minute lie-down is as good as a nap for refreshing you.

Look drawn out? Do a face-freshening makeup. Start with a face creaming, a skin freshener, a foundation with a glow, and use blusher lavishly—all around the outside of your face, including the chin, hairline, the area under the eyebrows, as well as the cheeks. Go warm with color. What you wear on your face—as well as on your figure—should be cheerful. In clothes, gray, black, or brown does nothing to lift your spirits or your looks. Some blues can turn you pale. Pink or rose in your clothing does most for a tired face because it casts a warm glow upward. Overbright colors, for their part, can outshine you. Use warm colors in your makeup. Pink blusher and a bright pink lip color will help turn you on. Have a rose note in your makeup base—especially for evening light. Repair your makeup often. Use blotter tissues and then gleamer for skin shine. Renew blusher —or treat your cheeks to pretty pink gleamer—and refreshen your lip color with a hint of pink.

Under-eye shadows? Understate your eye makeup to give light and shine to your eyes. Begin with a light foundation or highlighter under the eyes; then, with a cotton swab, apply highlighter directly below the brows. With a fresh swab, gently blend soft taupe shadow over the entire upper lid and a little above the fold of the eyelid. Use brown, not black, eye liner. And put mascara on the upper lashes only. If your eyes water from tiredness or cold, keep a cotton swab handy to erase mascara fallout. Moisten the swab with eye-makeup remover. Retouch the under-eye skin with beige or pale-yellow highlighter and a light coat of makeup base.

Straggly hair? Lift your looks and spirits with a fast redo. Lean forward from the waist so your head bounces freely in mid-air. This brings color to your skin and a tingle to the scalp. Brush all the hair forward for about 50 strokes. Straighten, and brush it all back. Then restore your hairdo with an instant set. Setting with quick-drying hair spray is one way. Or use any of the dry-set methods—curling iron, hot curlers. All give a loose, quick, becoming curl.

Need a lift? Let your hair go high on top. A lift at the forehead helps undo any downward droop of facial muscles. A straight-down hair style exaggerates it. Use a bow or barrette to tie up your forelock for this flattering touch.

Feel edgy? Be sure your clothing is comfortable. Tightness or any need for constant adjustment in what you wear is too much when you're tired. A well-fitted bra, a comfortable dress, and shoes that look trim but don't pinch are musts for feeling fresh, even when you aren't.

HAIR COLOR AS A MAKEUP KEY

You can harmonize your makeup to your hair color—or, if you change your hair color, you can use harmonizing makeup to key your skin tones to the new hair color. Brow pencil should also be keyed to hair color.

Redhead colors—Peachy skin tones, coral and orange-tone lip colors, and coral rouge; brow pencil—auburn with light brown.

Golden-blond colors—Pink skin tones, rose rouge and lip color; brow pencil—light brown with gray.

Ash-blond and light-brown colors—Pink tones for lips and cheeks and pink tone in the foundation help to avoid an all-beige look. Use brown brow pencil mixed with gray.

Brunette colors—Clear bright red in lipsticks, brightness in eye shadow, and a beige tone in the foundation color make for a total brunette look. For dark brown hair, brown with charcoal pencil.

Black hair—Clear bright colors are always dramatic (avoid blue tones) in lipstick; look for clear-bright greens and blues in eye shadows. Deep mauve shades can also be beautiful on the eyes. Lighten the brows with a brow powder for an eye-framing effect, Mascara in the color of the eye shadow—or tip off black mascara with color.

Gray-hair colors—The lip color should be neither dark nor light, neither blue nor orange. True rose red, clear coral, or clear red in lip color and clear green, turquoise, or blue-gray in eye shadow make for distinction. Avoid brown shadow and any brown tones in foundation. Instead, use foundation with a slight rose cast to give a fresh skin look. Brow pencil—charcoal or gray with light brown.

White hair—If your white hair is kept snowy white (no yellowish notes), you have the beautiful basis for dramatizing your skin tones and eyes with your makeup—the choice of delicate palest pastels if your skin is fair (be sure to add some pink notes so that you won't appear ghostly) to sun-tan makeups (gels preferably) if skin is brunette. Keep brows thin, but not too light.

Look Your Best In Daylight

If you're a blonde, you may look too pale, especially in daytime. How do you add glow? Don't go to a darker foundation. Instead, use a covering makeup as light as your skin tone (it can be your regular makeup) with translucent powder to help set the foundation and to protect the skin from wind and sun. Before powdering, apply cheek gel (pink) to a damp sponge and pat the sponge lightly on the cheeks for glow. Use powder blusher (after powdering) on the cheeks and also under the brows, down the nose and on the throat down into the hollow. Brush on lightly, just enough to give color. Strong eye makeup in violet and a red lipstick help overcome any paleness. To give a real outdoor glow, use brown or tan powder over your makeup; press on and brush off excess.

If you're a brunette with dark skin or have a good tan, you should let your natural color come through by using gel makeups. A deep-peach face gel, with pink-bronze cheek gel (pat it on so it won't streak) gives glow. A dusky plum shadow all over the upper lid (to the brows) with pale beige shadow in a wide band at the lash line above and below reverses the usual lid color pattern and makes the lashes show up more. Mouth can be a cheerful red with lip gloss in ginger brown for highlight and to mute color.

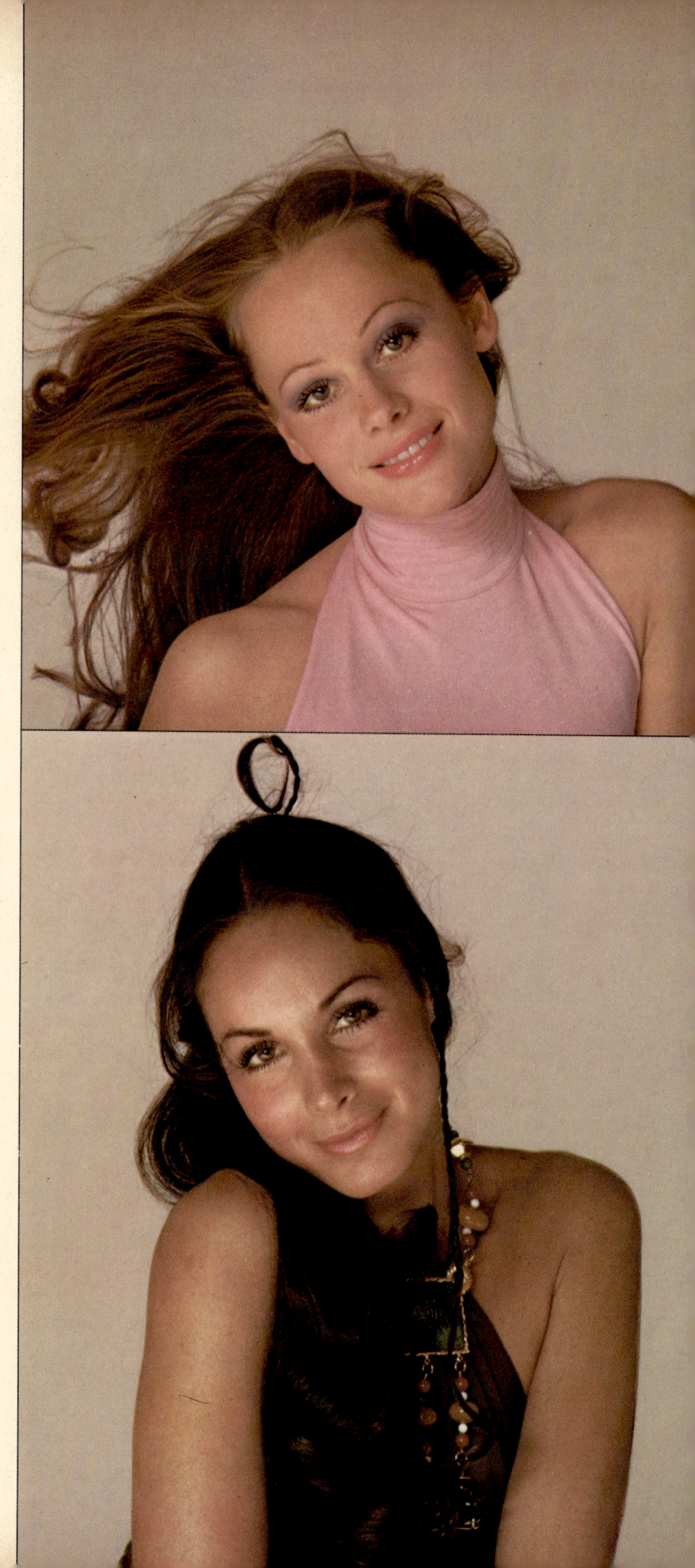

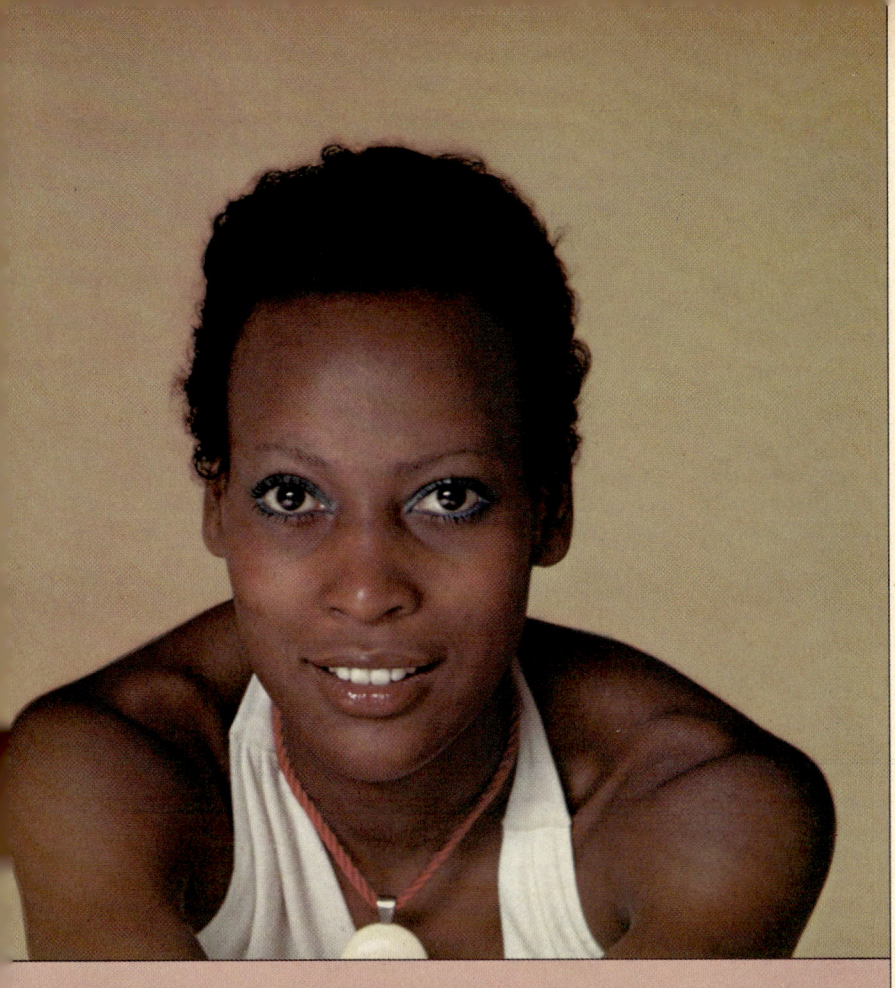

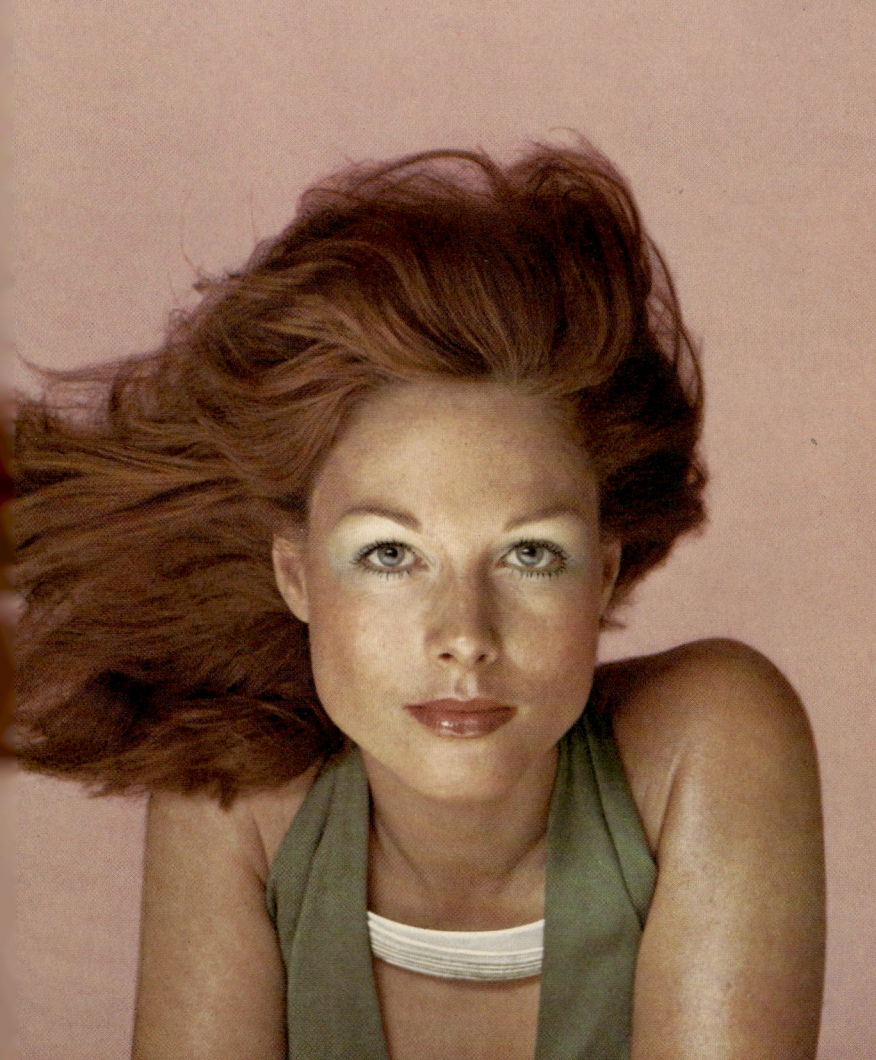

If you are a Black, with bronzy skin tones you need little foundation. You need makeup gel (in deep bronze) only to even the skin tone. (In summer, use a sun block under this to prevent uneven darkening of the skin.) Pat on a brown powder in the middle of the face, between the brows, on the nose and around the mouth, so the skin there does not appear gray. Pat on a very thin transparent cream rouge around the cheeks and eyes and above the brows and on the forehead to give a glow like that produced by sunshine. It beautifully balances a bright eye makeup—sea green. A gold-flecked beige makeup can be used under the brow and under the eyes to reflect the light. Do lips in a transparent chestnut with pink gloss.

If you're a redhead, you may have very delicate pale skin and freckle easily. You should not use lots of coverup—your freckles are probably becoming. A translucent shine-stopping base will give you a minimum of cover while providing some warmth and weather protection. Blend a tiny bit of ginger-tone eye gel (a drop or two) over the entire face. A golden blusher tone over the outside of cheeks and up under the eye (pat it on) gives a wholesome glow. Apply frosted yellow powder shadow (mix with water) over the entire upper lid down over the fold, and a frosted green below that—and even below the eye so the whole eye is wrapped in color. Redheads with pale lashes need liner plus mascara. In green, line outer three-quarters of the upper lid. Pale brown lipstick used with dark brown lip gloss looks great.

DAYTIME MAKEUP THAT LASTS ALL DAY

An all-day outing or going to the job calls for an all-day makeup. Do you know how to put on a really good face? A well-done makeup that lasts through a day—or an evening—with only an occasional lipstick touch-up and a patting of compact powder? Makeup that protects your skin as it pretties you?

❧ Before you begin your makeup be sure you're starting with a clean skin: Two coatings of cream, each tissued away. To get a thorough cleansing, use a clean makeup sponge (natural sponge). Soak it in water, squeeze the water out, and sponge-massage the cream into the skin. The sponge works the cream into the pores but it can't irritate. This is also a good way to get a facial massage. Always wash the sponge with soap and water after it's been used, so that it won't deteriorate. If you wish, follow creaming with a mild-soap-and-warm-water wash.

❧ For long-lasting makeup the skin also needs preparation: Pat on skin freshener with a thick pad of cotton. The thickness gives extra stimulation and helps tone the skin. Then smooth on moisturizer—freely around the eyes, sparingly over the rest of the face and throat—for all-day moisture retention. Once this is done, start the face-do that won't fail you:

Foundation—With a clean sponge, blend foundation makeup over face and throat. In color the base should match your skin tone. (Test for color on the inside of your wrist.) Once you have the matching shade, you can decide whether you want to add a warmer tone to your complexion; if so, choose a shade with a rose or peach cast.

Cover cream—Apply directly from the tube. It hides shadows around the eyes and offsets a tired look. Pat with fingertips to blend into foundation. Cover cream can also be used around the lips to prevent the lip color's filtering into vertical lines that cross the outline of the lips. Cover cream has more body than makeup base and forms a dam that prevents the lip color's fusing into these lines.

Cream eye shadow—Brush onto the upper lid from the base to the natural crease. Cream shadow is long-lasting and will not fade away during the day. Choose a shade to match your eyes or dress or simply to please yourself.

Powder—With a full puff, press loose translucent powder firmly onto the foundation (include eyelids and brows) till all the powder disappears. This pressing in of the powder sets your makeup for the entire day, so do it carefully. Brush any excess away with a powder brush. Brush in a downward direction.

Cake eye shadow—Intensify lid color by brushing on compressed cake shadow in the same shade as the cream. This gives long-lasting fresh color to the lids. As before, the color should cover the upper lid to the crease.

Liner—Line eyelids at the lash line—the upper lid more generously than the lower—with cake liner and a fine brush. Your eye liner will last longer if the brush is dipped in hot water instead of cold. (To help the white of the eye appear whiter, a white line can be drawn above the lashes on the shelf of the lower lid; continue outward to fill space between the extended lines of upper and lower lid.)

Brow pencil—Shape and touch up eyebrows with brow pencil so they will remain in shape all day long. If you tend to perspire freely, powder over the first application to set the color. Finish brows with tiny pencil strokes, following the arch of the brow.

Mascara—Darken and dramatize the lashes with waterproof mascara—cake or wand. Cake mascara can be more generously applied if brush is moistened with hot water.

Lipstick—Apply lipstick from the tube and then shape the outline with a lip brush. The moisturizers in lipstick help protect the lips as well as add color.

Blusher—Blush the highest part of the cheeks with soft color. Add it also to any other part of the face where you want shading or glow—chin, jaws, forehead.

Eyelashes—False lashes add glamour to the eyes and also help protect them from glare.

Compact powder—Touch-ups during the day need be no more than a light touch of translucent compact powder to nose, forehead, and cheeks and a freshening of lipstick. When you retouch with powder, always pat with the puff. If you rub, you disturb the foundation. Brush lightly with the puff to get rid of excess.

BEAUTY FOR THE TRAVELER

Today's tourist travels light, learns to limit her grooming needs and to keep makeup and personal items together in a compact portable kit. She finds useful new fresh-up aids and learns to value purse-size containers as an accessory to family-size packages. She protects hands, hair, and complexion from too much sun and wind, enjoys a variety of foods without adding pounds, tries to look at home anywhere and to be just a little dressed up. These tips for women-on-the-go can keep you pretty when you travel.

Be a beautiful tourist. Sightseeing? Be comfortable and casual but still look a little dressed up so that you can move becomingly from tourist haunts into town. Watch your posture and camera angles when your husband takes your picture—you'll be seeing yourself later as you look today. A small head scarf keeps your hairdo neat and lets you shake out your hair from time to time. For happy feet, shoes should be lightweight—flats or with a low broad-based heel. Don't weigh yourself down; have a light handbag to carry your musts. If you're a collector, take a separate souvenir basket—one you can put down while you stand and look.

❧ Cut the clutter. An overstuffed handbag wrecks the well-groomed look and contends with your patience. Keep a small, easy-to-hold-onto handbag neat with the fewest possible carry-alongs. Have the traveler's friends—small change and small bills—handy. If you need extra carrying space, a capacious swinging tote bag is for you.

❧ If sunglasses are important to you (or if you need glasses for close or distant vision), realize how prominent they are as a facial ornament and keep your other ornaments reasonably few. Keep eyeglass lenses clean and clear; smudgy lenses take the edge off your appearance as well as off your vision. When you put your glasses on, slide them over your side hair so as not to disturb your hairdo. When you don't want them on your face, push them up as a headband to hold hair in place in the wind.

❧ Kick discomfort with well-fitted stockings and shoes that look neat and new yet are easy to walk in and with a bra and girdle that adjust perfectly to motion. For the girl who wears no underslimmer for everyday, the going-out shaper should smooth and shape the figure and help clothes fit well but should not feel confining. Be sure the waistline of your dress or skirt matches your own; for easy walking, your hem line should be smartly short but flared so as not to ride up when you sit. Pants, which you may prefer, should fit comfortably.

❧ Retouch your makeup from time to time, but you'll need to do it very little if you start the day complete: Apply makeup base over the entire face—lips and lids included. Use a cream blusher over the base; then press on loose powder and remove excess with a brush. Mascara won't smudge if you brush the lashes well after mascara is dry; leave it off the lower lashes (make instead a line of dots between the natural lashes). Use powder blusher as a touch-up with pressed powder and lip-

stick during the day. If skin is oily, dry it first with small facial blotting tissues.
❧ A mini-makeup for the traveler is needed sometimes, too. Here is one: A freshly cleaned face treated to a touch of moisturizer, a little eye liner to pretty up the eyes, and a bright lip gloss to cheer the scene. If you need color in your face, rub gleamer on your cheeks, forehead and chin. This face can go anywhere, even to bed at night without recleansing, for there's nothing to stop the skin from "breathing."
❧ A mini-hairdo is needed, too. Curls do away with the bad effects of the most dragged out day. Quick-set your hair in hot rollers, and turn side curls against the cheeks for a happy look.

Off on an auto trip? You'll feel freshest if you start each day with a shower; for scent, use a long-lasting skin-soothing lotion perfume; sprinkle absorbent deodorant powder in bra and girdle and rub the feet well with it. A careful morning makeup will last all day with occasional blotting and touch-ups of pressed powder and lip color; if you ride in an open car, use a sun screen as a makeup base. A good travel hairdo is short, with blow-about bangs. Keep the rest of the hair neat with a scarf. Sunglasses protect eyes from glare, eye skin from squint lines. Wear gloves to keep your hands clean and to have a dressed-up touch when you stop to look or to eat. A full skirt or pants let you sit comfortably, get in and out of the car gracefully. For your travel bag, choose a plastic-lined beauty case that holds all your grooming needs and is convenient for rest-room fresh-ups. Carry along hand soap—in a soap dish, a tube, or as towelettes.
❧ Start out "finished." This means setting out top-to-toe-groomed. Don't tell yourself, "I'll fix up when I get there," for this means toting your grooming aids and likely forgetting a few real needs. Besides, no rest room gives the grooming advantages of home base.

Flying? Travel light. A little has to go a long way if you're an air passenger, and grooming aids should travel with you in the cabin. For foot-and-leg comfort while sitting, avoid an overtight girdle, if any; use the footrest or, if none, rest your feet on your cabin luggage; wear ventilated easy-fitting shoes and avoid crossing legs above the ankles; take advantage of any chance to stroll about the cabin. Travelers tend to eat often, and you can avoid adding pounds by eating light at each food break, tasting some of each dish but not putting away the whole in-flight dinner or other full-course meal.

Look at home in the big city. If your trip includes a big city or is tied in with your husband's business meeting or convention, bring at least one go-anywhere outfit and dress-up accessories. Send out items for pressing as soon as you reach your hotel. When you order hotel reservations, write ahead for a hairdo appointment; you'll probably want a manicure, so specify that too in advance. If you want a beauty break in a big-name salon, allow at least a week's time for them to fit you in. Start any trip with a short workable hairdo—and don't ask for a "creation" when you get styled. Instead, ask for something that you or your own hairdresser can handle.

Dining out. When—day or evening—shoulders are bare, blend makeup of face and throat into your body tan; tan blender added to your makeup base does the trick. Do your evening lashes create under-eye shadows? Wear only a half strip at the outer fringe of your own; and try to sit to the side of any lamp (not under it) or seek a lamp that is below eye level. Night light calls for more color in the face—rosier blusher, deeper lip color, shadow and liner to enlarge and brighten the eyes. One or more hairpieces worked together can give you glamour beyond belief. Balance height with a bouncy behind-the-ear curl or forehead fringe.

Be a considerate house guest. If you're visiting relatives or friends for overnight or longer, chances are you'll be sharing a bathroom with members of the family. If family members go off to morning work or school, ask about their starting time: "When does everyone get up, and what's a good time for us to appear on the scene?" Be sure your bathrobe gives you good coverage. Use the bathroom for the minimum of grooming needs—a shower is quicker than a tub bath—and do your skin care, makeup, and hair in your room. Have a compact case for grooming aids and keep it in your room so you won't be borrowing bathroom shelf space. Provide your own facial tissues and other personal needs—deodorant, cologne, and bath powder. If you need extra bathroom time, consult your hostess: "I'd like to wash my hair. What's the best time?"

Charm for the camper. The outdoors offers beauty plusses—fresh air, cold water, and exercise. But there are hazards too. Mosquitoes are attracted to the young and active, so take along a repellent and use it. Avoid scents and scented creams; perfume attracts or excites insects. For gathering firewood or other rough work, wear canvas gloves so your hands get home in good shape. A hat protects your hair and won't let it catch in low branches. Woods walkers today find sneakers or basketball shoes give sure footing, but change canvas footwear once or twice a day. Relief for tired feet? Dunk them in the chill water of a lake or fast-running stream.
❧ What helps the camper face her morning face? Waterproof mascara! Your eyes won't go blank if you don't completely remove your eye makeup the night before. When you clean your face, tissue gently across the eyelids. Then use a warm damp cloth all over. What little mascara is left on the eye skin is quickly wiped away with clean fingers and a splash of clear water. Skin that has been cleansed well and moisturized the night before looks pretty and soft enough when you wake up. Next, a quick brushing or combing and a headband for your hair. Rub gleamer on your cheeks and you can face the sunshine.

Boaters—take care. If your hair is long enough to be a nuisance or a hazard aboard, wear it in pigtails as did old-time sailors. Sun reflection from water is twice that from green areas. If out for long hours, use zinc oxide or other opaque covering on the lips, shade the face with a brimmed hat and keep the rest of the body covered.

Sunglasses. It is good to protect the eyes with sunglasses when in very strong sunlight—chiefly because exposure to daytime glare can lead to poorer vision in the dark and because we tend to squint to protect ourselves from glare. Dark lenses should not be used all the time, however, or worn indoors, as this could produce eye strain.
❧ Lens color should be chosen with glare in mind. Extra dark for times when one is on or near water, because water reflects sunlight. Lighter for other situations, such as walking and driving. Pale green or light brown is considered most restful. It is wise to buy unbreakable glass or plastic lenses for safety.
❧ Frames should flatter the face—but there are no rules at all about this. Most women like "dramatic" sunglasses because they are an accessory as well as eye protection. Some now are fitted to rest down on the nose so you can see over them. Frames should be well fitted so the glasses stay on during active sports and play.
❧ If you develop white circles around the eyes from wearing sunglasses, under-eye makeups—either powder or cake—in a beige tone work best because they are light in texture. Gels are too transparent, and foundations usually too heavy.

Outdoor Beauty

Your summer look changes with your body tan. You'll want your body beautifully gilded if not bronzed. Be too wise to give your face and throat much sun. Sunlight on unprotected facial skin is held a cause of skin aging; start young to protect your face against sunlight's ill effects by using a sunlight filter on face, throat, and hands as well as on body skin. In winter, look apple-cheeked healthy, but again, protect your skin against weather.

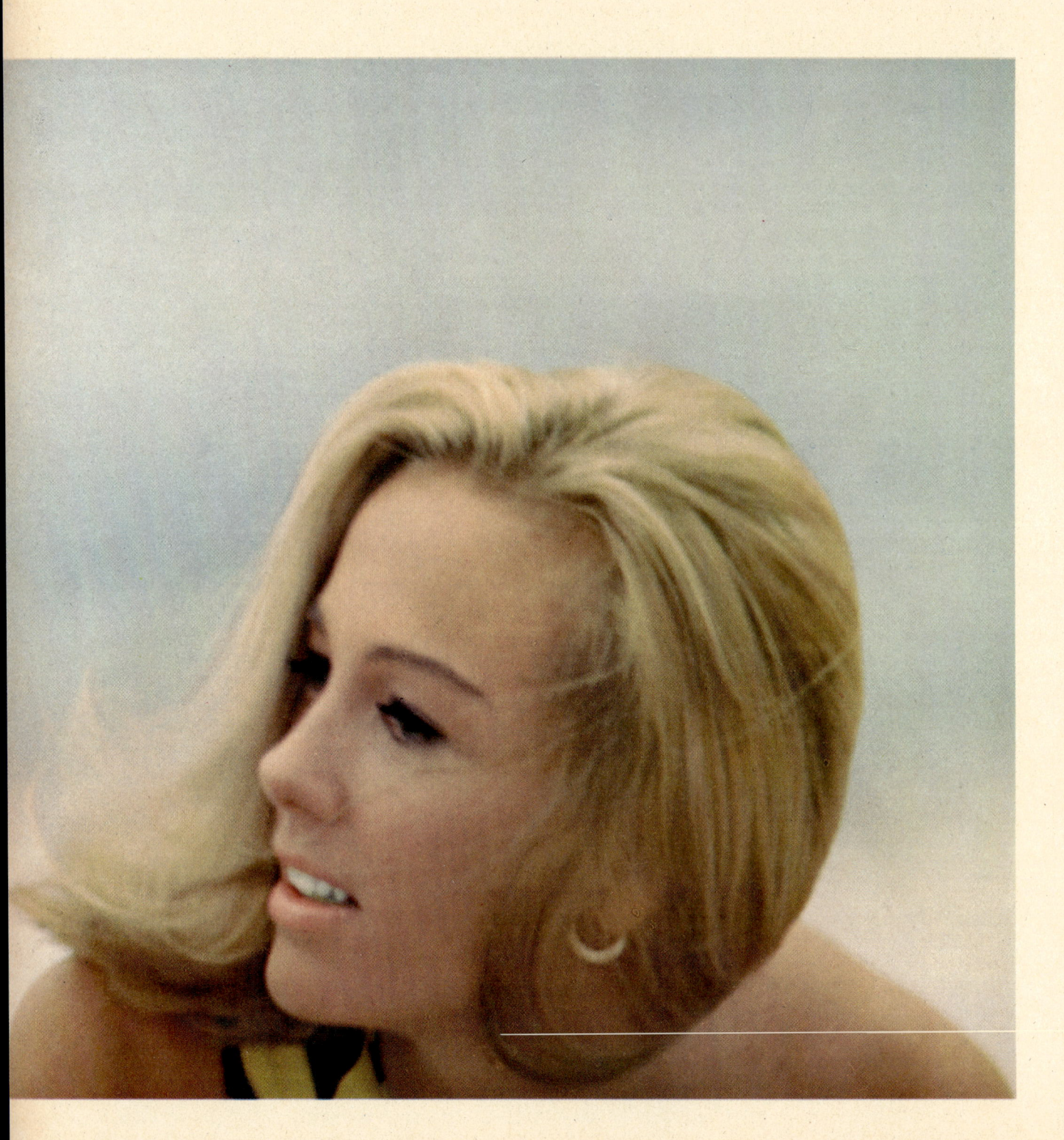

Your outdoor makeup. This is one defense against wind, sun, drying air. Let your face shine; keep it blushing; set your lips alight with luminous color and lip gloss. You needn't rely on night creams to keep skin supple; sleeptime is the time the skin's natural oils collect on it and protect it; daytime, when the skin is freshly washed and exposed to outdoor elements, is the time it most needs a cosmetic moisturizer.

Base—Start your makeup with a moisture base. A liquid or cream foundation is the smart choice; it goes on evenly and can be put on sparingly; it clings to the skin, creating a makeup that will stay fresh and look moist and clean through daylong activities.

♣ For summer, find a neutral beige tone that will blend your complexion color into your body tan—gold tone, tan tone, bronze tone. If you are deeply tanned, you face and throat, even with makeup, can be somewhat lighter than your body skin, but there should be no clear line of change from the made-up area to the natural skin when you go bare-shouldered or wear a low-neckline dress.

♣ Makeup is best applied with foam-rubber sponge. When sponge is used, makeup is removed as it is applied. The result is a smooth and even base. Put the makeup on with a gently rolling motion. Roll the base onto the skin of the entire face and throat, fading it out at the collarbone; remove the excess with fresh foam-rubber sponge.

Cream blusher—This is the secret of outdoor glow. Brush-on blusher works fine as a finishing touch, but for a makeup that is to stay fresh for a day and perhaps go underwater, cream rouge has staying power and a natural look.

♣ Smile as you apply the blusher—and keep it to the fleshy part of the cheek and away from the nose, not bringing it very far up the side of the face and never up beside the eye. Too near (beside or below) the rouge takes color away from the eye. Too near the nose, it makes the nose appear large. Blend the rouge with foam-rubber sponge for a natural pink look. For young skin, pink blusher is more natural-looking than orange or tawny.

Eyes—Begin your eye makeup with a line of brown pencil in the lash line below the eye. Start at the inner corner and bring the line to the outer tip and then lightly blend it with a fingertip till it is almost invisible. This makes the eye appear fuller and prettier in shape. Line the upper lid right in the lash line with a black or brown pencil; this line is not obvious but makes the lashes appear thicker. Pencil this lash line from the inner corner of the eye to the outer tip. Do not extend the line behind the end of the eye or upward toward the brow tip. Instead, keep the line on the lashes and stop at the last lash. This makes the eye appear large and open.

♣ Put shadow on the upper lid, starting at the inner tip of the eye and bringing the shadow across the upper lid to the tip, keeping it close to the lash line. Do not carry the shadow above the fold of the upper lid or fan it out at the end of the eye, toward the brow. Cover the lid only to the fold—or shadow only half the lid or even a fourth of it.

♣ The brows form a frame for the eye. Keep brows light; pencil as little as possible or use a brush-on brow color sparingly.

♣ Be belashed. Use mascara, lash-lengthener mascara, or false lashes. Take care, however, that extra lashes are beautifying. Sometimes false lashes make the eyes appear small or cast unbecoming under-eye shadows. For an open-eye look, clip off a short piece of false-lash strip and fix it to the outer section of natural lashes. Realize that even "waterproof" mascara or lashes cannot resist long periods of submersion. If you go underwater when you swim, it is wise to leave your lashes unretouched.

Lips—Lip gloss gives gleam to your lips and also protects lips against dryness and cracking. For active sports—especially for winter sports or underwater sports, beach, and boating—protect your lips by premixing lipstick with lip gloss or petroleum jelly and applying the blend with a brush.

Powder—When other makeup is complete, powder carefully with loose translucent powder. For summer this should be a truly no-color powder; pigmented (colored) powders tend to change in contact with skin oils and can soon look smudged and unfresh. A translucent powder is unchanged by skin oils and gives the soft luminous look natural to young skin.

♣ Use a puff for powdering, pressing it against the skin and then rolling it away from the face so that the powder clings but the makeup base is not smudged. Do not dab or pat except on the nose, where powder must be dabbed on and rolled off if it is to cling. Powder lavishly and then remove the excess in downward motions with a powder brush.

♣ Retouch lips and eyelashes—and you have a makeup that will stay with you all day. Your perspiration and skin oils can create shine through this makeup without its looking soiled; if you need to refresh it, blot carefully with special blotting tissue.

CHOOSE YOUR MAKEUP COLORS

Natural-look makeup—luminous, light—now gets new life. Color glimmers on lips and lids. And what marvelous color! If at first you find a new makeup hard to wear, don't give up, saying "Just not for me." Instead, learn the ways that will make these refreshing cosmetic colors appear just right for your face.

A fresh "new complexion" look is one secret of this new makeup; another secret is a bold bringing forward of the color on lips and lids. Here are clues to success with "hard-to-wear" makeup shades:

- Avoid anything that will let your skin appear sallow. As soon as a tan, for example, begins to fade, help it go. To pale prettily and quickly, give your face and throat a daily scrub with a stimulating cleanser; use a moisturizer round the clock to soften surface skin, and use a sun-screen cream as protection when you're outdoors in summer.
- Keep your makeup base neutral so your skin tones appear clear. The base should be a true beige—light, medium, or dark to complement your skin tones, but with no orange or yellow cast.
- Use a no-color powder (pigmented powder is likely to turn yellow or orange on the skin) to help the skin appear luminous and keep its neutral tone.
- Blusher should be pink to give a rosy glow. Avoid blusher with a yellow cast.
- Soften the eyes with brown mascara and keep brows light. You can choose the shade that matches your hair color, or use a light and a dark shade together for a natural look.
- The upper lid is only lightly lined and use liner in the same color as your eye shadow (but deeper in shade) or use a transparent liner in a smoky color. The line should be extremely fine and kept directly on the roots of the lashes.
- The lower lid is unlined or this line is in color and kept light and in the lash line, but the effect is prettiest when the line is softened by smudging it a little with a fingertip.
- To give color to the upper lid, use luminous cake eye shadow in two shades of the same color. With a brush, stroke the shadow in one direction only—from the inner corner of the lid to the outer—and only to the fold of the eyelid. Use the lighter shadow near the fold of the lid, the darker shade near the lashes.
- Use brown mascara for its softening effect. If you do not wear false lashes, use a lash-lengthening mascara. Stroke it first over the upper side of the upper lashes and then more lavishly to the underside of the upper lashes. Two or three coats are better than one. With the tip of the mascara wand, touch each of the lower lashes individually with mascara in the color of your eye shadow. Bring color forward on both lips and lids.
- The lips should glisten as well as have color. Be sure you fill out the mouth to the lip line.
- The bolder color is then put on the middle of the mouth—on both upper and lower lips—to give a bright flash. Apply lip gloss over all for added glimmer.

BALANCE YOUR FACE WITH MAKEUP

How can you look your prettiest? Once you find the key to your own beauty, you can make any little adjustments that keep you in style. Once you have found the right hairdo that will balance your face, brows and mouth should be shaped to create the total look. And color—your makeup—becomes the completing touch.

Mouth balance. If you have a small face, do not exaggerate your mouth, but if face is large or full, keep the mouth full, drawing the outline right on the outer rim of the natural outline.

- If face is long, keep width in the mouth from corner to corner rather than fullness from top to bottom. Avoid too deep an indent at the middle of the upper lip.
- If face is full but squarish, keep the mouth full.
- If face is full and round, keep the mouth full but not wide from corner to corner and make the outline of upper lip slightly angular.
- If jaw line is heavy, mouth should be wide and also full at the middle.

Shaping the mouth—For a pretty mouth follow a few simple rules.

- The highest points of the upper lip should always be within the area defined by the outer edges of the nostrils.
- Fullness of the lips should match at the corners and the color should meet exactly at the tips.
- To avoid droop at mouth corners, make sure color on both upper and lower lips meets exactly, that lower lip is not fuller than upper lip at the corners, and that the mouth—both upper and lower lips—has most fullness at the middle. This middle fullness makes the corners appear to turn up, thus putting in a smile.
- If some angularity is needed in the mouth outline, put it at the points of

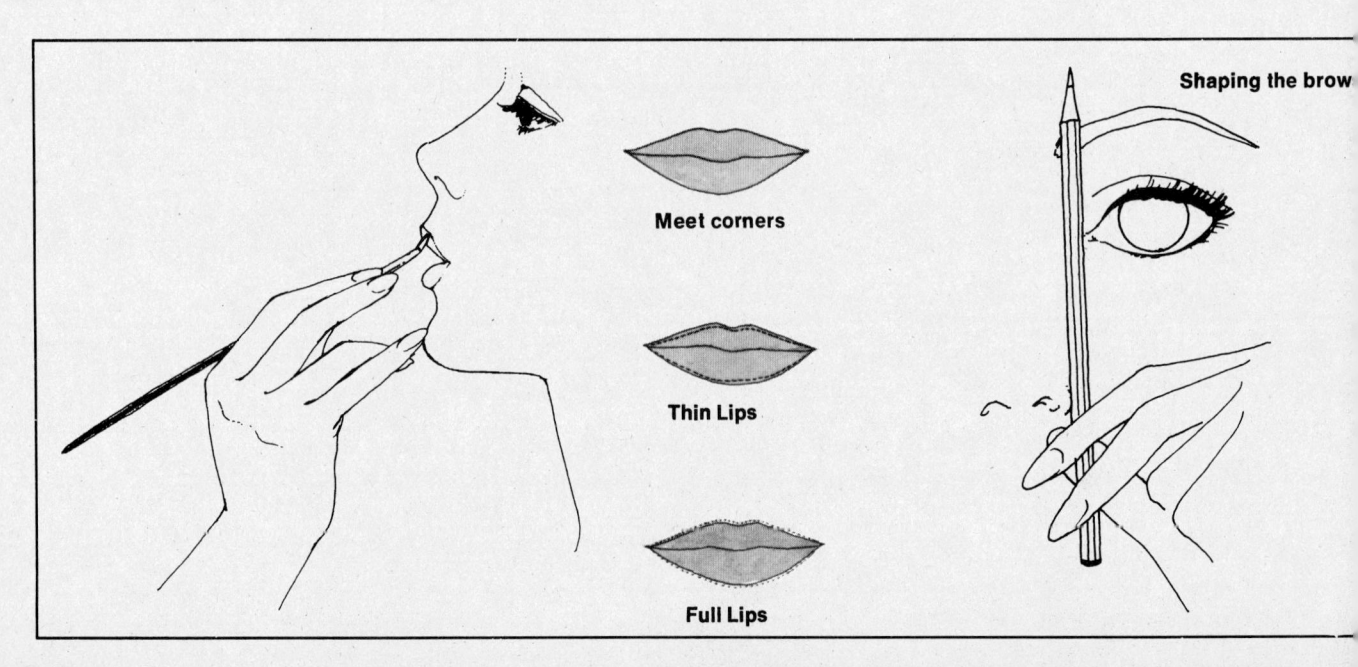

Meet corners

Thin Lips

Full Lips

Shaping the brow

upper lips, matching color at the corners.

☙ To make the upper lip appear fuller, shape the upper lip so that it is as full as the lower lip, making the middle dip shallow. Extend the tips of the upper lip slightly beyond the natural corners and then bring the tips of the lower lip up and out to meet the corners of the upper lip outline. Filling the indentation slightly and extending the highpoints a little to the outside also makes the upper lip more rounded and full.

☙ If lips are thick, keep the outline within the natural form of the mouth; if lips are thin, keep the line as full as possible while following the natural line of the mouth.

Mouth makeup—Lips should first be outlined; use a brush to give fullness and contour. The lip brush should be saturated with color for lips go on better as color collects in the brush.

☙ Holding the lip brush as you would pen or pencil, rest elbow on the table and rest the little finger against the chin to act as a pivot.

☙ Use a soft sable-tip brush with a long handle and use lots of color. It is usually better to use a medium or bright shade to outline the lips, a paler color within the outline.

☙ Be sure lips are dry to start; apply foundation to lips and then powder over the lips to give a base for the lip color.

☙ Start in the middle of the upper lip and outline one side. Then, starting again in the middle, outline the other side of the upper lip. Then outline the lower lip from middle to corners so that corners match exactly with the upper lip outline.

☙ Fill in with lipstick or with brush.

☙ Blot so that a full mouth imprint appears on tissue.

☙ Apply gloss in middle of mouth.

Shaping the brows. There are fashions in eyebrows just as there are in mouth makeup and hairdos; today the brow is light in color, natural in shape, and fairly thin. Heavy brows do nothing for any face—and detract from beauty when worn with full face-framing hair styles. Today's brow is beautifully groomed and definitely arched. Here are basic rules for shaping the brows:

☙ Find the natural brow line. Feel the edge of the bone that forms the upper rim of the eye socket; this is the natural line that the brow follows. Remove hairs only below this natural arch—and pencil the brows only above this line.

☙ Find the start of the brow line. Place a pencil against the widest part of the nostril and, holding the pencil straight, mark the point where pencil intersects the eyebrow. This is where the brow should begin. Do the same on the other side. Pluck stray hairs between these points.

☙ Find the end of the brow line. Set a pencil diagonally from the outer tip of the eye to the temple. Mark the point where the pencil crosses the eyebrow. Do not pencil the brow beyond this point.

☙ Balance the brow tips. Place a pencil along the eyebrow tip to tip. The inner and outer tips of the brow should be on the same level.

☙ Find the high point of the arch. Look straight ahead into a mirror. Note the position of the outer edge of the iris—the colored portion of the eye. The highest point of the brow arch should be directly above the outer edge of the iris.

Brow makeup—When drawing the brows, keep them in proportion to the size of the face and eyes and mouth. If changing the shape, keep penciling above the natural line. This raising and thickening of the brows with an outward flare at the tip makes the orbit of the eye appear large and the eye takes on an oval shape.

☙ Brush the eyebrows in all directions with their own special brush.

☙ Apply a little petroleum jelly.

☙ Then brush the brows outward and upward toward the highest point of the arch. Brush the tail of the brow outward toward the temple to give fullness here.

☙ Use two pencils, both fairly light in color—a brown pencil (do not use black) just a shade darker than the hair and a charcoal or light gray pencil.

☙ A wood-cased brow pencil should be sharpened to a flat blade edge; an automatic pencil to a short sharp point.

☙ The start of the brow should be penciled lightly because here the brow is usually sparse and should not look heavy. The thickness of the brow should be widest here.

☙ Pencil the brow with small hairlike strokes in a diagonal (upward and outward) direction—never in a hard continuous line—to the highest point of the arch. Beyond this point, pencil in almost horizontal strokes, bringing the lines out toward the temple. Never draw the brow down; taper width slightly at tip.

☙ Keep the width of the brow almost the same from inner tip to the highest point of the natural arch; tapering only slightly on the outer side of the arch.

☙ After penciling, smudge the brows lightly with the finger to blend the line and then brush the brow hairs to blend.

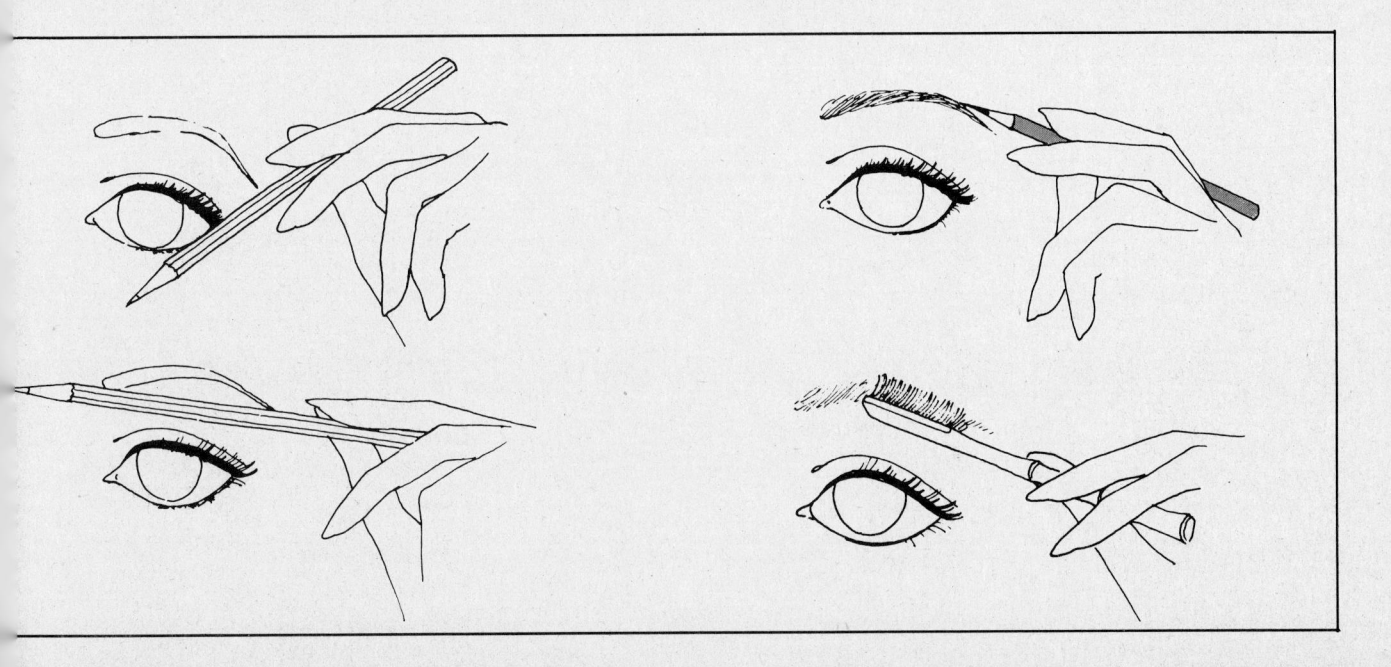

🍃 Avoid ending brows in a steep down curve, plucking brows too thin, hooking the brows too far in toward the eye at the inner tip; avoid, too, bushiness and an unkempt look, an exaggerated arch or too round an arch.

🍃 If you find it hard to draw eyebrows lightly, rest elbow on table, hold the brow pencil as you would hold a pencil to write with, and then rest the little finger against the cheek for firm support as you make your light feathery strokes.

🍃 Brow powder can be used to lighten or darken the brows. Brush the powder on the brow hairs, not on the skin, and brush after applying so the brows do not look dusty.

Improving your eye shape. Eyes are of many shapes and sizes. For the average eye the makeup should give the eye greater depth, an oval shape, and an appearance of being wider and larger.

Small eyes—Little eyes will look larger if you cover the lids and eye socket with a light foundation. Use bright-color shadow (blue or green or turquoise) just on the upper lid close to the lash line. Then draw a fine line along the upper lashes, not coming quite into the inner corner of the eye; lift the line a little here and extend the line at the outer corner. Draw a very light line in the lashes of the lower lid. Use lash lengthener or a small swatch of false eyelashes on the outer upper lashes to emphasize length.

Round eyes — Apply shadow slightly above the fold of the upper lid and bring the shadow out toward the tip of the brow. Extend the lash line just a little to lengthen the eye. Deepen liner toward outer corner of the eye and sweep the line upward. Keep mascara heavier on outer lashes.

Eyes too close together—Eye shadow blended and deepened on the outer side of lids will give width to eye area. A light foundation under brows will make eyes appear farther apart. Draw a thin line above upper lashes starting in about a third of the way along the upper lid. Mascara and lengthener should emphasize outer half of upper lashes; pluck eyebrows at inner tips to give eye width.

Eyebrow pouches — Drooping or fatty folds under the brow call for darker than usual foundation on this area plus light-color eye shadow on upper lids and just under the brow so that the pouch recedes and the upper lid is emphasized. Curl lashes upward and use lash lengthener mascara.

Protruding eyes — Apply dark shadow over entire upper eyelids right up to eyebrow area, this will make eyes appear to be more deeply set.

Deep-set eyes—Use a light foundation round the eyes and blend a light shadow on upper lid to the brow on the outer corner. Extend liner at outer corner.

Circles—Brush a light shade of makeup over darkened areas and then apply regular foundation over entire face. Blend rouge up and over edges of outer rims of circles.

How to make up the eyes. Apply foundation to the whole face, including eyelids, before starting eye makeup.

Eye shadow—For a subtle effect, pat on eye shadow gently with the tip of an index finger. To avoid unbecoming smudges on the sides of the nose between the eyes, gently stretch the eye skin away from the nose with fingers of one hand and pat the shadow on with a finger of the other hand. Starting at the inside tip and covering the upper lid to the fold, pat the shadow over the ball of the eye. At the outer tip of the eye, fan the shadow outward and upward to the eye bone, extending the upward curve of the lower lid toward the brow tip.

Eye liner—Again, stretch the eye skin away from the nose so the liner can be applied in an extremely fine line at the inner tip of the upper lid. Keep the line at the roots of the lashes to give an effect of lash thickness. From a hairlike line at the inner tip of the eye, thicken the line slightly over the middle of the lid and a little more at the outer tip. To line the eyes, use liquid liner or cake liner in a shade darker than your eye shadow but in the same color. While liner is still moist, blend it lightly with the tip of a finger to soften the line, but take care not to smudge it.

🍃 When lining the eyes, hold the brush parallel to the line of the eyelid. For a soft effect, you can make a broken line first and then carefully fill it in. Start the line at the middle of the lid, and line the lid all the way to the inner corner of the eye. Then, starting again at the middle, round out the outer side of the lid, keeping the liner in the lash line and drawing the line neither up nor out at the outer corner; instead, stop the line at the end of the lid.

Mascara—To apply mascara, pull the eye skin upward with fingers of one hand. Then apply the mascara all the way to the roots and bring the mascara all the way out so that lashes are evenly coated from roots to tips. Brush the lashes and then reapply mascara and brush the lashes again. Lashes should be brushed in the direction they grow—toward the nose for the inner lashes, away from the nose for the outer lashes, and straight ahead for middle lashes. To mascara lower lashes, use only the tip of the wand or brush, and lift the lashes individually as you apply the mascara.

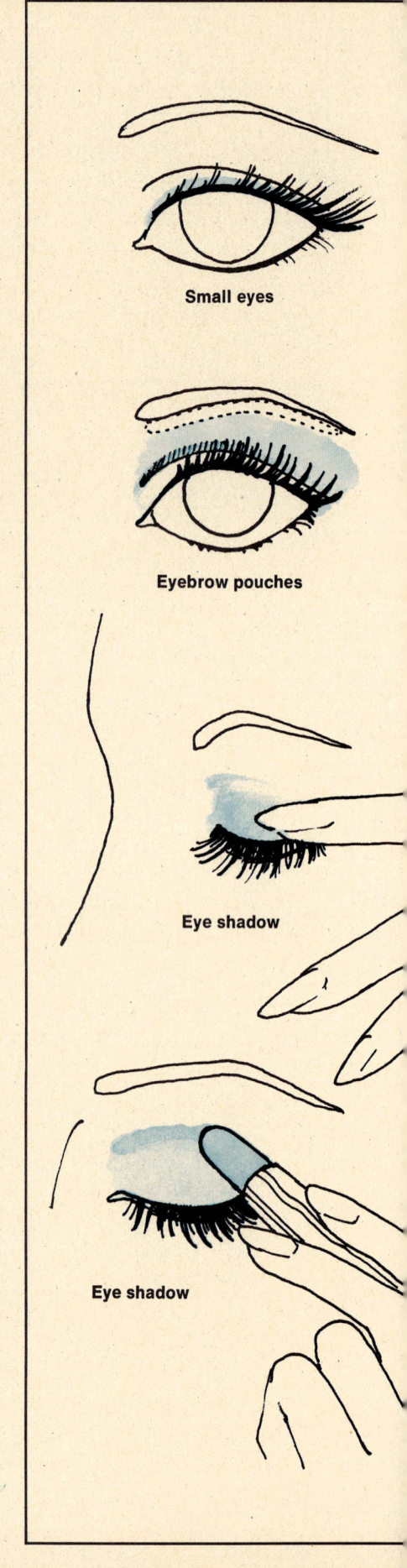

Small eyes

Eyebrow pouches

Eye shadow

Eye shadow

Round eyes

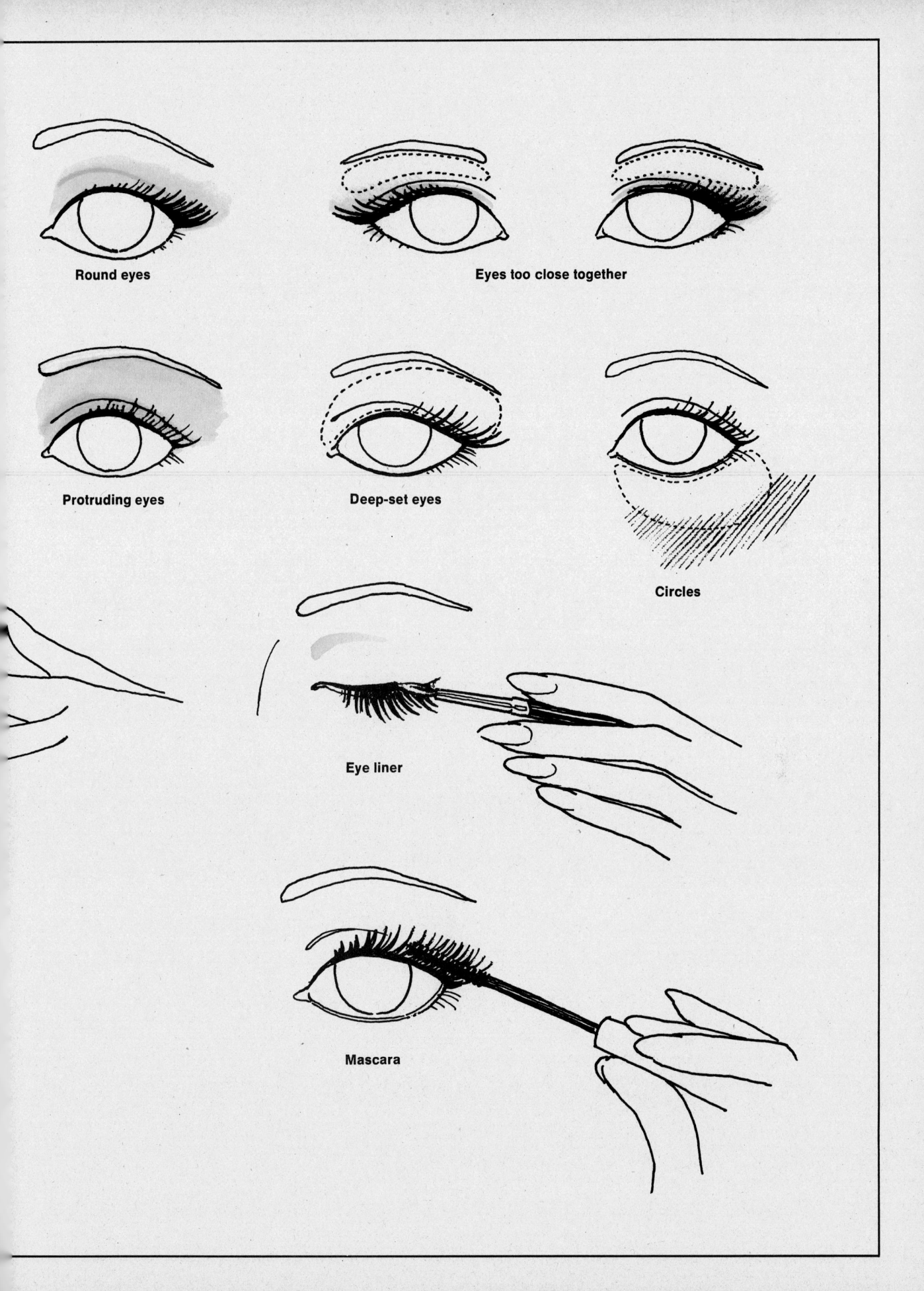

Eyes too close together

Protruding eyes

Deep-set eyes

Circles

Eye liner

Mascara

False lashes. Pastel (pale and pearly) eye shadows give the light and luminosity you'll want with false lashes. A thin black line is sometimes needed; otherwise, line the eye in a slightly deeper tone of the shadow shade you wear.

❧ For a perfect lash fit, try on the lashes—glue-free—for size and clip if needed from the outer (longer-lash) end.

❧ Start the lashes at the outer corner of the eye and never bring them so close to the inner tip that you cover the tearduct area. If the strip reaches that far in, it will be irritating—eyes will water a little, and the lash will be likely to loosen.

❧ Before using your new lashes, remove the adhesive that holds them to the container and apply fresh lash glue to the lash strip.

❧ Remove glue after taking lashes off, clean them, and then store them in their own case to keep them in shape.

❧ You may have to recurl your lashes from time to time: First moisten them in water, brush them into order, and put them between two small pieces of waxed paper. Roll carefully on a round pencil; fasten with a rubber band and let dry overnight.

❧ Positioning lashes on the lid correctly takes practice. Try placing them without adhesive a few times before you do it with glue. Use either an applicator, your fingers, or a tweezer to put them on.

❧ Look down into a mirror to apply the lashes. This relaxes your eyelids and puts your own lashes in a receptive position.

Applicator—Grasp false lashes lengthwise in applicator and position on your own. Place applicator over both and squeeze to fasten. To firm, tap lightly at the middle and both ends.

Fingers—Pick up lashes with fingers and position close to your own lash line. Pinch both sets together at middle and corners and pat along the whole length of lid. Hold briefly at tips.

Individual lashes—Use tweezers to pick up a clump of two or three hairs and dip end into a small amount of glue. Place

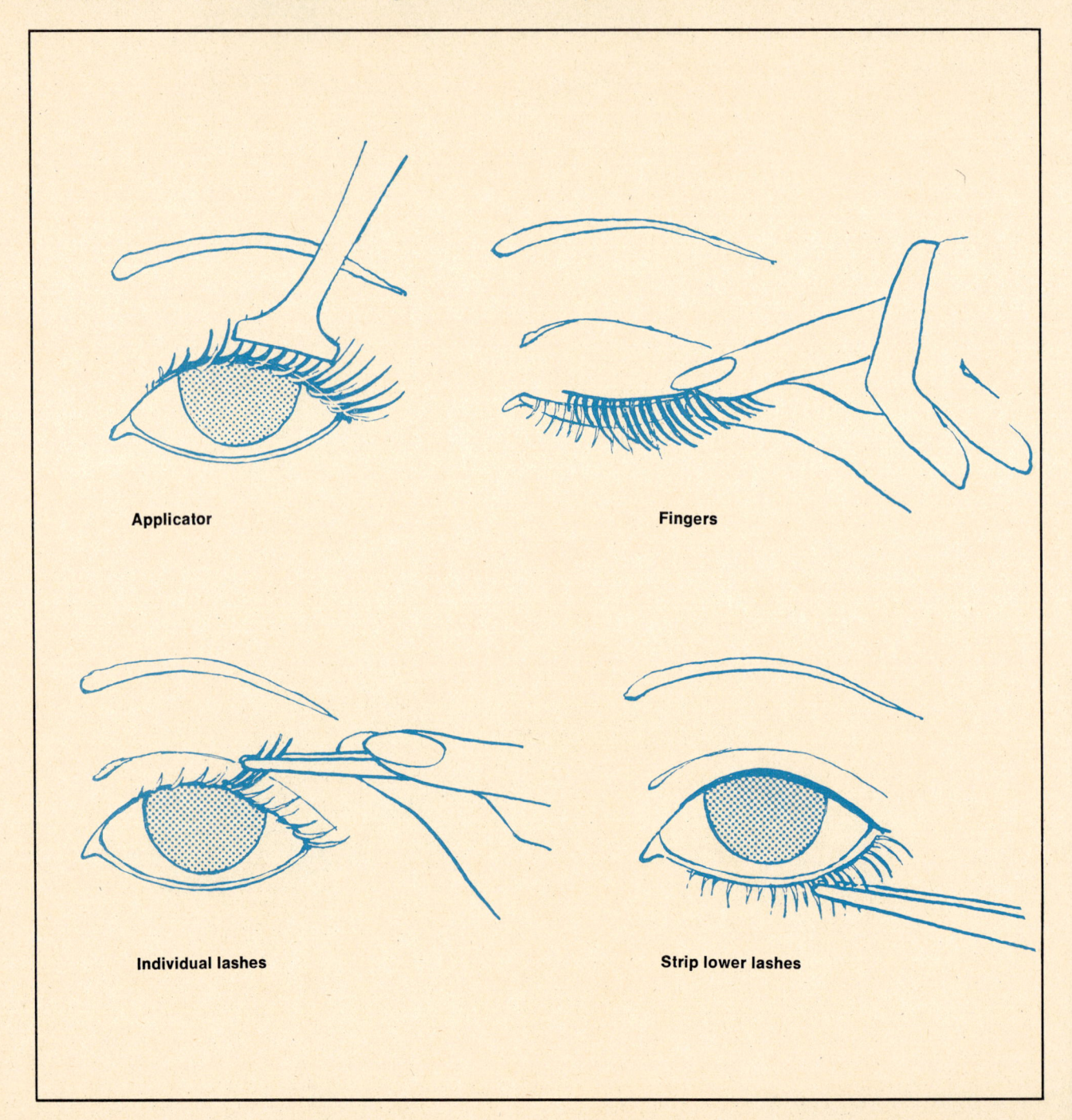

Applicator

Fingers

Individual lashes

Strip lower lashes

each clump on the lash line to fill spaces between your own lashes. Do upper lash line first. On lower lid, add three or four clumps toward the outer tip of eye as needed to balance the weight of the lashes above.

Strip lower lashes — Hold strip, curl downward, in tweezers and apply the glue. Look straight into mirror and carefully guide lash into position directly under your own natural lower lashes, the longer end at the outer tip of eye. Touch down firmly to set.

1. If your lashes are short and stubby (common with slightly protruding eyes and overhanging lids), use seven-eighths-length demilashes in a dark-brown shade with a slight curl and natural sweep. Push your own lashes up into the falsies.

2. Enhance very sparse, poorly placed lashes with individual falsies. You can cut a strip lash into clumps of two or so lash hairs, or use strip lashes on which the hairs are wide-set to look like individuals (available also as lowers).

3. Overly curly lashes often appear on a large prominent eye. Eyes can seem deeper and darker if a full sweeping lash to spread from tip to tip is added. The thin dark base gives the effect of the thin eye line that is otherwise needed.

4. For straight lashes with no curl, add a three-quarter-length lash that tapers from nearly nothing to a longish outer tip. Put a drop of glue on top of your own lashes and press them up into the falsies so they stick together.

5. If you have faded no-color lashes, pick false lashes of a color to complement your hair and skin tone. Variegated or streaked lashes look great with streaky hair. With the just-right lashes, eyes are enhanced—look glamorous.

6. Thin or missing lashes often accompany deep-set eyes. Set a half-size demilash to the outer corner of the eye to extend it an eighth of an inch and so bring the eye forward from its natural depth. You should not add mascara here.

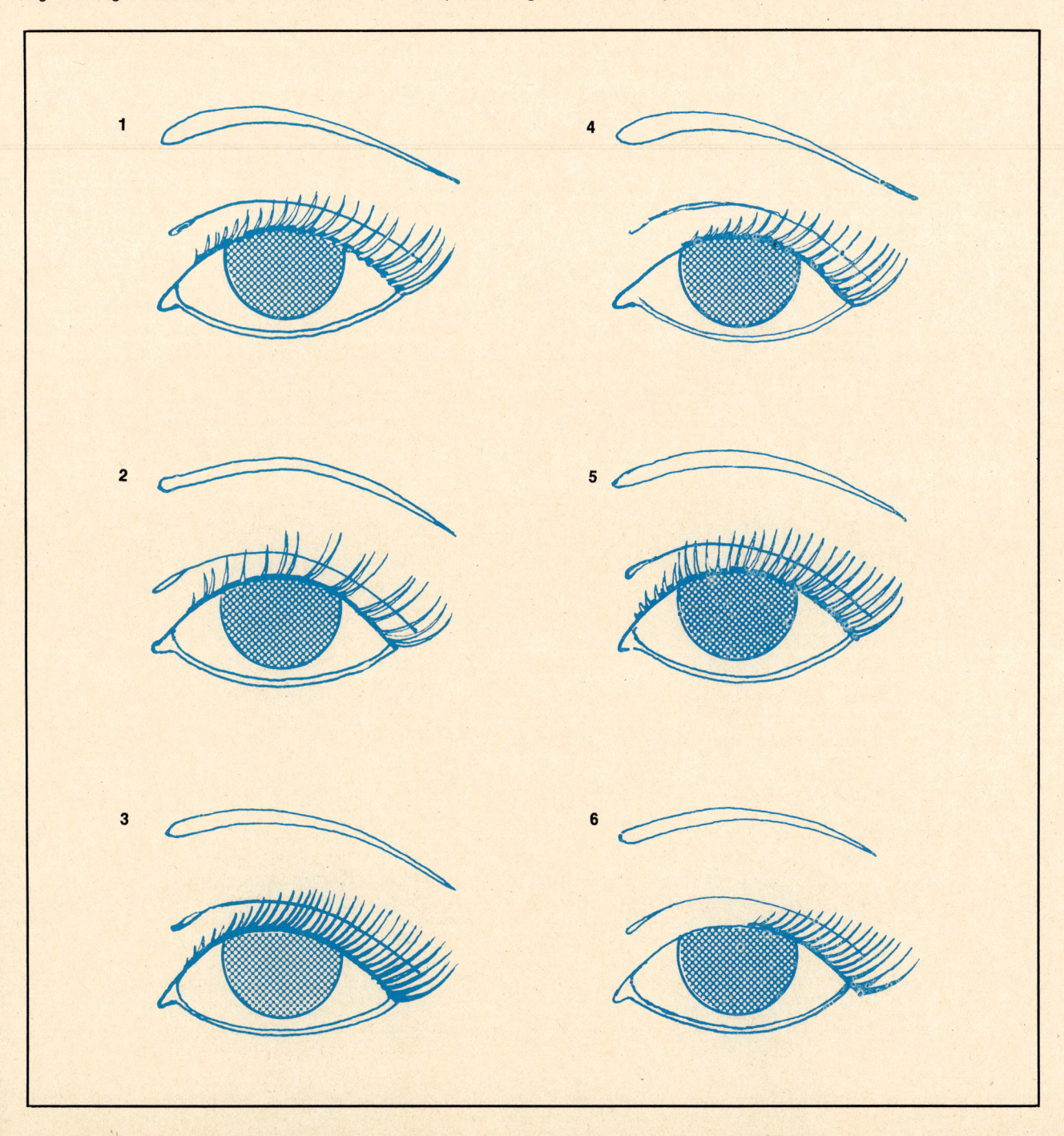

Wide face

Thin face

Round face

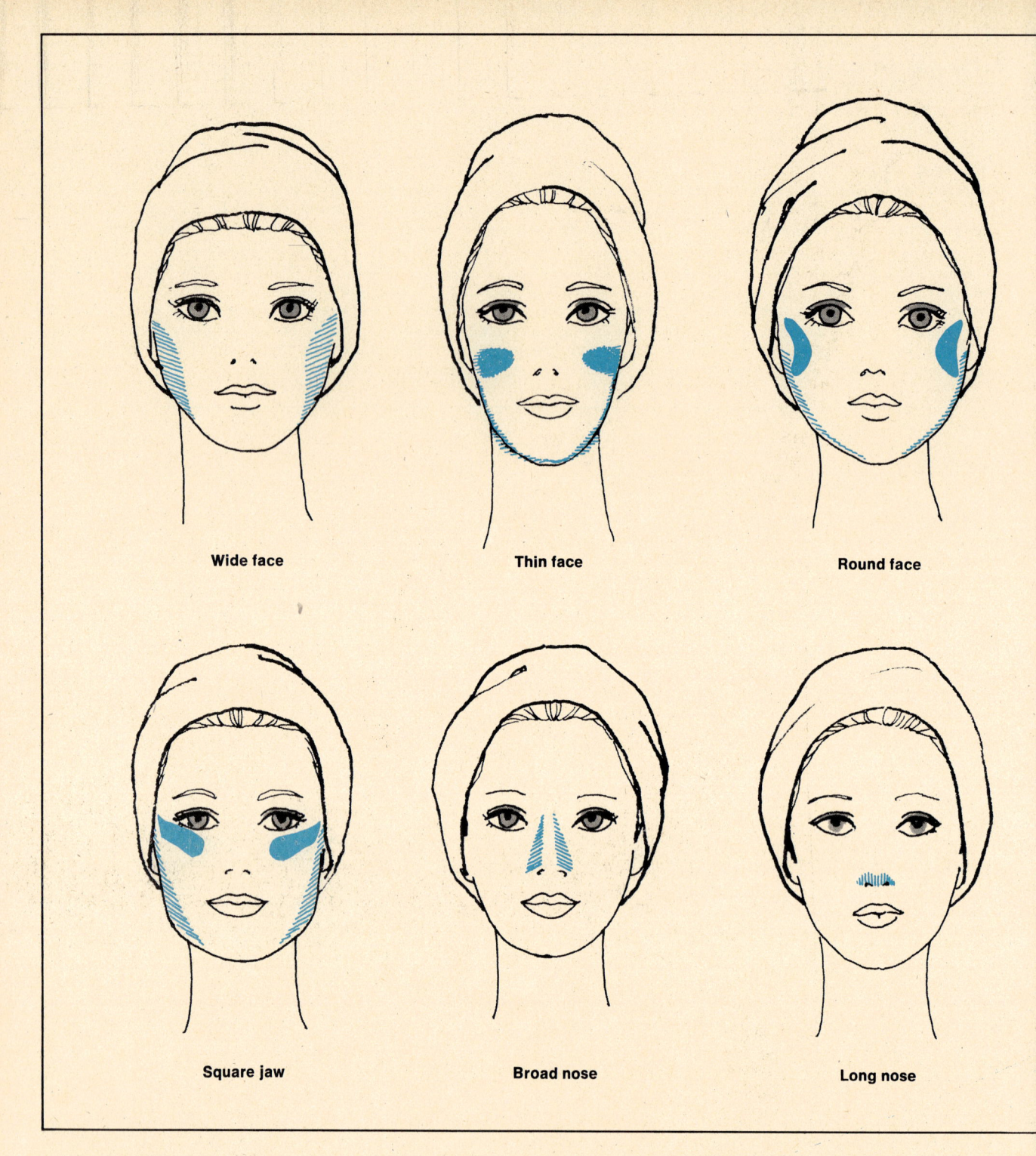

Square jaw

Broad nose

Long nose

SHAPE YOUR FACE WITH MAKEUP

You can use light and dark foundation to reshape the face. This effect is achieved because light reflection is cut down on areas where shading is applied and is picked up by light foundation. Be sure to blend the shading well into the foundation in the area where they meet so there is no visible change; if this area is carefully blended, shading can be quite dark toward the outside of the cheek or forehead. You may also use shading under the jaw line and along the chin to make the face stand out. Light foundation can be used in the eye area or toward the middle of the face and will also help hide deep lines, dark circles, and minor blemishes. Apply "darks" and "lights" with a damp makeup sponge.

Wide face—To make the face appear slimmer, use shading toward the *outside* of the face bringing the shading close to the line of the cheekbone. To make the face appear narrower, bring the rouge over the cheeks to the area directly below the middle of the eye and then down the highest parts of the cheek to about the level of the nostrils (but do not come very near the nose).

Thin face—Start on one side, blend dark foundation along jaw line, carry through to chin, and then to other side. Start rouge below middle of eyes under cheekbone, blend down and outward, keeping away from the nose. If you wish the face to appear wider, apply the

Hollow cheeks

Double chin

Receding chin

High-bridge nose

Narrow nostrils

Mouth lines

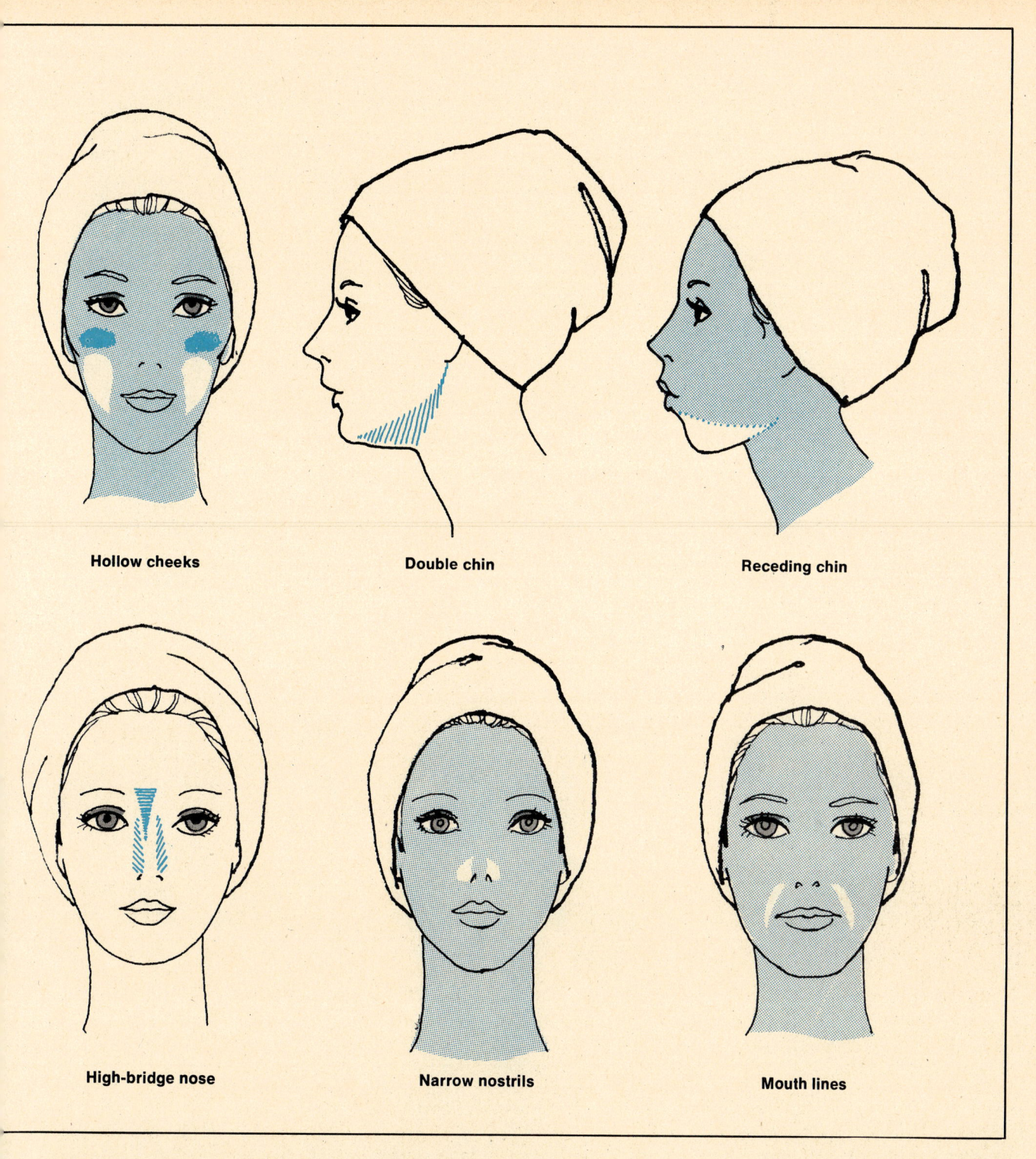

rouge only to the outside of the face, beginning at the temple and staying outside the eye bone.

Round face—Use shading along jaw line from ear to ear. Start rouge on outer portion of cheek under eyes, blending close to temple and downward to dark foundation on jaw.

Hollow cheeks—Use a light foundation in the hollows and a faint trace of rouge on the cheekbone and around the hollow to neutralize the natural shadow.

Double chin—Apply shading just under jawbone; blend from ear to ear along jaw line and under chin.

Receding chin—A triangle of light foundation over the chin brought from a point just below lower lip and extended along the jaw line to a point halfway from chin to ear will bring out the chin.

Square jaw—Use shading on outer sides of face and jawbone. Start rouge over the cheekbone, close to nose, blending carefully out to hairline and down toward the shaded area.

Nose too broad—Highlight middle of nose and play down width by applying two strokes of darker foundation down each side of nose. Blend well so change will not be conspicuous.

Nose too long—Blend dark foundation on edge of nostrils and under tip.

High-bridge nose—Blend a darker shade down bridge of nose, a lighter tone down each side.

Narrow nostrils—Apply a light foundation on sides of nose.

Mouth lines—Puff out cheeks and brush light foundation on lines; blend well.

65

Reshape your face

Well-groomed brows

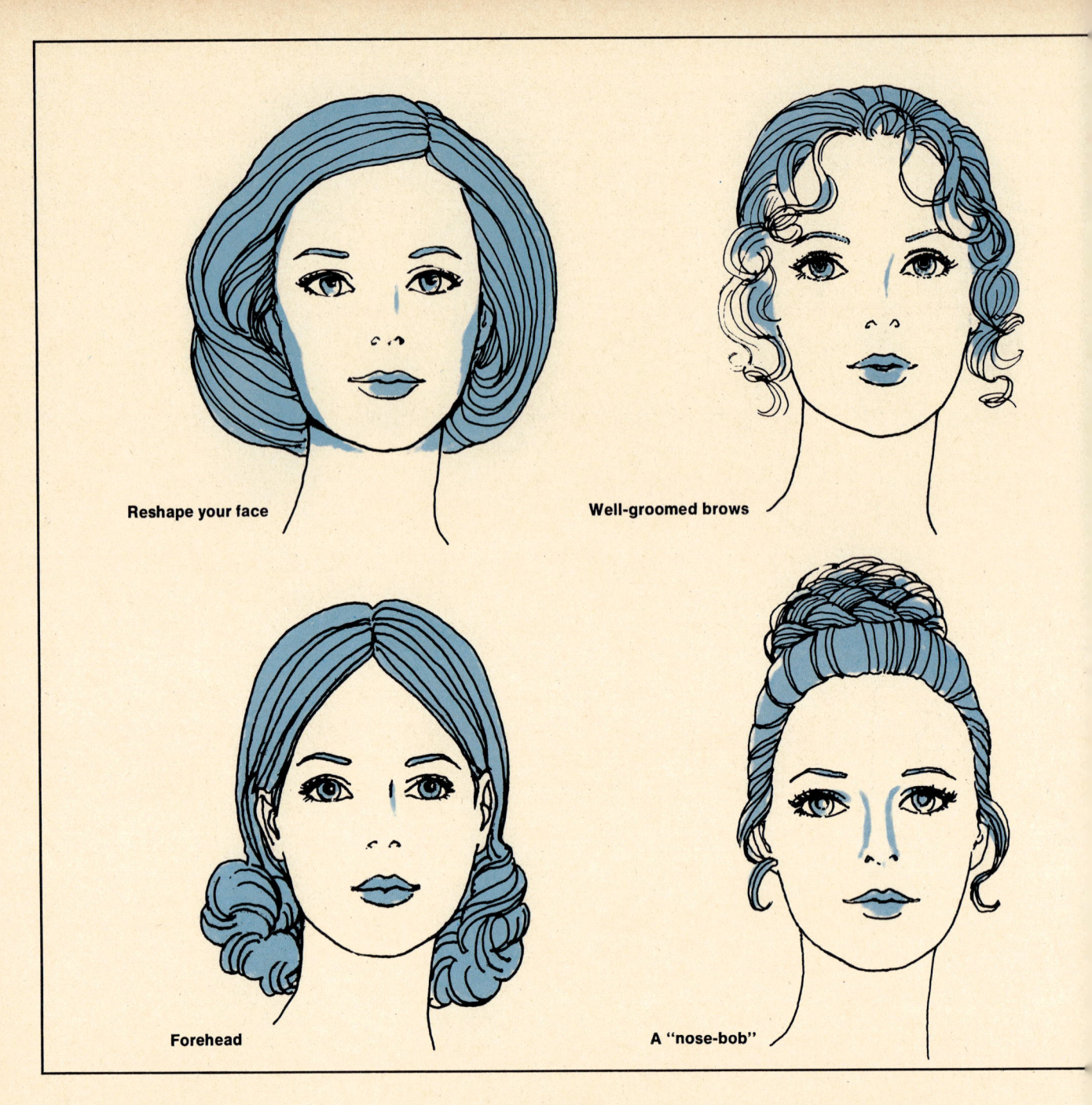

Forehead

A "nose-bob"

FACE-CHANGERS

Any face has its very own distinctive beauty that should be taken advantage of when you develop your look. If your face is angular, make use of the angles. If full, congratulate yourself on having one of the secrets of youth. There are few feature faults that can't be overcome with makeup and hairdo.

Then look for what could be a fault or a best feature. You have to work with your own bone structure—and create shadows where shadows would naturally fall for better facial contours. Highlights are placed where light is naturally reflected. Remember that dark makeup de-emphasizes an area; light makeup brings the area up. Before you begin to contour your face, decide what should be toned down by shading, what highlighted.

☙ Make flat cheekbones, a low or small forehead, or a disappearing chin catch the light by using a base half a shade lighter than the rest of the face on these areas, and avoid powdering so they will shine. For a prominent forehead, reverse —use makeup half a shade darker than on the face and powder the area well.

☙ Every forehead benefits from clean well-defined brows that, for today's look, are kept fairly light and thin. If brows are heavy or bushy, a good tweezing can help bring out the eye. Thin arched brows, lightened if this is necessary, are needed to avoid a furry look when hair is worn close to the face.

☙ A too-small nose looks less like a button if you highlight the top, lightly rouge the tip, and shade the sides.

☙ A deftly shadowed jaw line can give the illusion of a smooth-skinned neck, especially if a soft matte makeup is used on the face and the eyelids darkened to draw attention to another area. When a low neckline is worn, the makeup on the neck should cover all exposed skin in the same value and tone as the facial skin. With all feature fixing, the total picture is more important than any part.

Reshape your face. Try contouring makeup and sculptured hair style—a

Your mouth

Throat stretcher

Your eyes

Complexion woes

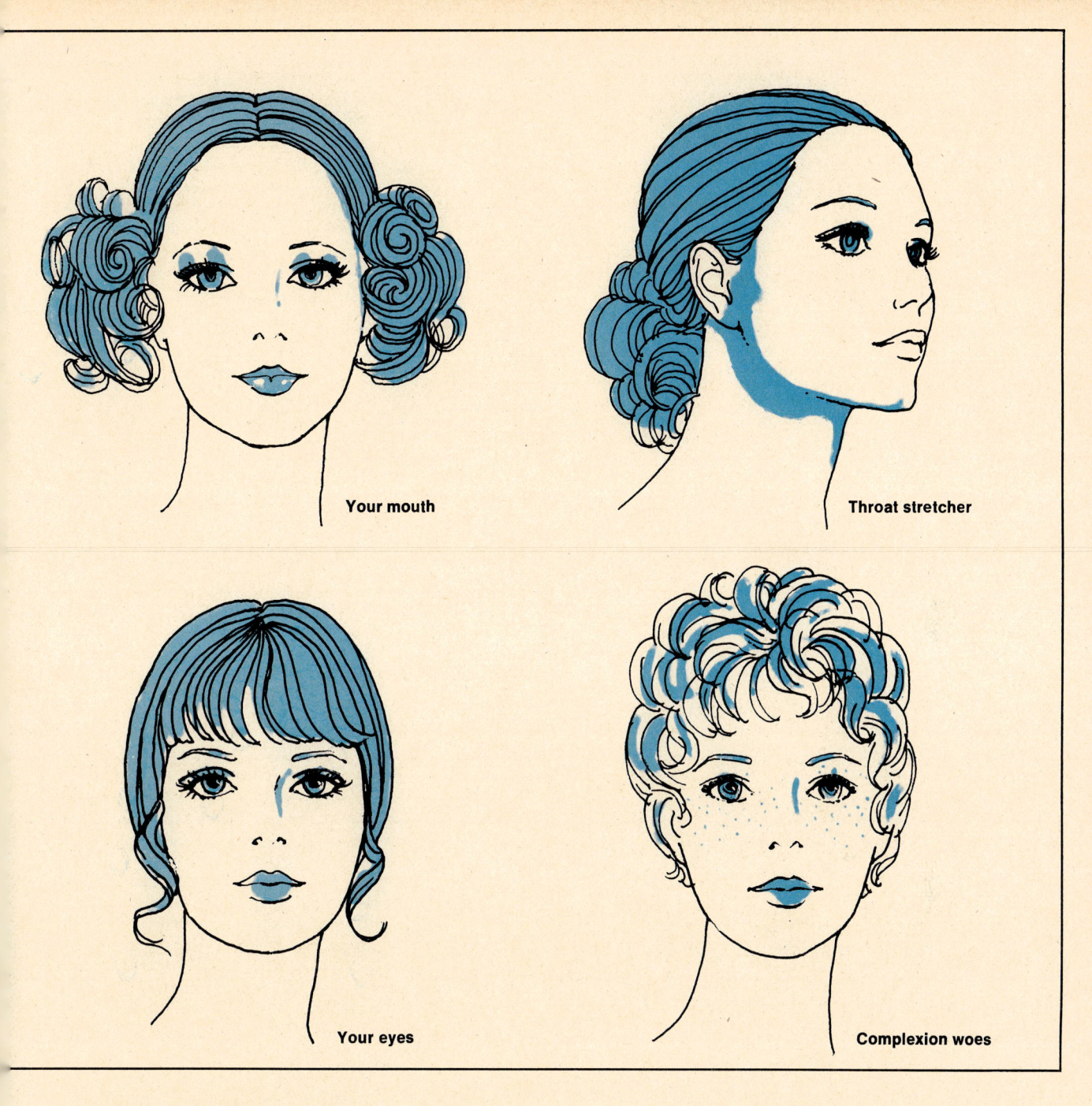

wide pageboy that slims by contrast. Shading in the cheek hollows knocks 10 pounds off a round face; below-the-jaw contouring disguises somewhat that extra half a chin.

Well-groomed brows. Lighten them if needed, to produce the clear look called for by airy tendrils of hair about the face. Leave enough space between the brows and lift the arch just above the outer rim of the iris; keep brow tips short and high to open up small or deep-set eyes.

Your mouth. Does it seem a bit thin and lips expressionless? Then create excitement with young color—real red —and draw the mouth full and pouty in a curved bow.

Throat stretcher. Shadow the jaw line, beginning behind the ear, extending the shading to emphasize the cleft in the chin, for the illusion of a longer, smooth-skinned throat.

Forehead. If forehead is prominent or high, use makeup base half a shade darker here and keep the area well-powdered to avoid shine. A bright lip color helps balance out the lower face.

A "nose-bob." It's yours with makeup that shades the sides and highlights the top. If hair is drawn back from the face and capped with a braided bun, a long nose is well-balanced; the eyes appear larger by such contrast.

Your eyes. They will loom twice as large if you use individual stick-on false lashes instead of strips. Rouge touched to the corner of the eyes (below the brows) makes them clear and beautiful. Brow-touching bangs and a light lip color enhance the all-eyes face.

Complexion woes. A summer-tan makeup sets the healthy outdoor glow that fools. Add-on freckles—dot them on with brown eye pencil and put a few on the upper eyelid, too—take attention from blemishes. So does streaked hair.

IF YOU WEAR GLASSES

When you start to wear glasses, you acquire a new day-in-day-out accessory—your frames become part of your face. Glasses aren't something to hide behind. They can be a fortunate added feature—a beauty-and-fashion accessory that enhances your look. But it's also true that, like your nose, your mouth, or your hair, glasses can create problems. Solutions to some of these take just a little know-how. Others you can solve right in the optometrist's office when you choose your frames and have the lenses put into them.

• Frames should be in proportion to the size of the face, but adjust your taste to changing fashions.

• The topline of the frame should be in harmony with the line of the brow so that the frames and eyebrow give the feeling of one line—not of two.

• To test for color, fold the frames and hold them against the cheek. Do they flatter the skin tones? Then try on the frames. Are they pleasing with the color of the brows and the color of the hair? Basically the harmony between brow and hair color and the frame color should be your guide, so a neutral—brown, black, gold, or sand—makes a good choice.

• If eyes are blue, blue frames with blue eye makeup create an appealing look. For green or hazel eyes, green frames do wonders. But think, too, of clothes colors when you choose. Avoid patterned frames—plaids, stripes, dots—because they cause confusion in the total look of the face. Red frames give a pink-eye look when others see you from a distance. Avoid over-ornamentation, too.

• Adjust your makeup to your eyeglasses. Pencil the brows only lightly (the topline of the frame should provide the emphasis). Wear "clean" eye makeup, minimizing shadow. Define the upper lash line with a clear line and make no line on the lower lid.

• Keep the mouth in harmony with the frames. Frames enlarge and emphasize the eye area; give the mouth all the width you can, but keep the color of lipstick light and soft.

• "Unbreakable" plastic or safety glass frames in both sunglasses and regular glasses protect your eyes and are worth the extra cost.

• If your eyes are "dropouts" behind your glasses, you may have frames with lenses too small. These mini-lenses were "in" a few years ago, but now (except in metal frames) lenses are large again. Whether you choose clear-plastic or shell frames, get as big a "window" for your eyes as the prescription permits and your face can wear. Wide-expanse frames are back again, just because they let the eye be seen behind the lens.

• The larger lenses also help avoid the exaggerated under-eye "gloom" that you get from small frames. By casting a shadow under the eye just where the natural hollow lies, small frames double dark circles. With any glasses, you need a makeup highlight in this natural hollow to bring the eye out. A pearly highlight just below it on the upper part of the cheek gives the eye area a similar prominence. And keeping lenses sparkling-clean also helps to make the eyes fully visible.

• If you wear mascara or false lashes, have them on when you pick out your glasses. Actually, the behind-the-lens eye shouldn't be made up so heavily as one that's exposed, because the lens, whether glass or plastic, tends to magnify. Anyway, makeup trends today are toward lighter, thinner, shorter false lashes or individual stick-on lashes that *do* look pretty with glasses.

Eye makeup behind glasses should not make the eye look smaller, nor should it create additional under-eye shadows—and this is what extra-long and extra-heavy strip lashes do. Any strip lashes—even of the mini type—tend to make the natural lashes droop just a little. To avoid this, touch a bit of the lash glue to the tops of your own lashes and pinch them up against the false ones to keep your look as wide-eyed as possible.

The first step in solving the eyelash problem, however, takes place in the optometrist's office. If you call the lash situation to his attention when your glasses are being fitted (and wear your usual eye makeup on this important day), he can have the lenses bowed slightly to accommodate the additional length. This extra curve must be included when the lens prescription is made up—and the extra curvature will not (in most cases) interfere with the vision correction prescribed for you.

• Frames don't take the place of eyebrows. In fact, well-groomed brows carefully made up (the secret here is shaping the line, brushing the brows smooth, and keeping the brow makeup on the light side) will usually help you to look great in glasses. (The exception is when brows are light and the frames somewhat severe; it may be appealing here to brush the brows up to look a little fluffy.)

Your best guide is that the line of the frame and the brow line should be in harmony. This doesn't mean they have to follow each other exactly. With an octagonal (eight-sided) or hexagonal (six-sided) frame, the rounded arched brow line may be most becoming. The brow line needs to be curved if the face and the frames are both angular. Seen straight on, the brows may be covered by the frames or appear above them, but from the side they are usually visible. Don't leave brows shaggy and unshaped just because you think they aren't seen. Shaping the brows also helps bring out the eyes—and this is what you want to do when you wear glasses.

Finally, try a touch of blusher *above* the eyebrows. It gives your eyes more sparkle and heightens the brightness of the entire face.

• Subtlety in makeup is the secret. Delicate pinks and lavenders as well as soft greens, blues, and browns, used correctly, look beautiful behind lenses. Cream or gel shadows—transparent pastels—keep the eye soft-looking and are much less drying than powders. Or, if you love your powder shadows, pat a creamy pearlized foundation on the lid before you brush on the shadow for a moist effect. Transparent eye liner is also great.

The eye behind the lens should be carefully contoured. Use highlights below the brow and as a reflector under the eye. The contour line in the crease of the upper lid and rising toward the brow gives the eye shape and depth. Contouring here can be in beige or pastel. On the upper lid to the crease, apply a pastel shadow with frosted glints so the lid will catch light. A soft line of pastel shadow in the lash line of the lower lid (used instead of under-eye liner) and a gentle brown eye line in the upper lashes are particularly becoming with glasses. True, with very thick lenses there can be some distortion of eye shape, but the eyes won't look strange unless the makeup is harsh or garish.

• With tinted pastel lenses, eye makeup will depend on the shade and strength of the lens tint. If it's a strong blue or green tint, the entire eye should be lightened with a frosted white shadow, including a faint touch of frosting under the eyes so the entire behind-the-lens area looks light. A thin line of iced navy blue shadow above and below the lash line makes the eye shape show up clearly through the glasses. Also wise with tinted lenses: A little rouge on the tip of the nose to brighten the face.

Keep to a cool-tone makeup with lavender lenses to avoid too much pink in the whole face. A combination of celery green and eggshell shadow—the green on the upper lid and near the lash line on the lower lid; the egg-

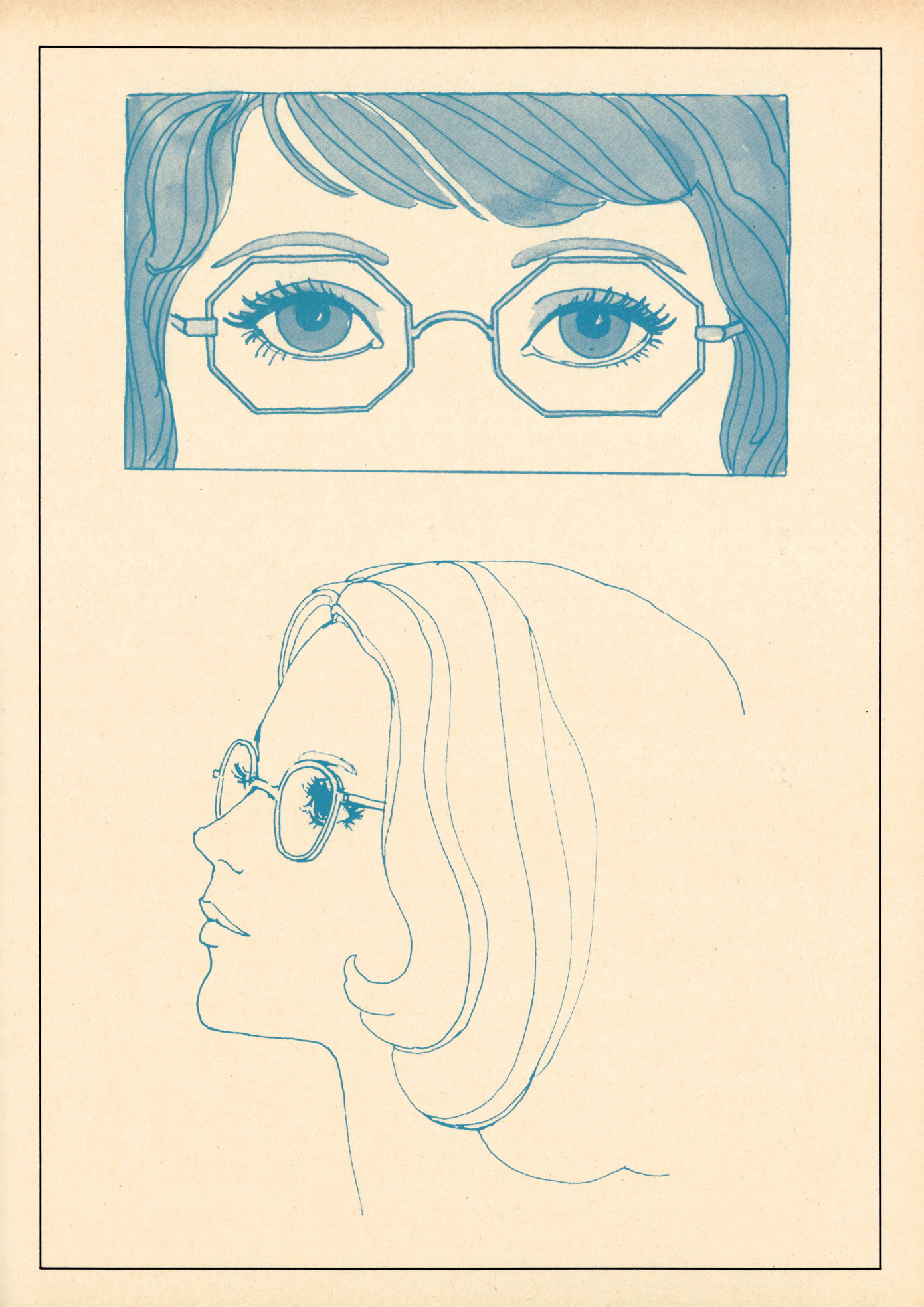

shell to lighten the entire area—keeps the eye in sight.

With pink lenses, make it violet shadow with either purple or blue liner and dark blue mascara, and a light dusting of purple powder shadow on the brows.

With yellow or amber lenses, a dark-brown liner and a taupe shadow give needed strength to the eye shape; keep the facial makeup in the corals and tans.

The smoky lenses require a clean, clear eye makeup that will not be grayed by the lens tint, but color is not changed noticeably by the smoke tone. Sure to be flattering: Pastel frosted eye makeup that picks up any mauve, pink, green, or bluish tone in the lens.

A good optometrist can help a lot in narrowing your choice of frames, for his experienced eye can see what will balance your face. Usually, though, you have to get things started by making your own "self-picture" evident to him. That is, you find a shape and color you like, and he improves on this choice by suggesting a somewhat smaller or larger size, a lighter or darker tone, and so forth—a suitable variation on your basic choice.

Shape, size, and color should harmonize with the same characteristics in your face. The larger the face, the larger the glasses that can be worn. A squarish face calls for neither square nor circular glasses but a harmonious something in between: Ovals are often the best choice, but hexagons, octagons, oblongs are possibilities to consider.

To find your own best shape, don't hesitate to try on a variety of frames. Then check the effect of various colors —pastels, light and dark shell, black— in the shape you select. The clear plastics in pastels—or even in strong reds, blues, greens—often look more feminine than do shell rims. Metal wire frames with large or small lenses, tinted or clear, can be a delightful change. In shell rims, choose frames for simplicity and size (big enough), in a tone that won't overpower your face. Select black only if you want your frames to look very bold. Blondes often look best in the light ambers; brunets, in the darker shell tones. Bypass frames that are ornamented if you wear your glasses in the daytime. Also steer clear of the kind that you think will be innocuous; the so-called invisible ones don't really disappear.

Examine the fittings, too. Some faces look best in glasses with the hinges set behind the frames; some need the width you get from hinges set out to the side. A raised nose bar is good with a high forehead.

Most important: Make your choice *standing* in front of a full-length mirror. Glasses are part of your total look and should be viewed this way from the start.

What hair style with glasses? Pull-back hairdos are great for glasses wearers because the style keeps your face uncluttered. Heavy bangs often close down the face too much. Wispy bangs, on the other hand, can be attractive and feminizing. Tendrils help soften the bare face look.

If your face is full and broad, glasses frames should be relatively large and the hairdo full to make the cheeks less prominent. For high cheekbones, round frames are becoming; with these the hair can be brought down from a center part in a cap that curves onto the cheeks.

With a square or angular face, the frames should not be similarly square but have an oval, oblong, or other comparable shape that gives some grace to the line. The hairline should be softened with tendrils, which de-emphasize the angularity of the face without detracting from its distinctive shape. Large oval glasses and a full-at-the-bottom page-boy hairdo flatter a wide jaw.

Overall, the rule to follow is: Some softness but not too much clutter in both hair design and accessories.

Not being able to see well without glasses when putting on makeup is a problem that women have tried to solve with magnifying mirrors, special out-from-the-face eyeglasses, and many other devices. Women who wear bifocals turn their glasses upside down and work below the glasses while looking up into the mirror through the inverted close-vision part of the lens. The best solution is to train yourself to put on the makeup by touch. After you have put on your makeup, check it carefully, with your glasses on, to be sure it is just as you want it.

WHAT SHOULD YOU DO ABOUT FACIAL HAIR?

Skin normally has a fine growth of hair, usually not noticeable on a woman's face, and this need not be interfered with. Even a noticeable growth of hair seems to be "normal"—perhaps an inherited trait—with some women. Even if hairs are coarse and dark on the upper lip, it is best not to pluck them, for plucking makes electrolysis more difficult in case you someday decide to have such treatment. A cream or wax depilatory for facial use is all right as a temporary measure; or scattered facial hairs or a growth of lip hairs may be clipped close to the skin. If hairs are dark, they may be bleached with peroxide or lemon juice or you can buy a facial hair bleach for this purpose. If hairs begin to appear after menopause or during treatment with some medications, endocrine factors may be involved, and a physician should be consulted. Electrolysis is the one recommended method of permanent hair removal and should be performed only by a competent operator. In many communities, but not all, these operators are licensed.

Electrolysis. Electrolysis is a medically accepted way of getting rid permanently of "unwanted" hair. Such hair is usually normal growth.

The human body has a downy coat of fine hair that is for the most part hardly noticed. On a woman's cheek, for example, there may be 5,000 hair follicles per square inch—but rarely are these potential "hair-raisers" all producing at one time. Sometimes, due to hereditary influences, such normal hair is dark, heavy, or peculiarly distributed—and is therefore "unwanted."

In electrolysis, a fine wire filament is introduced into the hair follicle (the depression from which the hair grows) and —by an electric current that produces a chemical reaction—the hair root is destroyed. The loosened hair is then removed.

Sensitivity varies—but the treatment usually produces only a mild sensation. Normal skin may be somewhat reddened, but this is a temporary condition and not a great problem.

Treatment varies in length. Individual sessions usually last 15 minutes, sometimes a half hour or an hour, depending on the condition and on the time and money a person can invest. Sessions usually are weekly or every two weeks to start and extend over a period of several months and sometimes a year or more.

There is a small amount of regrowth (usually from previously plucked or waxed hairs that are hard to treat), and an ethical practitioner will be the first to acknowledge this. There is also *new* growth from dormant follicles that awaken in their natural cycle during treatment and a reemergence of recently plucked hairs. It takes about three months for such plucked hairs to reappear on the scene and this is one thing that lengthens treatment time.

Rates for treatment vary. The frequency—once a week or every two weeks—depends upon the individual budget and needs, as does the number of months the treatment will span.

Dermatologists, family physicians, and dentists are usually able to make electrolysis referrals.

OTHER HELPS FOR YOUR LOOKS

For facial problems, such as acne scars, and fine surface wrinkling, "face planing," or dermabrasion, may be used. Here the skin is "frozen" and the top layers are removed with abrasive. Again, results are not always perfect, but improvement may be looked for.

※ "Face peeling," a process by which the top layer of skin is removed by applications of a caustic preparation, is used by some dermatologists to improve aged or weathered skin. This should be done only by a qualified physician.

※ Silicone foam is a means of filling out wrinkles and deep facial lines.

※ Cosmetic dentistry can also improve a receding jaw, hollow cheeks, denture lines round the mouth—as well as give you a sound bite.

※ Other medical aids may also improve facial beauty. Eyeglasses (or contact lenses) to bring vision up to par can help you to avoid the anxious expression, the squints, and the frowns that are often brought on by eyestrain. Sunglasses that protect from glare can also help avert squint lines.

※ Uncorrected hearing loss can often change the facial expression, leading to a look of anxiety as you strain to hear conversation or to a vacant expression as the sounds of life pass you by. A hearing aid or perhaps ear surgery can restore the zest of life to the hard-of-hearing and can consequently bring relaxation to the facial muscles.

HOW TO GET RID OF BEAUTY FLAWS

Has nature given you an unfortunate feature? Has time—or a bad habit—flawed your face? Does it bother you enough—and is it worth it to you—to spend the time and money for remodeling? Today, more and more of us are ready to do something about "my nose," "my chin," "my ears," even, "my breasts." Where do you start? First step is a consultation with a qualified plastic surgeon. If you have no reliable source of referral, names of plastic surgeons in your area can be had by checking the current *Directory of Medical Specialists*. This reference text should be available in any public library Or telephone your county medical society or a local hospital for a referral. With cosmetic surgery, you usually have to pay a consultation fee which may (not always) be applied to the surgery fee if you decide to go ahead. In the consultation, the surgeon will first find out what you want done. He will then examine you and explain to you what can be done or should be done and what results to expect. He will also discuss costs and hospitalization and recovery time. If you decide to go ahead, you will need "before" photographs. If the surgeon does not do these himself, he will send you to a medical photographer. The fee the surgeon quotes will probably include aftercare, but hospital costs and perhaps the anesthetist's fee are extra. Cosmetic surgery is not covered by medical plans, but is income-tax deductible as a medical expense (subject to the usual limitations). For the employed, time off from work must also be included in the budget. In most cases a patient can appear socially when swelling and discoloration have gone down—in three weeks or so—though full "recovery" (meaning your changed feature has assumed its new shape and consistency) may take considerably longer. Pain is not usually a factor in cosmetic surgery. but there is bound to be some discomfort and, as with any surgical procedure, some risk.

Nose. Reshaping the nose can be done as early as 14 to 16 years for girls—as soon as the bone structure is mature—or at any age thereafter. A thin hooked nose is relatively easy to correct; a bulbous nose, especially if the skin is thick, oily, with large pores, is more difficult to adjust; a hollow saddle nose or button nose may require silicone inplants. In most nose reshaping, work is done through the nostrils, so there are no visible scars. When there must be an exterior scar, incision is done where it is least noticeable—along the nostril folds, under the tip or, sometimes, at the floor of the nose. The anesthetic usually is a local aided by narcosis, a form of gentle sleep. Surgery takes one-and-a-half to two hours; hospitalization is from two nights to a week (average, four nights). A splint and bandage are needed for from three days to a week or longer. Swelling and discoloration (black eyes) go down within two to two-and-a-half weeks, but it takes six to ten months for the nose to assume its final shape and consistency. During this time, care must be taken to protect the nose from injury. In some cases an adjustment (minor surgery) may be required at a later date. Sometimes adjustment of the chin is needed along with the nose reshaping to keep the face in balance.

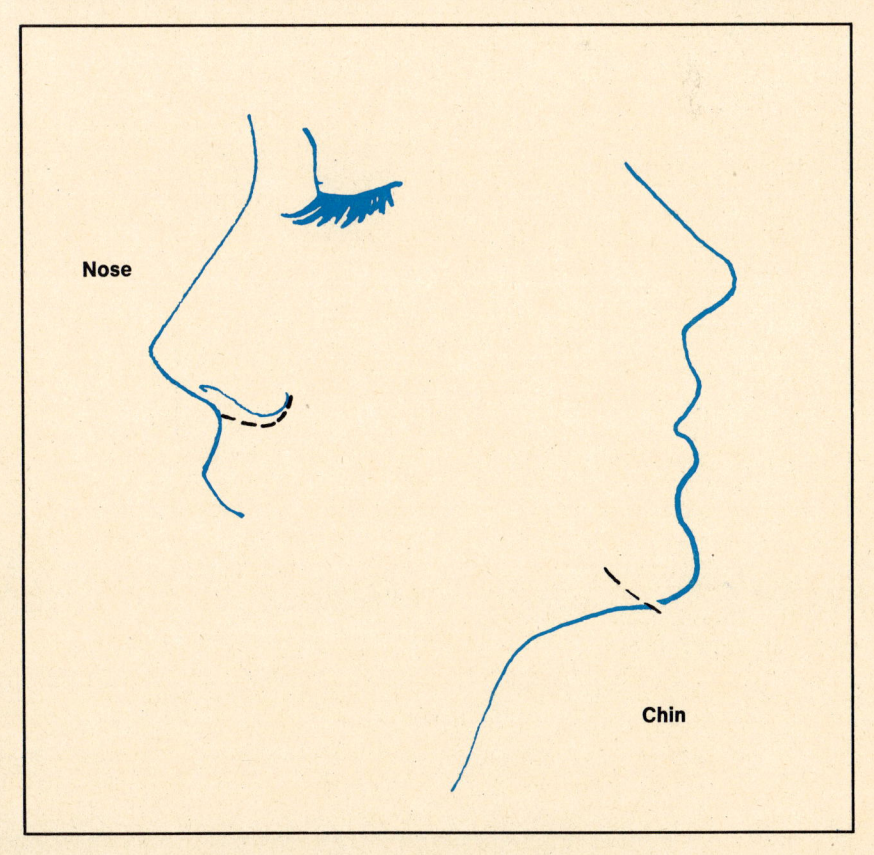

Chin. Reshaping of the chin can also be done starting in the middle teens, once bone structure is mature, or at any later date. Any needed dental restoration should be done before the chin is worked on. Incision may be inside the mouth (no exterior scar) or by an exterior incision, depending on the judgment of the surgeon. In the latter case, it is made just under the chin, where it will be least noticeable. For enlarging the chin, silicone implants may be used; for reducing the chin size, bone is removed. Surgery takes about a half to three-quarters of an hour for simple augmentation; local anesthesia and narcosis is used, with three to four nights of hospitalization. Stitches come out in five to seven days. Discoloration and swelling go down in two to two-and-a-half weeks; complete recovery takes six to eight months. Reshaping at a later date may be needed (implants can be removed and replaced). Operations are sometimes done to remove a layer of fat and skin (double chin) beneath the chin line, but these leave a visible scar. A double chin often develops because of frequent weight change; sometimes the angle between the chin and neck predisposes one toward a double or triple chin. A full face-lift to draw up the loose skin in this area, as well as elsewhere on the face, may be preferable.

Eyelids. Surgery can be done as soon as face structure is mature, but usually is not needed till after age 30. Baggy lids or puffy eye skin can be due to fluid retention or other systemic problems, so a physical examination is advised before the situation is surgically corrected. Usually the operation is done on both lids, upper and lower, and both eyes to keep the face in balance. To minimize scars, incision is made in the fold of the upper lid, just under the lash line of the lower lid, and is sometimes extended into the folds of the crow's feet, or wrinkles, at the side of the eye. This operation can be an office procedure, but is usually done in the hospital under local anesthetic, with the patient kept in the hospital for two nights. Stitches can usually be removed in four to six days; discoloration and swelling last two weeks. Sometimes, after lid surgery, there is a slight pulling down of the lower lid (especially in the elderly) but this, given time, is usually self-correcting.

Lips. Reduction of overly thick lips can be done at any age, but is usually done in the teens or thereafter. Incisions are made inside the mouth to remove excess tissue, so there is no exterior scar. Local anesthetic is used, and hospitalization is usually for three days. Lips tend to swell a great deal and reduction of swelling may take two weeks or more. Correction of drooping lips or other flaws that require working from the outside is usually discouraged because the scarring is external and hard to hide.

Ears. Correction of lop, or protruding, ears can be done from age seven and up. Overlarge ears or oversize or drooping lobes can also be corrected. Incision for lop ears or overlarge ears is at the back of the ear; at back and under the lobe, for reduction of the ear lobe. Sometimes this can be an office procedure. Local anesthesia is used for adults, general anesthesia for children. Hospitalization is usually two nights. Recovery is about one week, during which time the ears are bandaged. Stitches come out after two weeks, but it is usually recommended that a scarf be worn around the head while sleeping for several months after surgery.

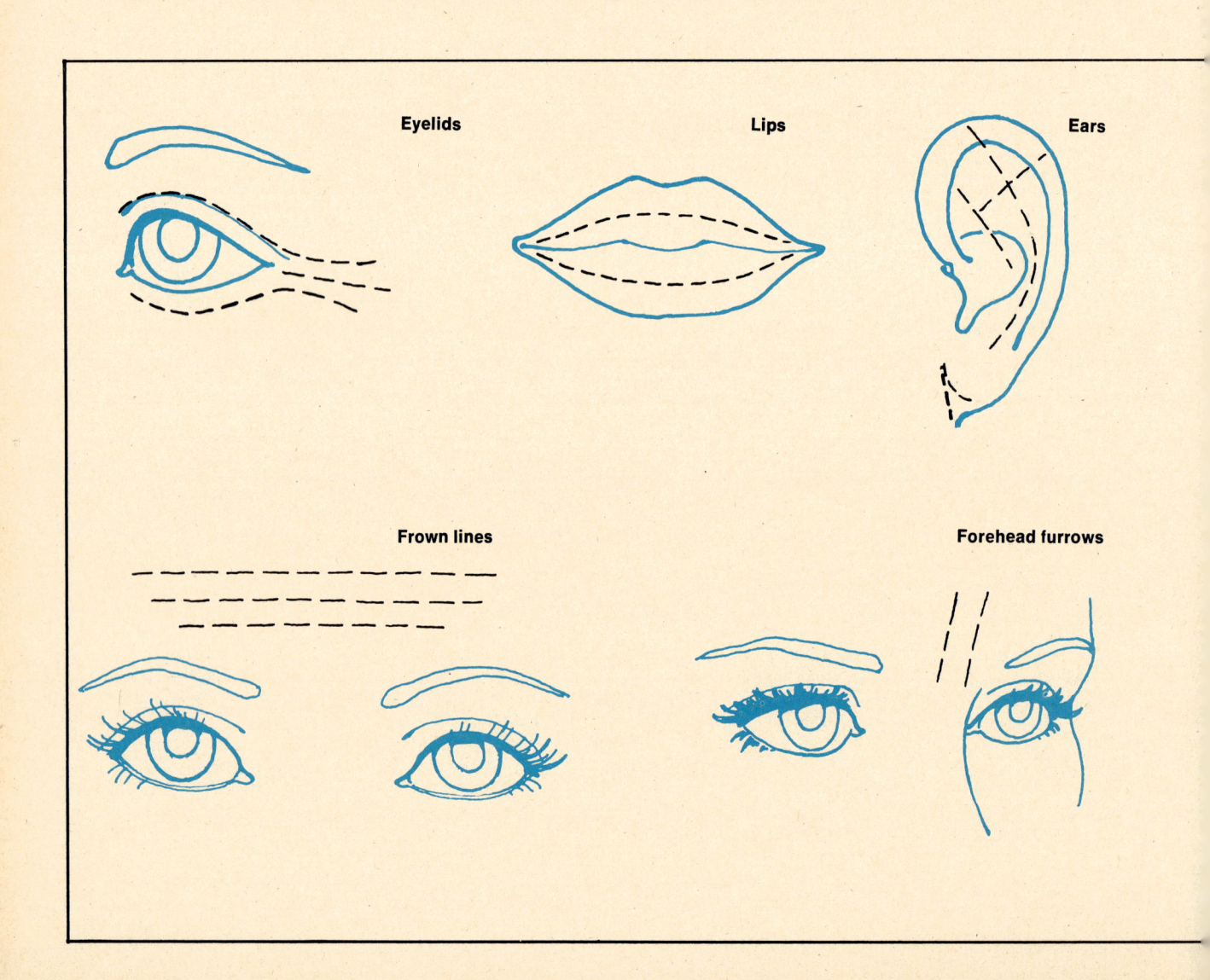

Eyelids **Lips** **Ears**

Frown lines **Forehead furrows**

Frown lines. Deep frown lines can be modified by making an incision between the eyebrows and filling in with fatty tissue. The surgery (under local anesthetic) can be done at any age, with hospitalization usually two nights. Stitches are usually removed after five to seven days and complete recovery is rapid. Many cosmetic surgeons discourage this operation because there are always visible scars.

Forehead furrows. These are hard to correct because any incision to erase them produces a scar that is hard to hide, even if it is in the forehead hairline. Usually the plastic surgeon prefers to deal with this problem, working from the side, in a complete face-lift.

Face-lift. Usually this operation is done at age 40, but it can be done as early as age 20 for improvement of deep acne scars that cannot be satisfactorily reduced by dermabrasion—skin-planing. The incision is made above the hairline, and the surgeon works through the hair (without shaving the scalp), along the side, in front of the ear to behind the ear and to the region above the hairline behind the ear. The only visible scar (not concealed by hair) is just in front of the ear. The skin is then undermined (lifted away from the underlying tissues) and drawn upward to the side and redraped, with the excess skin removed at the line of the incisions. This draws up and firms the whole face. General or local anesthetic may be used. The operation may take from four to five hours when done with the eyelids. Hospitalization is five to seven days. It usually takes four to six weeks (depending on the age and condition of the patient) for swelling and discoloration to go down and for the patient to be socially ready again. A major face-lift sometimes needs to be revised after several years; the mini-lift, or little tuck above the ear, is often successful as a revision of a major face-lift but is not recommended as a substitute for a major face-lift when this becomes necessary, though it appears to be an economy.

Breasts. Reshaping to enlarge or firm the breasts is usually requested by younger women (late teens and up), and breast reduction by older women (over 40). Incision is under the breast; for enlargement, a solid silicone implant is inserted under the skin of the breast to lift the natural breast tissue. In reducing the breast size, fat, breast tissue and skin are removed. Reshaping the breasts to firm and beautify them without enlarging them is often the more satisfactory kind of surgery for women with normal amounts of breast tissue but a drooping contour. Incision is a T-shape from below the nipple and along this fold. Operation takes two-and-a-half to three hours. General anesthesia is used, and hospitalization is usually three to four days. Stitches are removed in two to two-and-a-half weeks, and recovery is complete in six to eight weeks; it is recommended that a nursing bra be worn day and night for several months. Breast implants, if unsatisfactory, can be removed or the breasts refirmed with different implants.

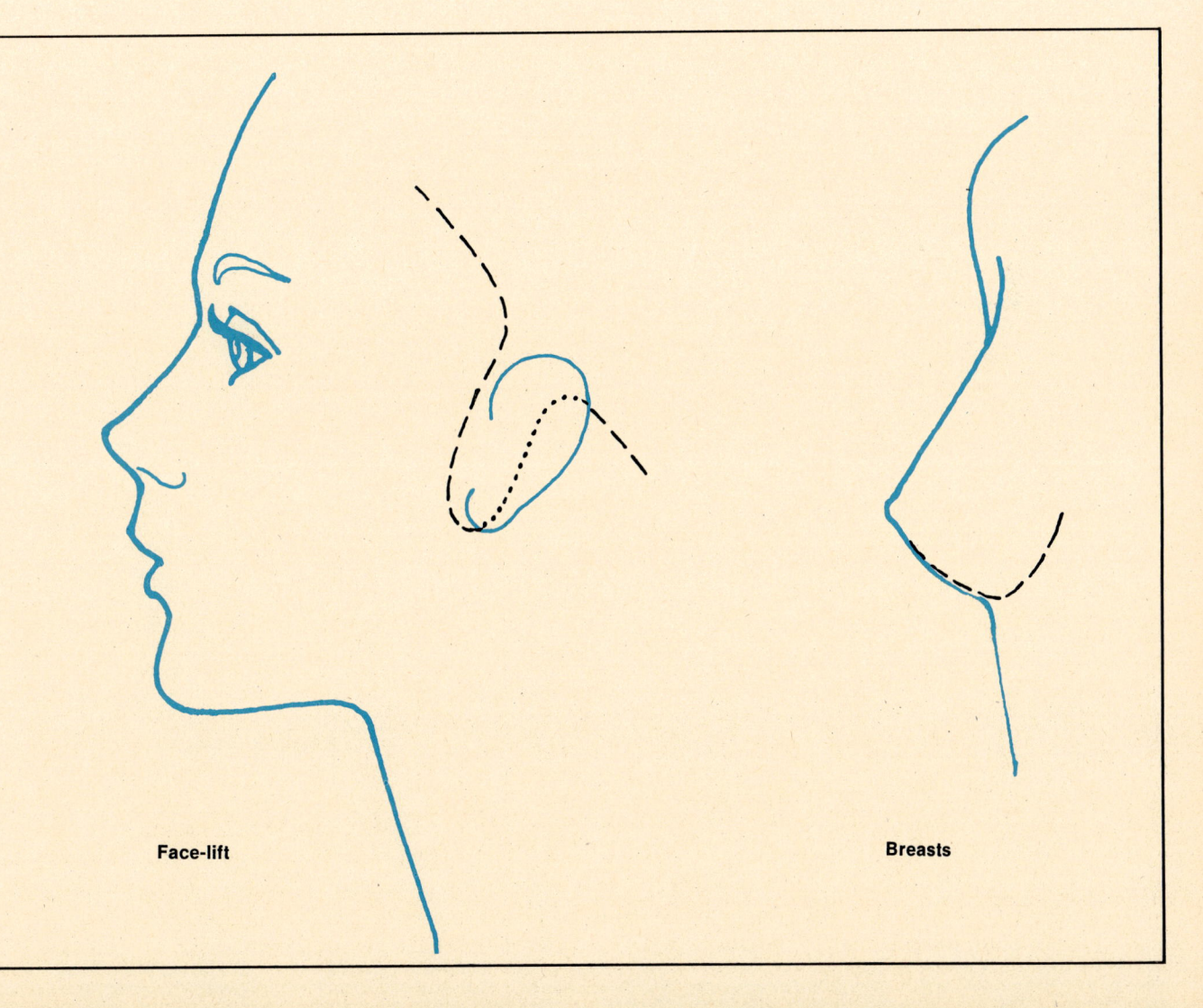

Face-lift

Breasts

FACE-SAVING FACIAL EXERCISES BY SARA MILDRED STRAUSS

To defer lines and wrinkles on the forehead and between the brows; to stimulate muscles of the scalp.

Hold head still; look straight ahead.

- Raise eyebrows and forehead skin as high as you can so that you feel the movement of the scalp and the muscles around the ears; then bring the brows down as far as possible into a deep frown.
- Repeat energetically—up and down, so that you feel the scalp muscles move.

At start, 10 times; increase to 20 times.

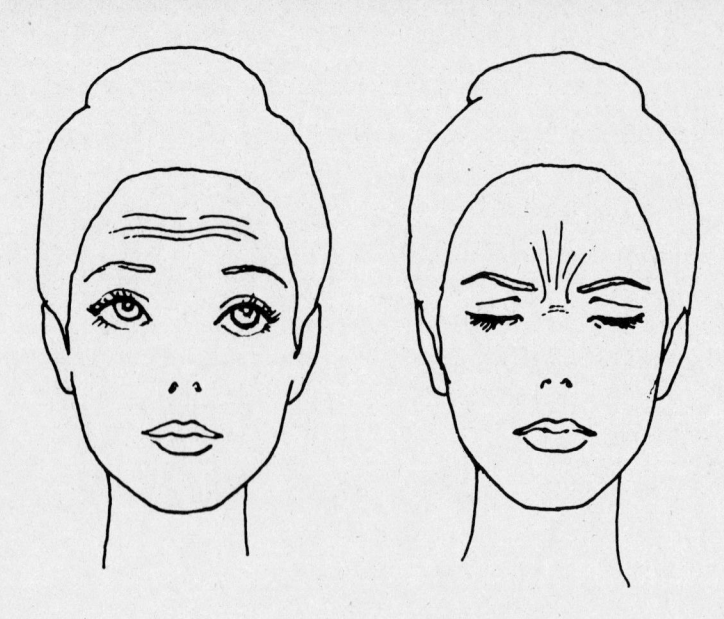

To strengthen and firm muscles of mouth, chin, cheeks and to stimulate skin circulation.

Keep chin in, head still.

- Stretch mouth open as widely as you can—as if you were ready to cheer—and then bring lips back together in a tight pucker.
- Alternate the movements slowly at first, using all the muscles around mouth, cheek, and chin as deeply and fully as you can.

Repeat 10 times to start and increase to as many times as you choose.

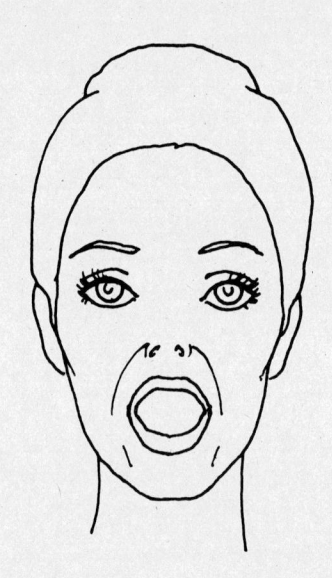

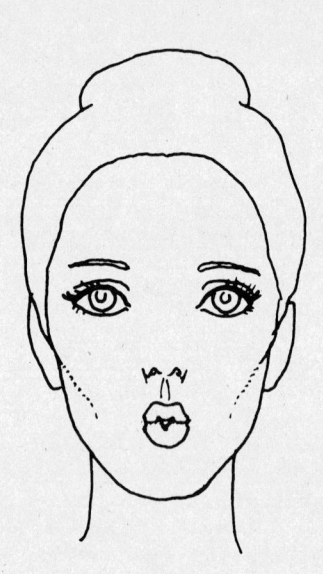

To strengthen and firm muscles around nose, chin, cheeks, and mouth and to stimulate circulation.

Keep mouth closed.

- Draw lips and nostrils upward as far as you can, wrinkling the nose in an enormous sniff.
- Then pull mouth down, still keeping it closed, to make the nose as long as possible. Do this slowly at first till you feel that you are using all the muscles in and around the nose.

Start with 10 and increase to as many times as are comfortable.

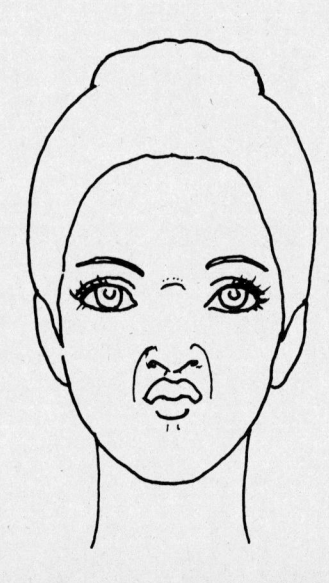

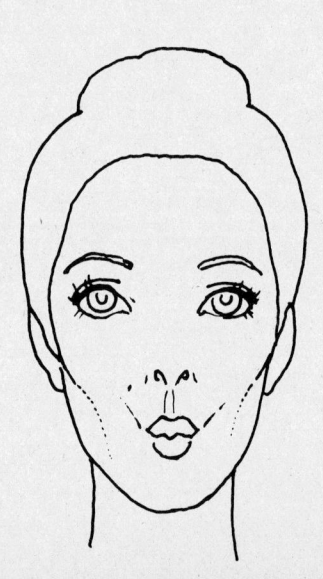

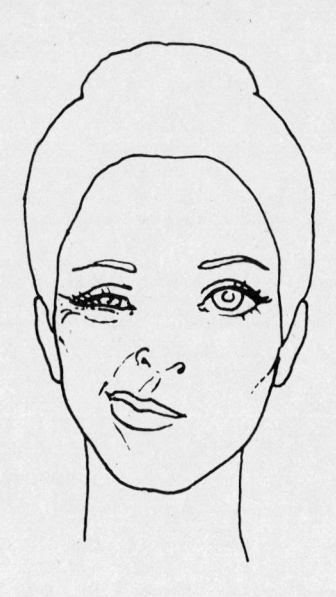

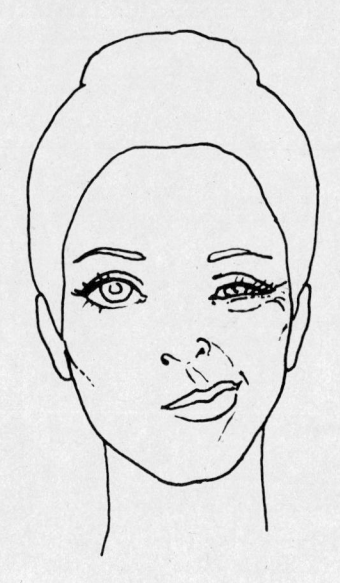

To strengthen and firm the cheek muscles; to stimulate circulation in the facial skin.
Hold head still, face without tension.
- Raise mouth and cheek of right side so high that right eye closes. Repeat to left.
- Do this strenuously so that you will be using as many muscles as you can in your huge "winks." At first these muscles may not be responsive, but gradually they will "come alive."

Do 10 winks to start; increase to as many winks as you like.

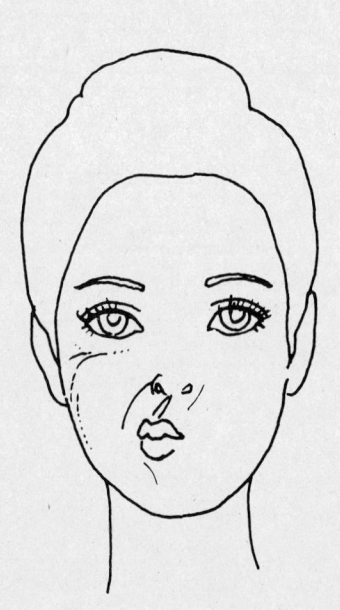

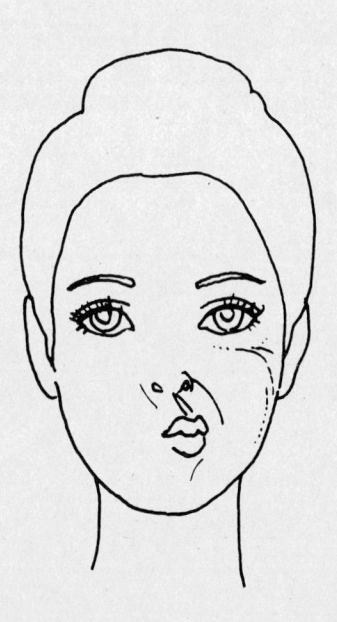

To tighten and firm up the flesh beneath the chin; to strengthen muscles of mouth, chin, and the lower cheeks.
Bring lips together in a tight pucker.
- Slowly circle this "kiss" to the right.
- Stop and then circle to the left. Make these movements vigorous (may be difficult at start).

Try eight chin firmers and increase gradually as the muscles strengthen.

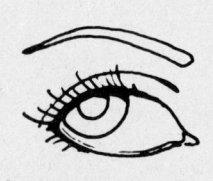

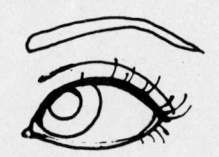

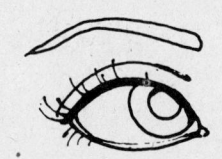

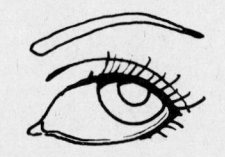

To strengthen muscles behind the eyes and to reduce lines and wrinkles around the eyes.
Keep head still, face without tension.
- Look straight up; then down.
- Look far to right; then to left.
- Make a slow circle with the eyes, starting from right—up, left, and down; reverse, starting from left.

Do this exercise only a few times to start so as not to tire eye muscles; slowly increase to 10 times.

Preliminary practice to gain awareness of the lower eyelid muscles.

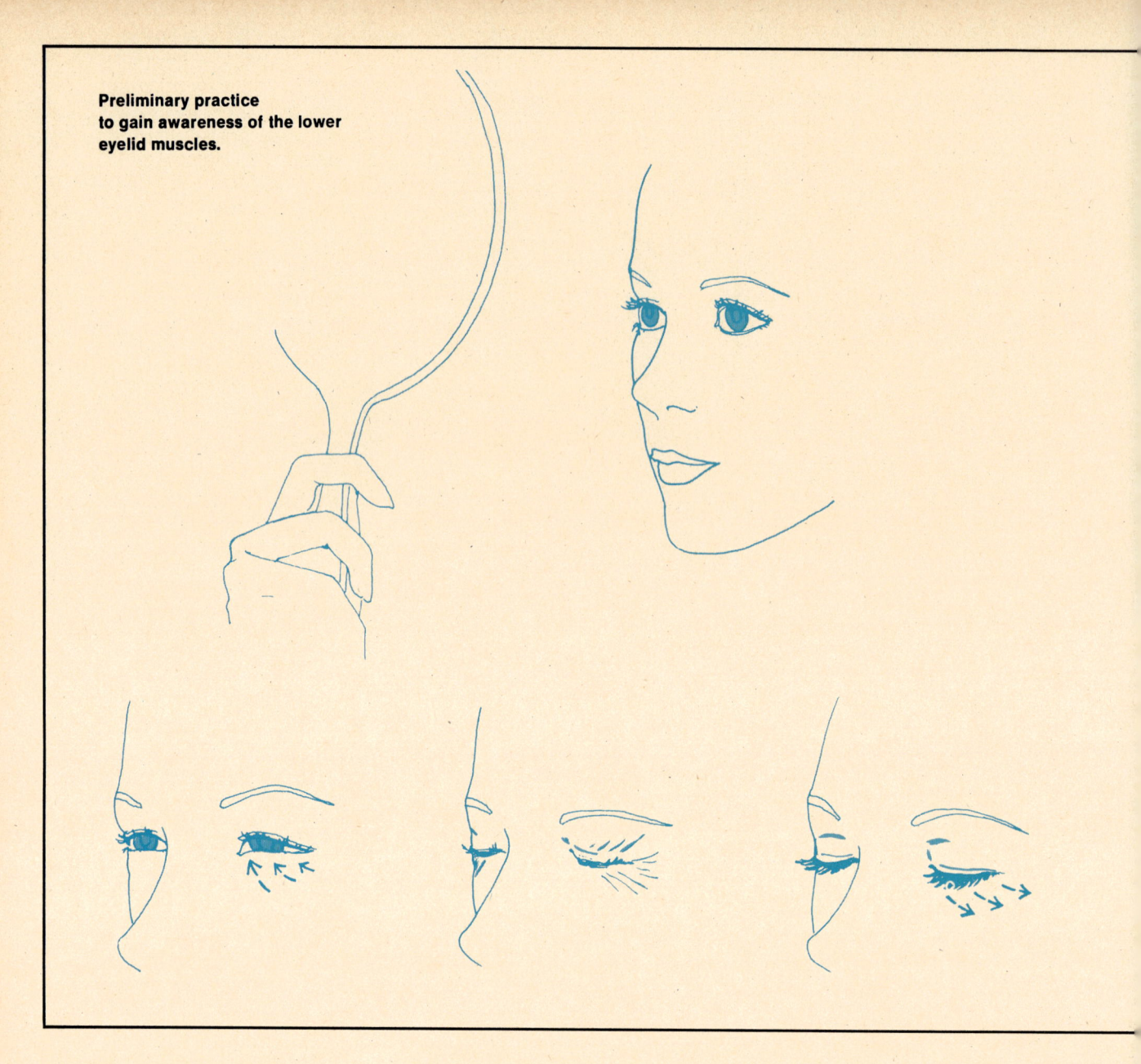

UNDER-EYE CIRCLES—
HOW TO RELIEVE THEM
BY SENTA MARIA RUNGE

Circles beneath the eyes aren't necessarily due to age; *young* women can have them, too. Their underlying cause may be a systemic disorder or tiredness. Or they may be hereditary.

Some people are born with circles shaped by the surrounding bone structure and these, like other physical features, are inherited. In many cases these circles are camouflaged till the end of the teen years by soft cushions of baby fat—fat which then gradually diminishes. Such circles cannot be removed, only concealed by makeup. Apply a corrective stick, cream or liquid two shades lighter than foundation makeup over the under-eye area. If you use blusher on your cheeks, apply it somewhat up over the edge of the circles, only more faintly than on cheeks.

If the circles are due to a systemic disorder—a rundown condition or other health problem—restoring your physical well-being is the cure.

Other under-eye circles—probably the most common—are due to lack of sleep or general tiredness. For these, we *can* offer help.

Preliminary practice to gain awareness of the lower eyelid muscles. This exercise can be done sitting or standing before a mirror. First, apply cream around the lower eyes.
1. Look straight into the mirror.
2. Lower head somewhat so that you have to look *up* slightly to see your eyes in the mirror. Do *not* raise eyebrows.
3. In even movements, raise lower lids to the middle of the eye. Notice that you can move each wrinkle individually or all together—every wrinkle in the lower eyelid is a muscle. Also observe that each of those wrinkles moves upward diagonally toward the nose.
4. Close upper and lower lids so they meet in the middle of the eye. Close tightly and hold tightness for three counts. After each count, breathe deep.
5. With both lids closed, lower eyelids as if you were slowly falling asleep.
Purpose of exercise—To move lid muscles freely and without tension to their fullest range.
Note—Do not push the lower lid muscles with your cheek muscles. Every muscle or muscle group has a certain range of movement. You will find it easier to expand a muscle in one quick movement than in several slow movements. Slow movements impose much more work on muscles than quick movements.

Isometric exercise

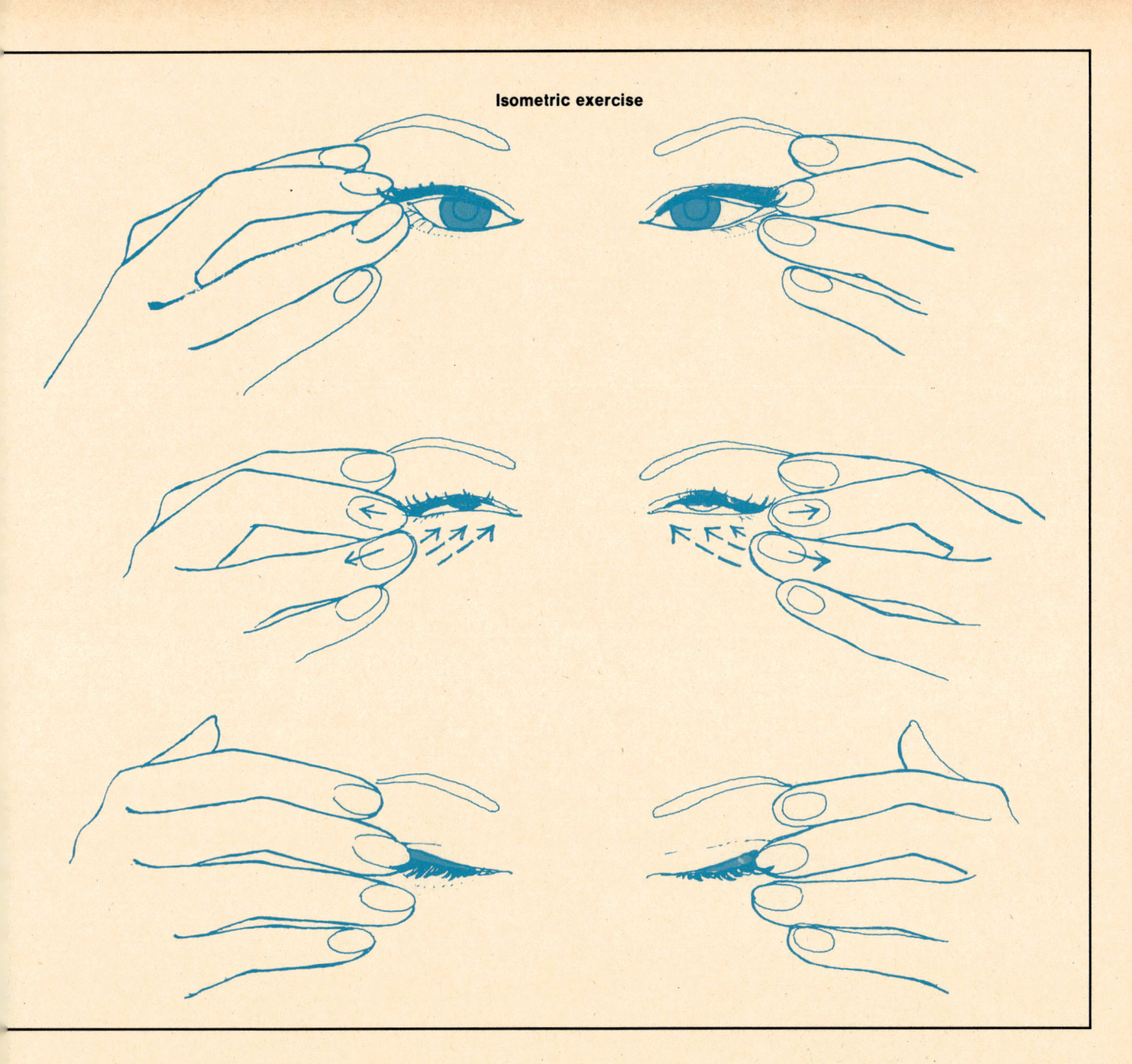

Start out by expanding the muscle section in one movement, which is the easiest way. Once you have learned this, divide the expansion into two even movements. Then into three. And so work up to the number of steps prescribed for each individual movement.
Aim—To open and expand muscles in 10 steps; keep eyes closed for three counts; return muscles in 10 steps.
Frequency—Once or twice a day three times in succession.

Isometric exercise. Do not attempt unless Preliminary Practice has been mastered. Do this exercise in sitting position with a mirror before you. Apply cream around lower eyelids and crow's feet area. Wrap tissue around fingers to prevent slipping.
1. Lift eyebrows and place tip of middle fingers flat against edge of bone and push muscle skin back somewhat. Hold fingers in this position as a resistance. To do this, elbows must be lifted to eye level. With ring fingers, grip muscle skin beneath the eyes and push it back somewhat. Hold it there firmly against underlying bone (including edge of bone) for resistance. With the index fingers, hold the muscle skin in the upper eyelid in resistance by pressing the skin there firmly against the bone.
Note—The proper finger position gives you the shape of Oriental eyes.
2. While you hold all the muscles beneath your fingers for resistance, look upward and gradually move the muscles in the lower eyelids upward diagonally toward the nose.
3. Once you have reached the middle of the eyes with the lower lid, close eyes tightly and hold this position while counting to three.
4. With eyelids closed, return upper and lower lid muscles gradually downward.
5. Now release resistance and remove fingers; open eyes.
Purpose—Expanding muscles freely to their fullest range.
Note—The idea is to hold each line in the lower lid by its end against the bone beneath the skin in firm resistance. Then slowly work the muscle (line) in its performing direction through the action of blinking upward in gradual steps. In this way, each line in the lower eyelid may be removed individually.
Aim—10 steps upward and keep eyes tightly closed for six counts; return muscles in 10 steps.
Frequency—Once a day three times in succession. Fingers must be removed and results observed after each performance. Apply cream before each exercise application.

To eliminate crow's feet

Isometric exercise

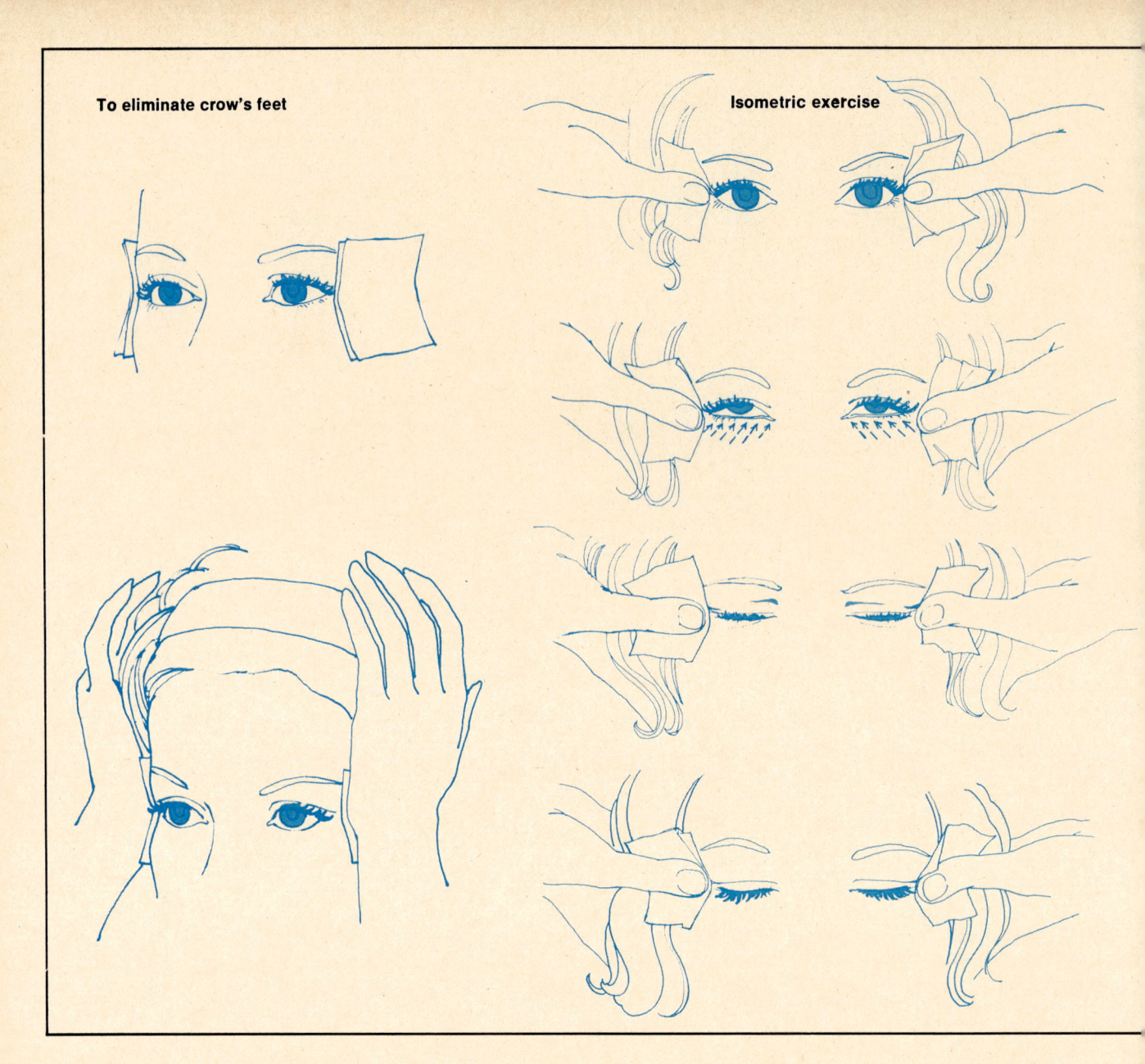

TO ELIMINATE CROW'S FEET

Crow's feet are lines caused by habitual squinting. The lines may be only "skin deep" and, therefore, can be ironed out of the skin by the principle of ironing a wrinkled cloth. However, if the crow's feet involve contour of the eyes, we have to restore the muscles involved through an isometric exercise. An overlapping upper eyelid may also appear in the form of crow's feet. However, as these particular lines are caused by elongated upper lid muscles, they can be eliminated only by exercising the muscles. Do this exercise in sitting position, elbows resting on table. Look into mirror. Apply cream over the crow's-feet lines. Place a folded tissue over the creamed area.

Note—The wrinkled skin is our cloth which we have moistened with the exercise cream. The ironing board is a firm bone underneath the wrinkled skin. The iron itself is a flat and firm pressure by our hands.

1. Lift eyebrows somewhat and place flat part of hands or thumb beside eyes, covering the wrinkled skin area, including the edge of the bone.
2. Press, starting softly, increasing to utmost firmness, while you count slowly to 15.
3. Release pressure gradually to the count of 10.

Frequency—Once a day three times in succession.

Aim—If done properly, lines will be diminished. Remaining lines indicate insufficient flat or firm pressure in this area. Treat such lines separately.

Note—Squinting has, of course, to be avoided. What good is it to iron out wrinkles when you put them back in?

Isometric exercise. To remove crow's feet from the contour. Do not attempt unless Preliminary Practice has been mastered. Do in sitting position. Look into mirror. Apply cream on skin in crow's-feet area. To avoid slipping, cover the creamed area with a tissue, cut in one-and-one-half-inch square.

1. Lift eyebrows and fit tip of thumbs or palm of hands flat against the bone beside the eyes, including the edge of this bone.
2. Press softly then increase to utmost firmness for five counts and keep this position for resistance.
3. Release eyebrows.
4. Against this resistance, lift lower eyelids slowly to the middle of the eyes, as in the Preliminary Practice, while looking up without frowning.
5. Close both lids tightly at middle and keep them closed for three counts.

Isometric combined eye exercise

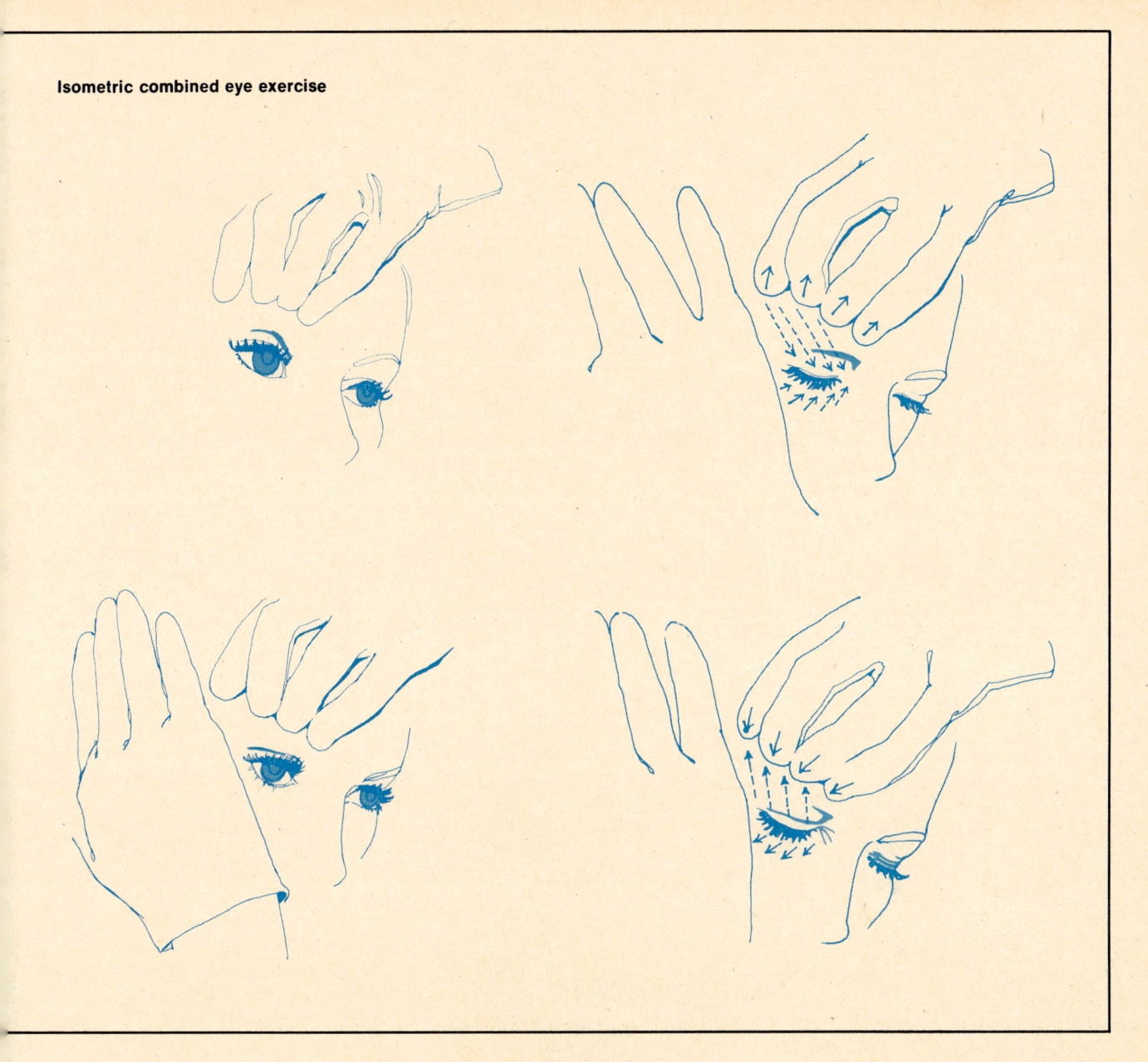

6. With closed eyes, return muscles downward.
7. Now release and remove resistance.
Purpose—Expanding muscles freely and to their fullest range without tension or help by other muscles.
Note—Guard against scowling during muscle performance.
Aim—20 steps; keep eyes tightly closed for six steps; return muscles in 10 steps.
Frequency—Once a day three times in succession. Hands must be removed and results observed after each performance.
Results—A remaining line indicates that you either have not resisted this particular muscle or you have not moved it.

Isometric—combined eye exercise. Do in sitting position, elbow resting on table. Look into mirror. Apply cream and folded tissue to lower eyelids. Do only after you have mastered previous exercises. Wear cosmetic glove on the hand that is holding eyebrow.
Note—This exercise can be done only on one side at a time. When exercising on right side of the face, wear glove on left hand. When exercising the left side of face, wear glove on left hand.
1. With fingertips of left hand, lift the right eyebrow upward and hold this position for firm resistance. Skin must be evenly taut.
2. Resist lower eyelid and crow's-feet muscles by pressing muscle skin in this area against the bone underneath. For firm and steady pressure, apply part of hand to the area as in preceding exercise.
3. Raise lower lid upward to middle of eye slowly for 10 counts (as practiced previously).
4. Close lids very tightly in middle-eye position.
5. Slowly return the muscles to position in 10 steps.
6. Remove resistance.
Purpose—To expand muscles freely and to their fullest range, this includes the muscles of the lower eyelids, crow's feet and upper eyelids.
Note—Resistance must be held steady throughout the exercise.
Aim—10 steps, with eyes tightly closed for six counts; return muscles in 10 steps.
Frequency—Once a day three times in succession. Remove the hands from the face and observe results after each performance.
Results—If performed correctly, the eyebrow must look lifted and the lower eyelid appear refreshed from each performance of the exercise.

SKIN BEAUTY GUIDE

Your skin condition depends partly upon heredity. Whether you are fair or dark-complected... whether the skin is fine or coarse in texture... whether it is sun-resistant or sun-sensitive... whether facial hair is dark or invisible... whether the skin is basically oily or dry—all these are to a great extent decided by your choice of ancestors.

Skin beauty is also affected by the feminine sex hormone estrogen; estrogen deficiency may lead to dryness and scaling; so can other glandular upsets. The female complexion is ordinarily more finely textured than the male, and facial hair is inconspicuous; sometimes endocrine imbalance can change both these conditions.

But you still have much to do with the health and beauty of your own skin.

Good diet. This is essential to skin beauty. Include in your menu each day both green and yellow vegetables; fresh fruits; meat or fish or eggs or other protein, such as cheese; milk, whole or skimmed; some cereal; some fat. If skin is oily or troubled, it is good to avoid fatty foods (including nuts) and fried foods; in some cases chocolate is to be avoided. If you are on a reducing diet, include *some* fat in the menu so that skin does not become deprived. Drink enough water to prevent dehydration. Much of our water intake comes from foods; when food intake is cut, drinking water (about four glasses a day) should be increased—but the once-famous "eight glasses a day" is now considered excessive.

Daily outdoor activity. The fresh air you breathe and the increased circulation that comes with exercise improve the skin tone. Exercise tones the entire body, aiding elimination and generally keeping all muscles, including those of face and eyes, in better condition.

Relaxation Sleep and rest and daily periods of relaxation—lying with the feet higher than the hips and the hips higher than the head—are restorative to the complexion. Bending down and bobbing the head toward the floor will also increase circulation to the face.

Protection. This is an important factor in skin beauty. Overexposure to sunlight and loss of moisture to the air are major causes of "aging" in the skin. Avoid overexposure; use creams or lotions as protection against weathering.

Gentle handling. Handle your skin carefully. Some skin damage is due to improper handling when creams are applied to the skin. You can exercise the skin muscles—*not* using massage—to prevent muscle sag.

Tension. Nervous tension is an enemy of skin beauty, and many skin problems, such as itching and scaling, can result from tension as much as from other causes. To avoid tension lines, try these suggestions:

❧ When tension is wrinkling your brow, try to become aware of those forehead lines. To ease the tension, simply stroke a hand across the forehead; furrows immediately relax.

❧ If you have a tendency to frown, simply place the tip of a finger firmly on the forehead between the brows. This eases the tension and lines relax.

❧ To relax the eye muscles, close both eyes, cup a hand over one,

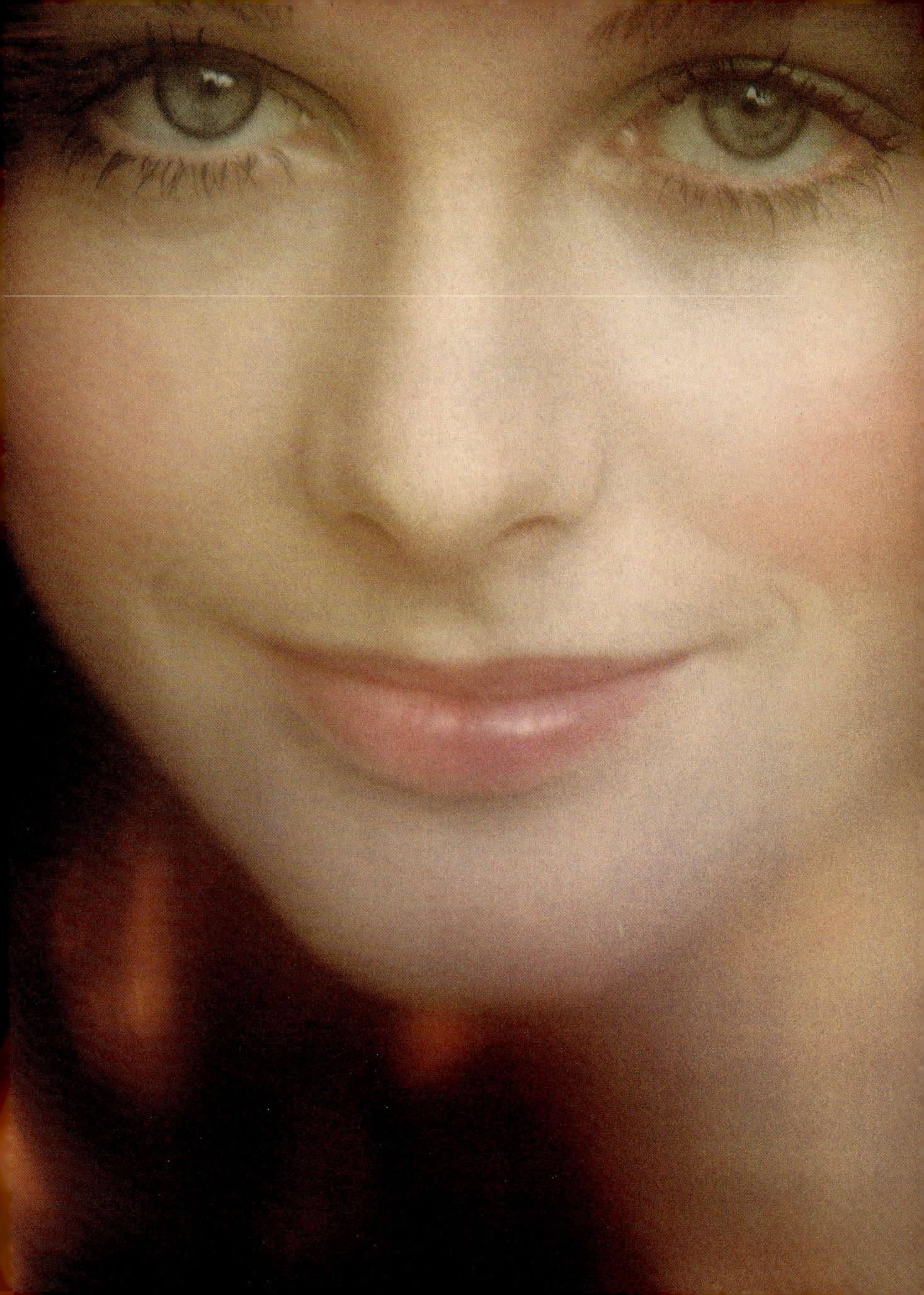

and then (both eyes closed) circle eyeballs first in one direction and then in the other. This helps prevent squint lines.

✻ If pursing your lip is a worry habit and tiny lines are appearing round the mouth, smooth them with this exercise: Close the lips without tightening them (all lines must be relaxed; use a mirror to make sure) and blow gently without opening the lips. Force air in to fill cheeks and space under upper lip. The pressure of the air helps to firm lip muscles.

SKIN-ANALYSIS CHART AND KEY
Find your present skin condition by checking the characteristics of each separate skin area

Forehead
- 4—Wrinkles ☐
- 2—Dryness, Flakiness ☐
- 1—Enlarged Pores ☐
- 1—Pimples ☐
- 1—Blackheads ☐
- 1—Acne ☐

Eyes
- 3—Crow's Feet ☐
- 3—Wrinkles ☐

Cheeks
- 1—Enlarged Pores ☐
- 1—Pimples ☐
- 1—Blackheads ☐
- 1—Acne ☐
- 1—Shininess ☐
- 2—Dryness, Flakiness ☐
- 5—Flabby Tissue ☐

Nose
- 1—Enlarged Pores ☐
- 1—Shininess ☐
- 1—Blackheads ☐
- 2—Dryness, Flakiness ☐

Mouth and Chin
- 1—Blackheads ☐
- 1—Pimples ☐
- 1—Acne ☐
- 1—Shininess ☐
- 2—Dryness, Flakiness ☐
- 5—Deep Lines ☐

Neck
- 5—Crepiness ☐
- 5—Wrinkles ☐
- 5—Flabby Tissue ☐

SKIN-ANALYSIS KEY

1. You have symptoms of an oily skin if you checked *all* items coded 1. In any part of the face where you checked a 1 symptom, you have an oily area.

2. Your skin has dry symptoms where you checked a 2 item, but if the area appears with open pores, blackheads, or pimples, the dryness is usually only top-layer dryness, and the skin is probably basically oily.

3. If you checked one or both 3 symptoms, you need lubrication under the eyes, for this is one area that is lacking in natural lubrication regardless of skin type. Pat cream in gently, starting at the outer corner of the eye and moving inward. Do not rub or massage eye skin, for you may stretch it.

4. If you checked the 4 symptom, you frown too much and will have furrows here regardless of skin type. Smooth these parallel creases between your brows and on the forehead by firmly pressing on the wrinkles with your fingertips. This relaxes taut muscles and helps stop the frown.

5. If you checked 5 symptoms, you can use some exercise to help strengthen tissues and combat wrinkles and flabbiness. Crepiness of the neck can also be forestalled by a faithful application of cream. To counteract neck creases that come with poor posture, lift the body tall from the tips of your toes. Place hands under jaw line on each side and jut the lower jaw forward, lengthening the throat. Relax and repeat. To firm the chin and to tone the entire facial area, pretend to chew gum vigorously while the head is bent back as far as possible.

WHAT CARE FOR YOUR SKIN

Whatever your skin type, your skin care should include four steps—cleansing, toning, conditioning, and protecting. With each step, handle your skin gently, working up from the collarbone over the face to the hairline and over the back of the neck and over the ears and back of the ears.

Cleansing. This also stimulates circulation and keeps the skin looking healthy and alive. Cleansing action also helps do away with sallowness and improves many skin problems.

Toning. Follow cleansing with skin freshener to remove residue of the cleanser. Freshener also acts to close pore openings slightly; astringents are more drying. Use the cotton square with which you apply the toner to pat upward and outward over throat and face or use "piano-playing" finger action to stimulate the skin.

Conditioning. Use the conditioner suggested for your individual skin type, applying it with the motions suggested for correct skin handling.

Protecting. Use a sun-screen preparation during exposure to the sun, an emollient during dry weather, a moisturizer to protect against evaporation of skin moisture at any time. The eye area is dry at every age, so use special eye cream day and night; if the throat needs attention, give this area special care as well.

HOW TO CLEAN YOUR FACE

In cleaning the face we remove both soiled makeup and the day's collection of grime—and also the skin's own protective coating that helps keep it healthy. For this reason cleansing should always be followed by toning and conditioning.

When cleaning the skin, work all the way into the hairline and over the ears and behind the ears and over the back of the neck. To protect the hair, wear a headband whether soaping or creaming the face.

Makeup removal. Cleansing cream is ordinarily used for makeup removal, but the woman with dry skin may also use her cleansing cream, if she chooses, to *cream-wash* her face. There also are creamy lotions, washaway cleansers, and specially formulated cleansers for oily skin. If cream should not be used—on excessively oily or troubled skin, for example—medicated lotions will serve to remove makeup.

Cleansing cream or lotion is designed to remove makeup oils and pigments as well as surface dirt and to *lift* any soil from the face once the makeup has been softened by the cream. The effect after creaming should be one of skin freshness, not of oiliness or stickiness. Use freshening lotion if necessary.

Detergent cleansing lotion and washaway cleanser dry up the skin oil as they remove soil and makeup.

❊ Dot makeup-removal cream or lotion over the face and throat.
❊ Working up from the collarbone, smooth the cream lightly over the face so as not to rub the cream into the skin.
❊ Let the cream set for a few seconds so it picks up the soiled makeup.
❊ Remove cream with a terry cloth or tissues, lightly lifting the cream from the face with upward and outward motions.

Cream washing. If skin is dry, repeat the cream cleansing, leaving the film of oil from the cream on the skin as a lubricant.

❊ If you like the feeling of water on your face, take a clean washcloth, dampen it with warm water, and lightly remove the film of oil with a warm-water rinse before toning.
❊ Washaway cleansers are also followed by a water rinse to remove the residue.

Soap-and-water wash. Many of us do not feel comfortable without a soap-and-water wash; unless the skin is over-dry or sensitive, we can usually enjoy this method of skin cleansing at least once a day—preferably at bedtime. For oily and troubled skin, soap-and-water cleansing is often recommended.

Soap is an excellent cleanser, but it has a tendency to be alkaline while the skin is naturally slightly acid. Cold-cream soaps, super-fatted soaps, and "soapless soaps" (bar-form cleansers that lather but lack the alkaline property of soap) are suggested for dry or aging skin. Medicated soaps are also available for those who have skin blemishes.

❊ Splash the face with warm (not hot) water and then rub the side of a wet bar of soap lightly over the skin in upward-and-outward motion.
❊ Gently film the soap over the face as you would a cream.
❊ Rinse the face thoroughly and then repeat the soaping in the same manner.
❊ Rinse again, being sure to remove all soap residue.
❊ Splash the skin with cool water.
❊ Dry with a soft terry towel, using a gentle blotting action in upward-and-outward motion. Do not rub or scrub—roughness won't help your skin.

Deep-pore cleansers. Detergent lotions may be used instead of a soap-and-water wash.

❊ Apply the lotion with a cotton ball or square, working over the face and throat from the collarbone to the hairline, over the ears and the back of the ears, and the back of the neck.
❊ Repeat the cleansing over each face area, using a cotton square, till no sign of soil appears on the cotton.
❊ For an even more thorough cleansing, steam the face under a very warm towel or over a basin of steaming water after using cleansing lotion. This will make the pore openings more accessible to the cleanser.

Cleansing grains—These grains act like an abrasive to work into the tiny openings of the pores and also to flake off surface skin and to bring out the fresh layer of new skin below. The grains have a stimulating action and bring up a good pink color. This cleanser is useful for young oily skin but should be applied gently and without pressure.

❊ Rinse the face with warm water.
❊ Apply dots of the grainy cream or lotion over the face (except for eye area).
❊ Work the grains gently over the skin with upward-and-outward motion.
❊ Let dry.
❊ Rinse off with cool water.

Stimulating cleansers—Skin has normal "flora"—bacteria—that need not be disturbed for good skin health, but when pore plugs and surface-caused acne become a problem, antiseptic or medicated cream, soap, lotion, or cleanser will help hold down infection.

❊ Stimulating cleansers—and neutral soaps too—have an acid-alkali balance close to that of the skin. Thus they leave the skin feeling comfortable.
❊ Stimulating cleansers are excellent for the woman with oily or troubled skin. The skin will not, however, produce *less* oil when these cleansers are used. The cleanser is detergent—it frees the pores of plugs if used consistently and so lets the natural oil flow freely from the pores onto the skin surface. There the oil serves as a natural lubricant.
❊ The clean fresh feeling is due to various cooling agents, such as menthol. Astringents, such as small amounts of alcohol, produce the tingle. Their stimulating action speeds blood circulation to the skin.
❊ Many of these cleansers include an antiseptic that helps prevent infection. Once a pore becomes plugged, it may rupture, and this lets infective bacteria find a foothold. The result—a pimple. The antiseptic helps.

Detergent masks—These also act as deep-pore cleansers.

83

Handle Your Skin With A Light Touch

Every step of your skin-care routine—even if it takes just a few minutes a day—should help you maintain a healthy, glowing complexion. To turn these daily tasks into a daily beauty treatment, follow these basic exercises for firming with a "light touch".

"Light-touch" rules.

🌸 Avoid touching your index finger to the face. The touch of this finger becomes too forceful and can damage delicate muscle fibers. Instead, use the balls of the second and third fingers in a gentle *rotary* upward-and-outward movement to roll on cleanser, creams or makeup.

🌸 Avoid rubbing your face with the knuckles or strongly pushing and pulling your skin with cleansing tissue, washcloth or sponge.

🌸 Keep your elbows high. If you tend to make your touch overly forceful, keep your elbows high when touching the skin. This is especially important when working around the eyes and mouth.

🌸 Keep your face relaxed. It is safe to manipulate your facial skin if the muscles are relaxed. Don't ever apply creams, makeup or a facial mask when the muscles are stretched or tensed.

Cheeks—Use the balls of the second and third fingers with a rotary motion on the cheeks. Start at the chin, move up the face, outward and upward.

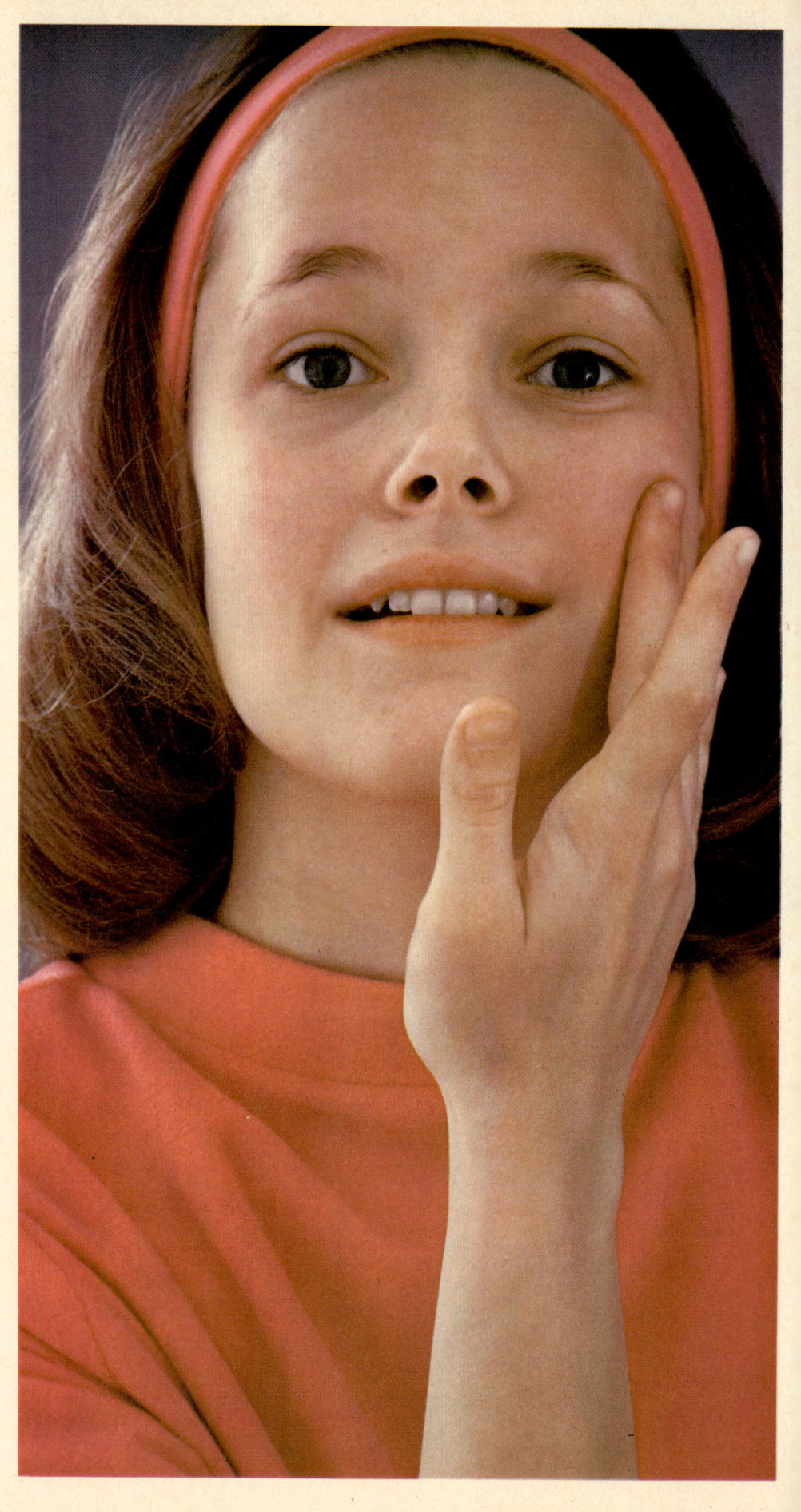

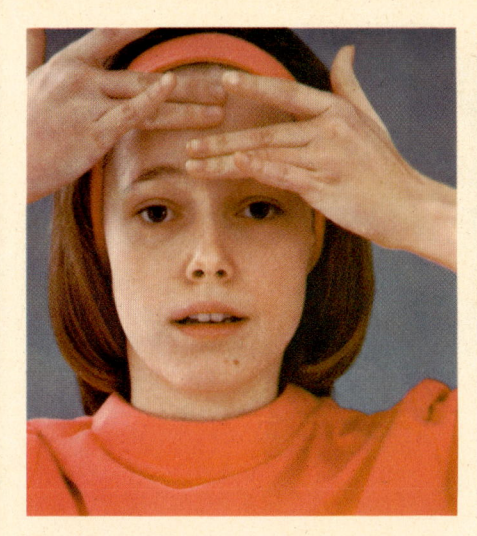

Forehead—Work up the forehead in three sections—middle and both sides—with the second and third fingers of both hands, gently rotating the balls of the fingers on the skin.

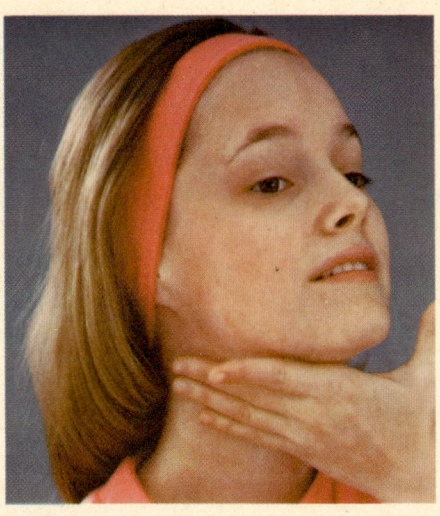

Throat—With the flat of the hand and the fingers, stroke upward from the base of the throat to the jaw on both sides and up the middle of the throat and up under the chin.

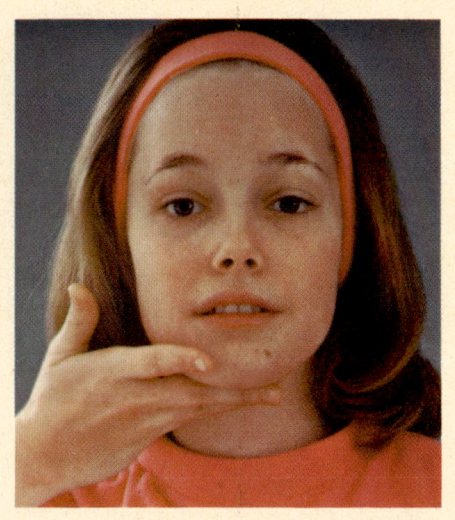

Chin—To help avoid flab or a double chin, look straight ahead, keeping the chin level, when stroking under the chin. Don't tilt the head back—that stretches the throat muscles.

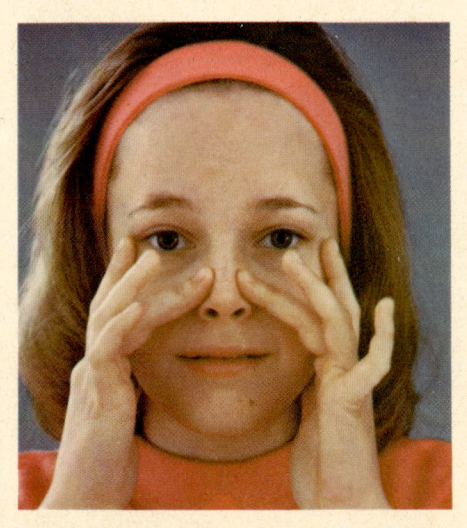

Nose—Work *down* the nose and in a rotary motion around the nostrils. This area is very important in cleansing oily skin. Again, use second and third (not the index) fingers.

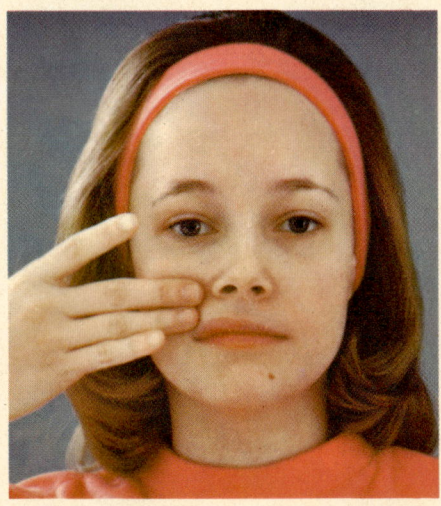

Mouth (1)—Work around the mouth in a rotary motion (using the second and middle fingers) across the upper lip and then around, circling the mouth in both directions.

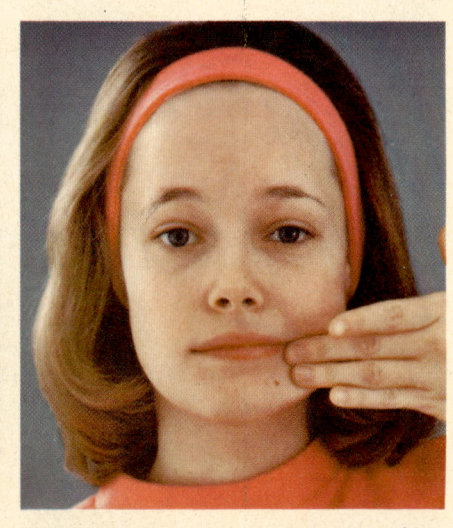

Mouth (2)—The rotary motion helps keep the lip area firm and avoids tiny lines. Keep the mouth relaxed and hold elbow high to avoid too much pressure from the fingers.

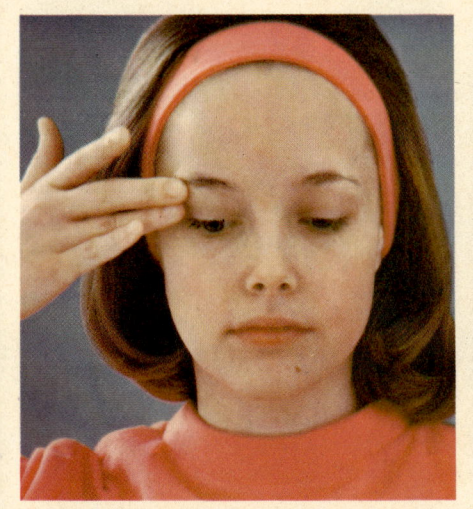

Eyes—Be very gentle on the eye skin. Use a light patting movement across the upper lid from the inner corner to the outer; on the lower lid, pat from outer to inner corner.

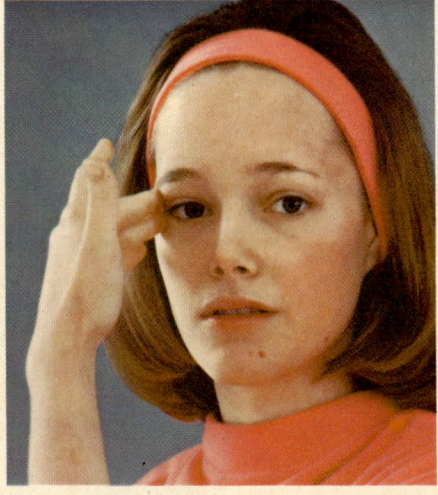

Eye spread (1)—Spread the outer corners of the eyes to help avoid tiny wrinkles in this area. Begin by resting the balls of the second and third fingers against the skin at outer eye.

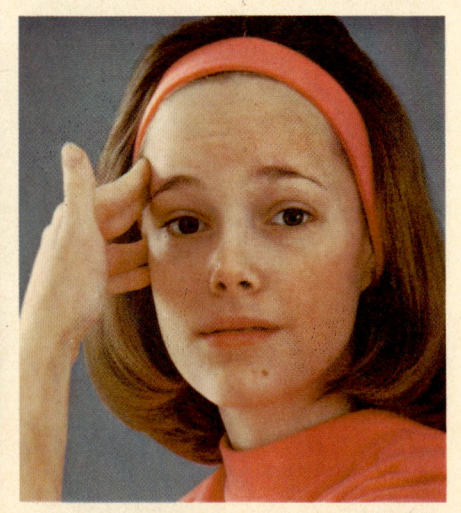

Eye spread (2)—From the resting position, delicately separate the fingers to spread the corner of the eye slightly. The touch and movement here should always be very gentle.

85

Rotary motion (balls of fingers)

Pat (balls of fingers)

Stroke (fingers) both directions

Stroke (fingers) in direction

Stroke (hand and fingers)

Cream removal (1)

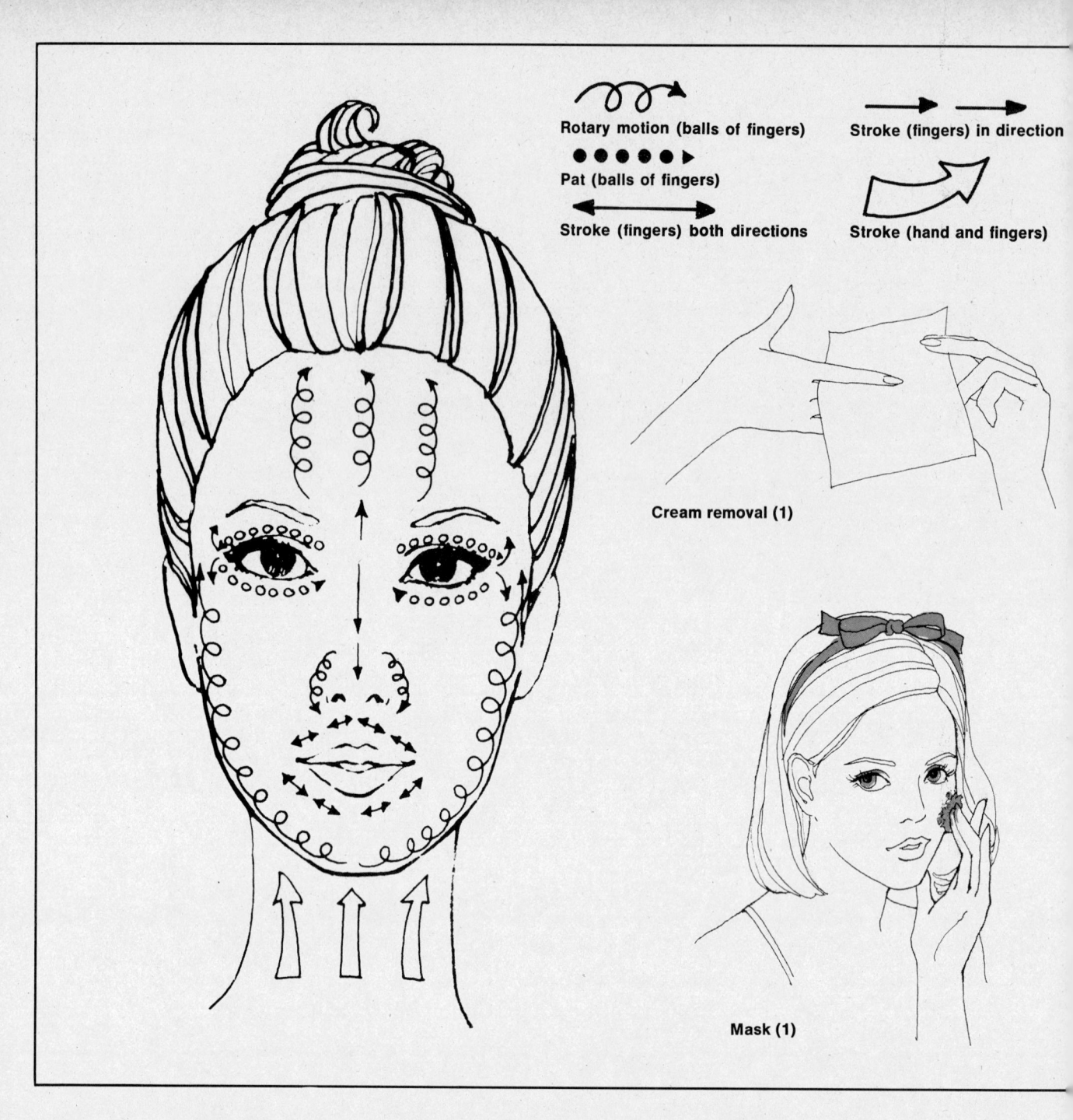

Mask (1)

Basic cleansing. Use the step-by-step "light touch" exercises (preceding pages and above) keeping the "light touch" rules in mind. Remember: Cleansing with creams is just like cleansing with soap and water. First you "wash" with the cream—then you "rinse" with a solvent or toning lotion to remove cream residues. The solvent is especially important in morning cleansing because you are also removing leftover night cream. On oily skin, particularly, residues that aren't removed can build up. This can attract bacteria, which, in turn, often causes blemishes.

Day care. With oily skin you probably will not need a moisturizer under your makeup. Most makeup today is light in texture and quite transparent. *Dry* and *normal* skins require a moisturizer to protect the skin from actual contact with makeup and to insure the proper moisture balance. Choose one with little (if any) perfume, because the moisturizer lies right on the skin, and a sensitive skin may react to perfumes.

✤ If your skin is well-cleaned in the morning, and a moisturizer and light makeup are used, you need not redo your face during the day. If makeup needs refreshing, splash your face from time to time with cool water. This is better than repowdering, which tends to give the makeup a dull heavy look.

Night care. Bedtime is the time to give yourself a mask treatment or fast facial to help create a natural glow.

✤ First remove makeup by using the basic cleansing method.

✤ A mask treatment will help clean your skin from the inside as well as from the outside by stimulating circulation of blood to the skin. It's very good for the woman with oily skin. For her, the mask should step up circulation as well as refine the pores. An organic mask, made with vegetables, herbs, clay, and no perfume, is best. For dry and normal skin, the mask should firm,

Cream removal (2)

Cream removal (3)

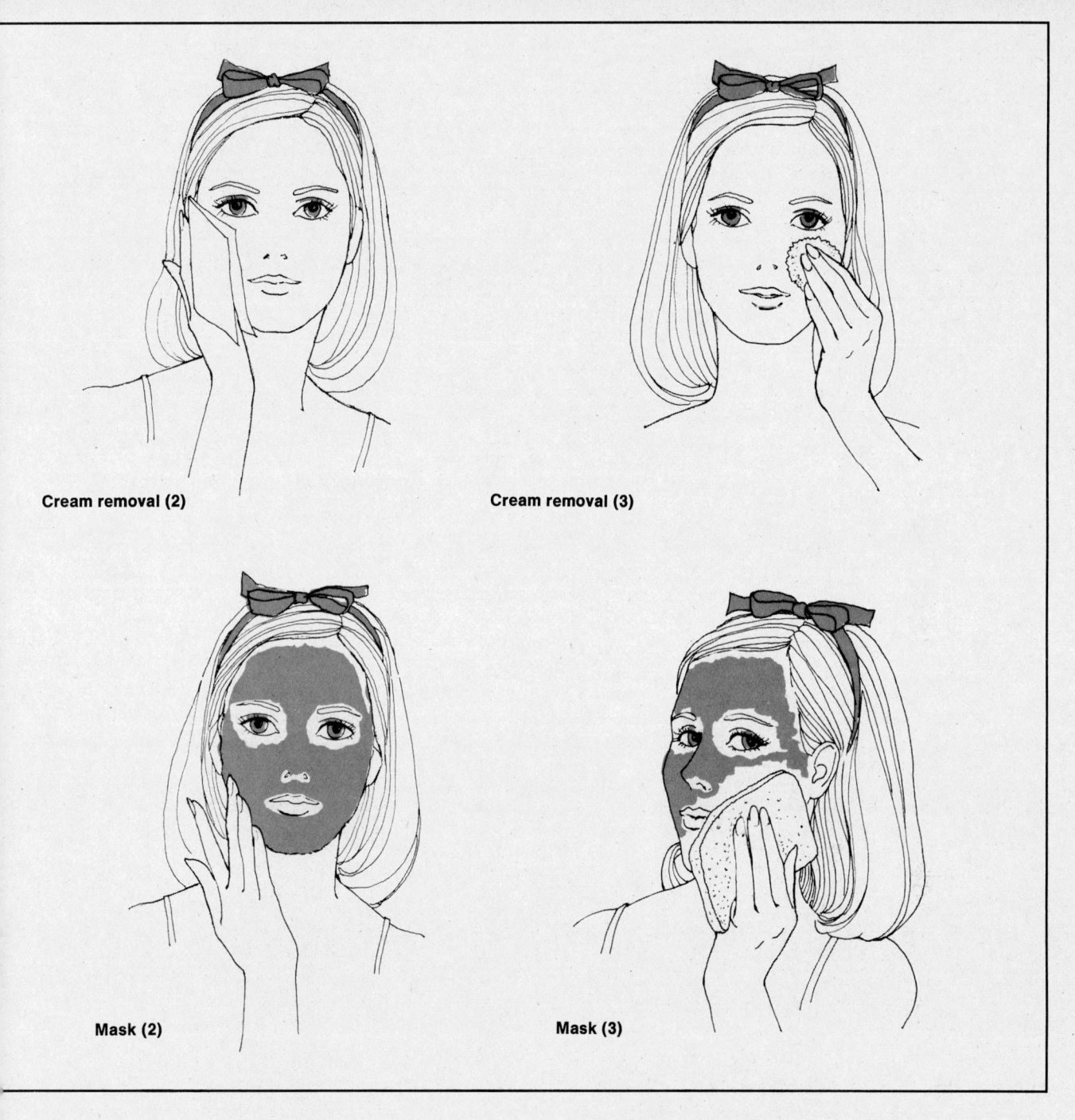

Mask (2)

Mask (3)

tighten and relieve any puffiness, but should not be drying. If your skin is naturally dry, use a mask only once a week; if oily, two or three times a week.

❧ Night cream is one of the most important parts of skin care. If skin is oily, choose a cream low in oils and light in texture. For normal to dry skin, choose a cream with some vegetable oils and one that is *very* light in texture. On the eyelids, a light oil is helpful.

❧ It is while you are applying the bedtime night cream that you can give yourself a fast facial. Use the "light touch" movements to exercise the skin, but now do it by a counting method— 10 times for each motion. Avoid the nose with night creams. Even a dry skin produces more oil in the area of the nose. Tissue off excess cream before bedtime.

Cream removal (1)—Fold tissue over three fingers, holding it in place with the index finger. Again, this finger should not touch the face—it merely holds and guides the tissue.

Cream removal (2)—Tissue cream away gently with the same upward and outward movements (rotary around the nostrils and mouth) on face and throat, keeping the facial muscles relaxed.

Cream removal (3)—A solvent (toning lotion) removes cream residues. Moisten a large piece of cotton and pat against the skin firmly as you do in other face-touching.

Mask (1)—A firming and tightening mask can be used once a week or oftener. Apply with fingertips, patting it on, keeping facial muscles relaxed. An organic mask is good for most skins.

Mask (2)—The mask should cover this area—keep away from eye skin. While the mask dries, try not to talk or even move face. It's best to lie with feet higher than the head.

Mask (3)—A moist sponge helps in mask removal. Be very gentle—the purpose of a mask is to firm and mold the skin, so take care not to stretch or pull skin during removal process.

How To Do A Home Facial

Moisturizing? Conditioning? Beautifying? Is that what a facial is all about? Frankly, no! Basically, it's cleaning your skin and helping it function in a healthy way—whether it's dry, oily, medium, or mixed. In a salon, a facial treatment lasts at least an hour—often longer— and 80% of this time (about 50 minutes) is spent in cleaning the skin. A salon facial involves use of a number of mechanical devices to do the job—brushes, suction cups, galvanic stimulators, mist-makers, jet showers. At home you can choose whether to use facial tools and mist-makers along with the skin preparations available for cleaning, stimulation, and protection. Look out, though, that you don't do wrong things: Don't over-stimulate oily acne skin—it will only produce more oil. Don't overcream dry skin—this makes scarce and lazy oil glands even more sluggish. Never overmanipulate any skin.

❧ First, makeup and surface soil are removed with cream. A liquid cleanser of the strength required for your particular type of skin is applied with loose pieces of cotton till the final piece shows no soil.

❧ Then, with a towel covering your head, hold your face over a bowl of steaming water to which mixed herbs have been added (rosemary, sage or fines herbes) and steam the face for about 10 minutes. This helps to bring impurities to the surface.

❧ Deep-pore cleanser—a "gritty" preparation—is worked over the skin to cleanse it further.

❧ Then a mask (the one used depends on the skin type) to tighten the pores. After 10 to 15 minutes remove the mask with cotton moistened with cold water.

❧ When the mask is off, apply cream around the eyes, dotted on from the temple bone inward toward the nose.

❧ Pat on skin freshener.

❧ Acne lotion may be used wherever there is an eruption.

Your home facial goes better with vibrating tools to do the work. Keep motions upward and outward (circular on forehead, chin, and nose), as you would with your fingers.

1. Mist helps cream penetrate (or use it before creaming to flush pores).

2. Cream-cleanse the skin to remove makeup and then use makeup-removal brush to lift residue from the skin.

3. A soft-bristle cleanser brush (lather the brush, not the skin) gives you a soap-and-water wash.

4. Rinse and then cream the skin; work cream in with massage tool.

5. Close pores with a cold pack (dip metal massager in ice water to chill). A beauty mask can be used with the home facial.

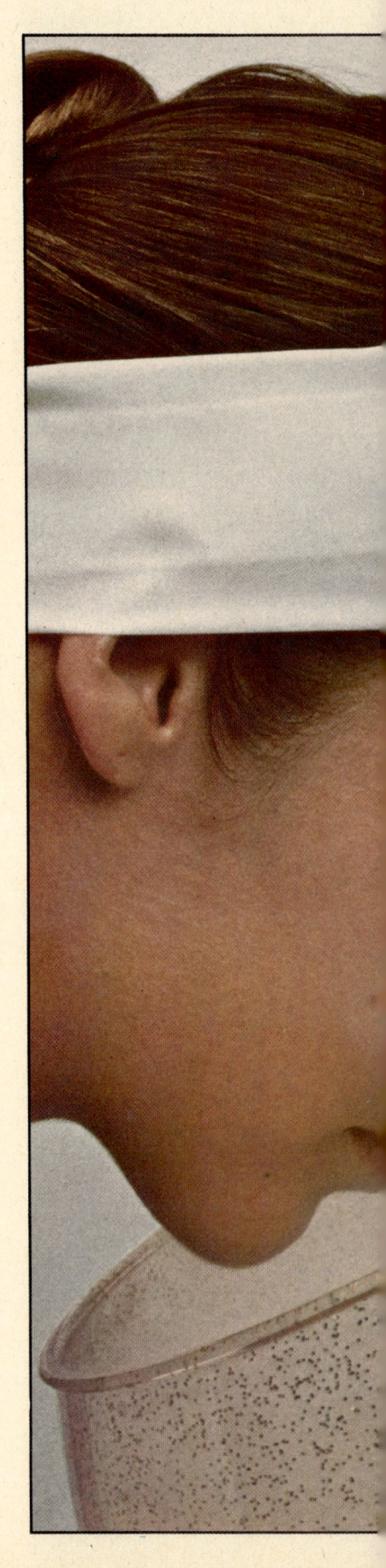

89

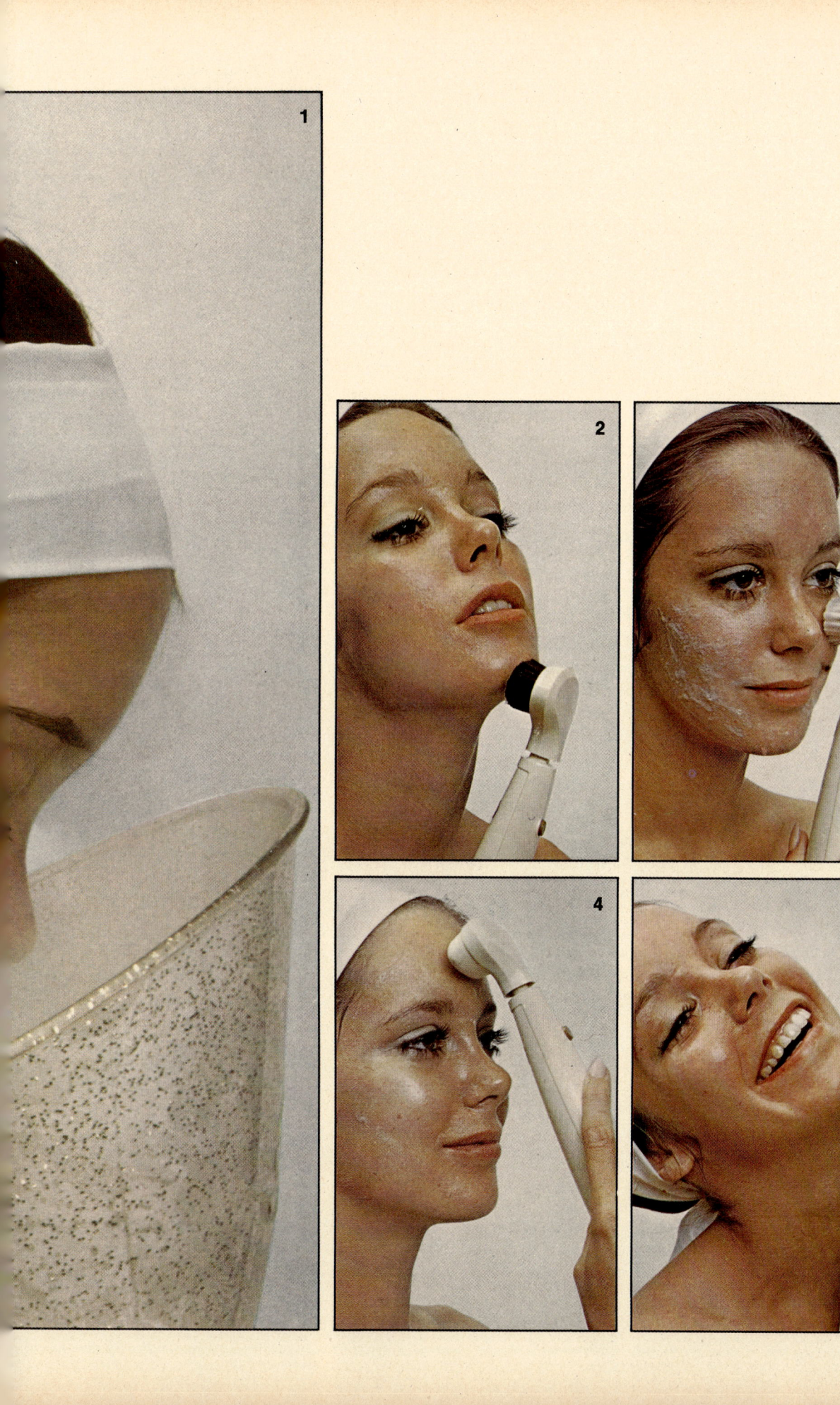

Try a water facial. Because water is so much a part of this fresh-washed feeling that our skin-care habits call for, a water facial can become part of your new-skin look. Try this special drying method with your water facial:

✳ Instead of rubbing or patting your skin dry with a towel (this may abrade the skin surface and even cause pore ruptures), let your skin dry at room temperature after rinsing. If the room is reasonably warm, chapping is not a hazard. It takes only two to four minutes for the skin to dry naturally, and the effect seems to be good, particularly for those with tender or sensitive skin.

Dry skin—Apply a generous coat of dry-skin cream to face and throat. Leave on for one to three minutes (longer if you have time). Remove the cream gently with a damp washcloth so that a slight film of cream remains to lubricate the skin. Or tissue off the cream and splash the face with fresh water. Let the skin dry at room temperature.

Normal skin—Rinse the face with tepid water. Apply a stimulating cleanser. Leave on for one minute only. Rinse face and let skin dry at room temperature. Apply a moisturizer or a light film of dry-skin cream.

Oily skin—Apply a stimulating cleanser directly to the skin. Leave on for two to five minutes. Rinse off with cool water, let the skin dry at room temperature.

Combination skin—Apply a generous coat of vanishing cream to oily areas. Leave on for one minute. Remove with a damp washcloth and splash the skin with fresh water. Let face dry at room temperature.

Troubled skin—Apply your stimulating cleanser directly to the face skin. Leave on for two to five minutes. Rinse off with cool water. Let the skin dry and then apply medicated lotion or stimulating cleanser to troubled areas.

ANY AGE SKIN CARE

AGE 16 TO 24

Normal skin. Wash your face with soap and water once a day—not more. Over-washing dries out oil and does nothing for skin. Do this once-a-day soap-and-water wash in the morning. Rinse well.

✳ Wear a moisturizer all day.
✳ Use makeup on top of the moisturizer (this helps protect the skin).
✳ At night, remove—*really remove*—the makeup with cleansing cream or lotion; clear off with tissues.
✳ Follow with toning lotion (on a cotton ball) to clean skin thoroughly.
✳ Splash with cool water (no soap).
✳ No night cream needed.

Very dry skin. Do not use soap on the skin—instead, clean with lotion or cream in the morning and then splash your face with cool water.
✳ Dry the skin thoroughly.
✳ Always use a moisturizer (never put makeup directly on the skin).
✳ Use a cream makeup very lightly.
✳ Otherwise, follow the routine for normal skin.

Very oily skin. Wash with soap and water *twice* a day (morning and night). Rub soap on the washcloth and go over your face, especially nose and chin, with circular motions to really clean the skin. Rinse thoroughly.
✳ Do not squeeze blackheads; instead steam your face over hot water or use a facial sauna, then gently press the blackheads out with a damp cloth (never with fingers or metal instruments).
✳ Otherwise, follow the routine for normal skin.

AGE 25 TO 44

Normal skin. Wash face once a day (in the morning) with soap and water. Rinse skin well.
✳ Use an astringent to smooth pores.
✳ Apply moisturizer and let set for five minutes.
✳ Apply makeup
✳ In the evening, remove makeup well with cleansing cream or lotion.
✳ Apply a good nourishing cream, massaging it into the skin with circular movements, and leave it on during bath or shower. Remove cream at bedtime.
✳ Once a week, give yourself a mask treatment to clean pores.

Very dry skin. Use no soap. Use cleansing cream or lotion morning and night.
✳ Splash face with cool water.
✳ In the morning, after cleansing, apply moisturizer and makeup. (Do not use an astringent in the morning.)
✳ Remove makeup once during the day with a mild astringent and feed the skin with a rich cream (just a little). Massage the cream into your skin. Remove with tissue before reapplying makeup.
✳ At night, use an astringent to complete cleansing.
✳ Once a week, use a nondrying mask.
✳ Otherwise, follow the routine for normal skin.

Oily skin. In the morning, wash face with warm water and soap.
✳ Follow cleaning with an astringent.
✳ Clean face once during the day, removing makeup and using an astringent. Reapply makeup.
✳ In the evening, after removing makeup, wash face with soap and water. Rinse well.
✳ Apply a cream for oily skin, but remove before going to bed.
✳ Once a week, steam your face and apply a mask. Pay special attention to oily areas, nose and chin.

AGE 45 AND OVER

Older women often have good skin because they take better care of it than do younger women. Give your skin the same kind of care recommended for the 25-to-44-year-old woman, but feed and exercise the skin more.

✳ After cleansing in the evening, massage the skin, using a rich nourishing cream, for five to 10 minutes—till circulation is worked up and face feels warm. Remove cream before bedtime.
✳ Exercise your face frequently before a mirror—saying "Q" and "X" very strongly is good.
✳ You also need an eye cream: Leave it on overnight. It's around the eyes that most lines appear.
✳ Stay out of sunlight as much as possible and wear sunglasses on bright days to prevent squinting.

OUTDOOR SKIN CARE

Medical men believe that "weathering," or overexposure, is the chief menace to skin youth. To judge the situation for yourself, compare facial skin (or skin of the back of the hand) to skin of body areas that are ordinarily protected by clothing. It is the "exposed" areas that show "age."

The face is always *out*—bared to summer sun and winter wind and to outdoor and indoor air day and night throughout the year. Daily protection from effects of exposure—loss of skin moisture as well as the damaging effects of sunlight—should be part of your beauty routine.

✳ Wear a protective cream chosen for your own skin type whenever you go outdoors.
✳ If you use a cream or liquid base, your makeup gives some protection to the skin. If you are not wearing makeup, use a protective cream indoors as well.
✳ A protective conditioner, if skin is dry, should be applied at bedtime and after five minutes tissued off.
✳ If skin shows signs of "aging," take even greater precautions by avoiding the overuse of soap—soap changes the skin's natural protective chemistry.
✳ Wear a brimmed hat in sunshine; a scarf or hood to cut off wind from the face in winter.
✳ Be sure that the air in your home is of the correct humidity both summer and winter.

Chapping. Chapping is the result of excessive dryness in the surface skin, which flakes off, exposing underskin that is sensitive, and looks and feels "raw." Skin that chaps readily should be well protected in dry and windy weather. Once the skin is chapped, it will heal by itself if it is protected from further exposure with chap cream, lubricant, or medicated ointment.

❧ To avoid chapping, be sure to rinse away all soap residue after face washing. Dry the face gently and well, patting it dry with a soft terry towel, and apply a protective cream or lotion as soon as you have dried the face.

❧ Never expose damp skin to the outdoor air; wear moisturizer under your makeup on snowy and rainy days.

Tanning. It is not commonly realized that the sun's rays actually penetrate the skin, but they do. When certain of these rays enter the skin, they stimulate the development of *melanin,* the skin pigment that some of us know as a tan, others as freckles, and many as simply their brunet coloring. With continued exposure, the melanin rises to the skin surface to create a screen that filters out harmful rays of the sun and so protects underlayers against damage.

Tanning gives some protection against burning but tanning also toughens the skin surface. Continued overexposure can result in a skin that is parched, wrinkled, discolored, and thickened; and toughening and thickening make "use lines"—those from facial expressions—more apparent.

Moderate seasonal tanning of the body skin is probably desirable as a protection against burning if you are enjoying a great deal of outdoor activity—but the body skin is ordinarily covered by clothing and so gets much less weathering. The face is always vulnerable, so make these your sun rules:

❧ Use a sun-screen preparation that is also an emollient, or lubricant.

❧ Keep the face, throat, and back of neck well lubricated between exposures.

❧ Keep the face, throat, and back of neck out of the sun as much as possible; a wide-brim hat, a beach umbrella, a spot of shade give protection. Your face will get some "color" from reflected light and ordinary daily exposure.

Freckles. In people (usually the fair-skinned) who do not tan easily, the pigment that normally would create a tan appears scattered over the skin in the tiny spots called "freckles." Freckles may be bleached by use of lemon juice or peroxide or freckle cream, but usually it is better simply to live with them. Bleaching is temporary at best, and the treatment may be drying or irritating. Use a sunblock (not a tanning lotion) on freckle areas.

Sunburn. Make every effort to avoid sunburn and windburn, particularly on the face; carefully limit exposure to be sure you are not damaging your skin. By the time skin shows redness, the skin is already slightly burned. Sunburn is a real burn—the same kind of burn you might get from a hot oven.

❧ If sunburn develops, treat it like any burn—with ice water, medicated ointments, and soothing lotions. If the burn is severe, see a doctor.

❧ Sunburn peels because the surface skin has been dried and damaged by heat; this "dead" skin is then shed. The new layer of surface skin will often be pink and sensitive; treat it to an emollient cream and protect it from exposure to the sun.

Perspiration. Sweating is a normal function—part of the skin's cooling process—and is *not* drying to the skin. In fact, perspiration helps to protect the skin against drying by distributing natural skin oils and maintaining the normal skin chemistry.

❧ Facial perspiration is usually heaviest on the forehead, nose, chin, and upper lip; to absorb moisture without disturbing your makeup, blot these areas with tissue when they feel moist. Antiperspirants should *not* be used on the face.

❧ Perspiration can wash away your skin-protecting sun-screen preparation, so reapply the preparation frequently even if you don't swim.

❧ Excitement, nervous tension, physical activity, as well as warmth, may stimulate perspiration. Excessive perspiration may have an internal cause; a physician should be consulted.

Sensitivity. Skin that reacts allergically—with burning, itching, or a rash, for example—to sunlight or to various creams and other cosmetics or even to soap, should be protected from irritation. Skin tests by an allergist can tell you what to avoid. Most cosmetics are formulated to screen out the common skin irritants; some hypoallergenic cosmetics screen out still others. An individual may, however, be allergic to *anything;* treatment by a physician may desensitize you if the irritant cannot be completely avoided.

❧ Air pollution — dust and soot and chemicals in the air—are common skin irritants. Again, your protective cream and makeup, if used consistently, will be of great help.

WHAT GOES ON IN A SALON FACIAL?

Here from the Christine Valmy Salon, New York City, is her facial step by step.

The type and texture of our skin, Miss Valmy reminds us, are determined by heredity, just as our eye color is. The purpose of facial treatment is to help any skin function well—to bring it into good condition, regardless of type. If you thoroughly clean your skin, oily or dry or mixed, you get improvement in the way it works.

❧ The skin is cleaned with a cleansing preparation, and then three types of massage (each takes five to seven minutes) are used to remove surface dirt and dead cells and to stimulate circulation: A kneading massage, a caressing massage, and a massage that combines both types of hand action. The kneading massage requires special training to be done correctly, but you can use caressing movements—upward and outward—and tapping movements (as if you were lightly playing the piano over face and throat) to soothe skin nerves. With acne skin, no massage is given because it only overstimulates the sebum (oil-producing) glands.

❧ Spraying with a lukewarm mist that brings oxygen to the skin and softens surface cells and is also germicidal.

❧ Brushing with a soft-bristle rotary brush removes dead surface cells as an aid to further cleansing.

❧ An electric treatment that softens the sebum (skin oil) in the pores and makes it easier to extrude.

❧ After this the skin is massaged by hand to work the sebum plugs out of the pores, or a suction cup is used to draw out pore deposits.

❧ This is followed by a lotion spray—like a jet shower—which acts as a massage, stimulating blood flow to the skin.

❧ By this time the skin is thoroughly clean and ready for appropriate treatment—pore-tightening for oily skin or pore-penetrating preparations for dry skin. (High-frequency current with tingling ultraviolet light helps penetration.)

❧ One of a variety of masks (some 40 are available) is also used on the skin after the third massage.

❧ Next, the skin is sprayed with a lotion of plant extracts (which one depends on what the skin needs) for soothing, pretightening, constricting of tiny veins, and so forth.

❧ The last step is a protective lotion that contains silicones for a natural film of protection against irritants in the outside air. Or, for those who want some color, a light foundation.

Action pictures of a salon facial appear on the following pages.

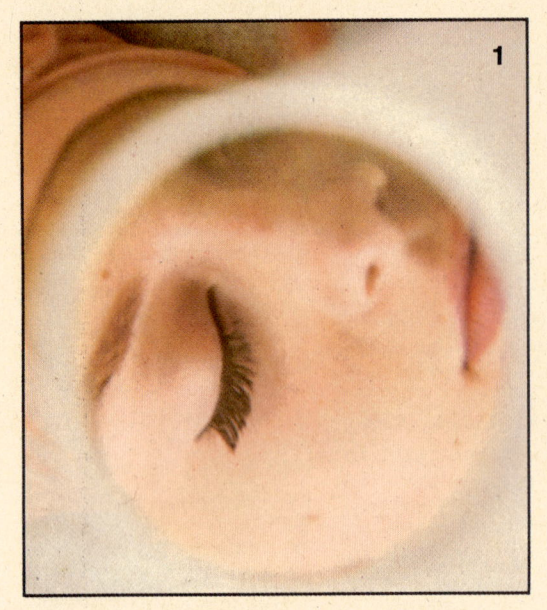

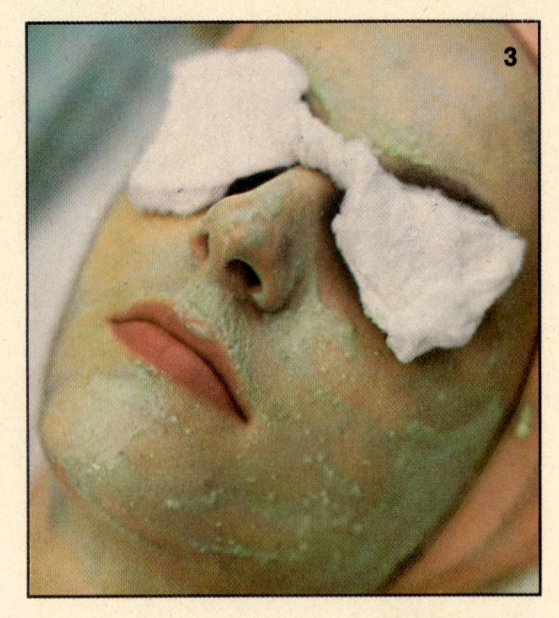

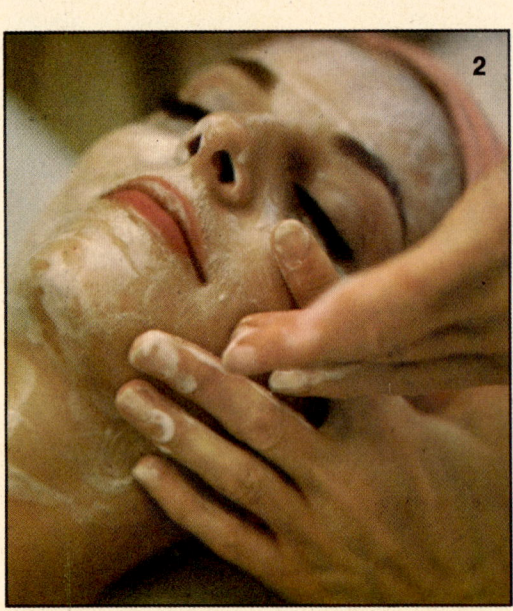

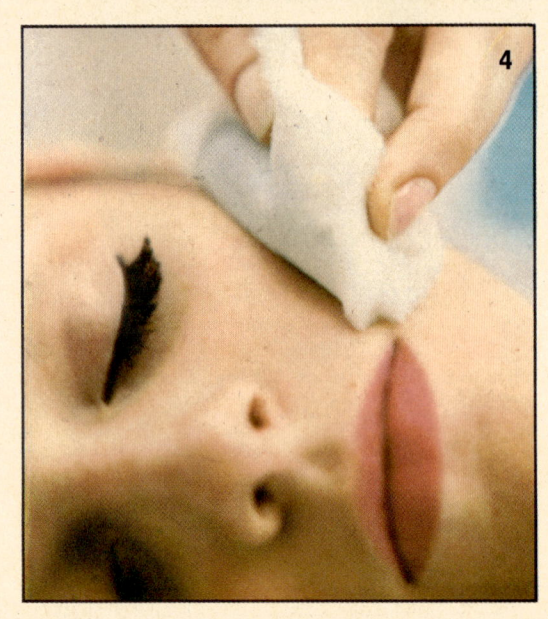

Salon Facial

Lying relaxed in a chair is an important part of the salon facial. A vibrating chair is often used.
Cleansing and relaxation. Hair is covered; and you recline, knees raised, while the vibration of the chair and the manipulations of the treatment encourage relaxation.
❧ Cleansing lotion is applied, starting at the collarbone, working hand-over-hand over the throat and with rotary and smoothing motions over the face.
❧ The skin is examined under a magnifying glass to reveal any problem areas (**1**).
❧ A new application of cleansing lotion, with manipulation to promote skin stimulation and to induce relaxation, follows. During this period problem areas are worked over, muscles are stimulated with manipulation, the mouth is relaxed with circular motion (**2**), and lotion is delicately applied to the eye area.

Deep cleansing. The knees are straightened to lie flat, and the vibration of the chair is lowered. This is a period of deep relaxation.
❧ The second lotion is removed with stimulating manipulation.
❧ A series of three towels, wrung out of very hot water-and-herb solution, is applied to the face.
❧ A mask (**3**) is put on. It may, depending on the skin type, be a nutritional mask or a gentle drawing mask to remove surface impurities. The whole face is

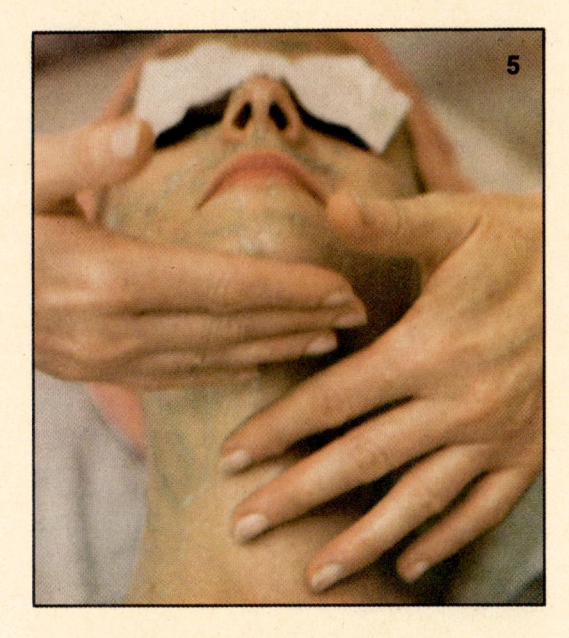

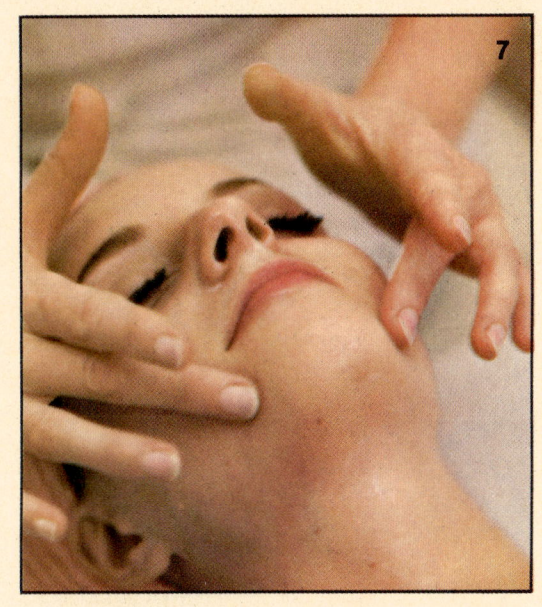

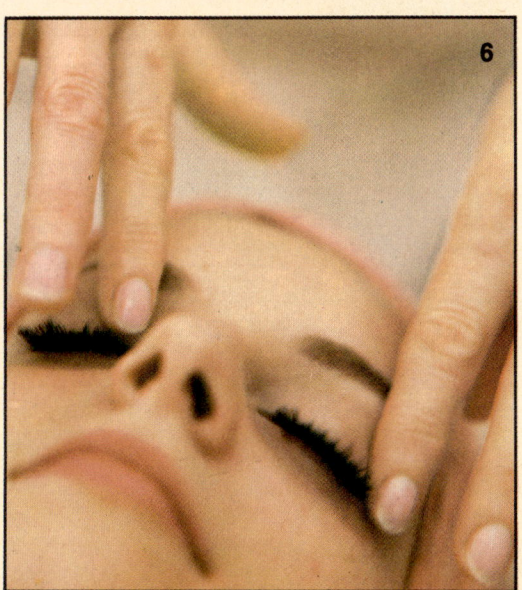

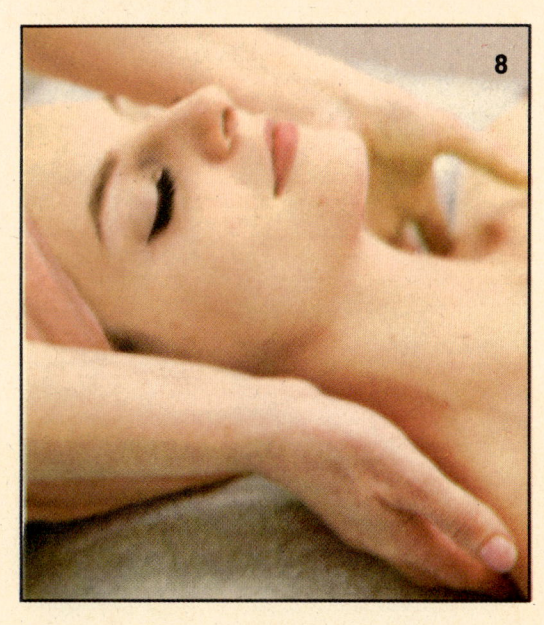

covered, except for the eyes, which are protected with eye pads, and this mask is left on for 15 minutes. While the mask works, hands and arms are gently massaged to stimulate circulation to the face.

🌿 The mask is removed with warm water.

🌿 A series of three warm towels is applied.

Toning. A freshening lotion is applied to close the pore openings slightly (**4**).

🌿 A mask stimulator is put on with stimulating motions (**5**). Cool pads cover the eyes.

🌿 A series of three very *cold* towels is used to remove the mask.

🌿 Skin is toned with an antiseptic lotion, smoothing gently over eyes (**6**).

Stimulation. Chair vibration is now at a minimum.

🌿 A mask is applied to close the pores as much as possible. This mask is very taut and takes 15 minutes to work; the face must be held immobile during this time.

🌿 Mask is removed with a series of three very cold towels.

🌿 Tightening action of the mask is eased by firm touches in eye, mouth, and nose areas.

🌿 Freshening lotion is applied from chest over throat and neck and ears and into the hairline.

🌿 Circulation to the skin is stimulated with "piano-playing" finger action (**7**).

Conditioning. Moisture lotion is freely applied from shoulders to hairline (**8**).

🌿 The scalp is given gentle manipulation.

WHAT'S YOUR SKIN TYPE?

Knowing your skin—where skin is dry and where oily and whether dry areas are dehydrated (lacking cell moisture) or sebum-poor (lacking natural skin oils)—is important to good skin care. If you know what your skin needs for good health, you can help it be healthy.

IS YOUR SKIN DRY?

How to recognize dry skin. There is a feeling of tightness—a lack of "give," or elasticity.
- Skin chaps easily; powder flakes.
- Skin looks parched, reacts readily to heat, cold, and wind.
- Skin feels drawn and tight after soap-and-water washing.
- The skin may appear glassy.
- Perspiration is scant.

What causes dry skin? Skin dryness is due specifically to lack of moisture, not lack of oil, but oils play their part in keeping the skin moist. Dry skin produces little natural oil and perspiration is slight, so any oil will be poorly distributed over the skin. Unprotected by oil, the outermost layer of skin loses water through evaporation of moisture into the air; this dry layer then flakes off easily, and new exposed skin in turn becomes vulnerable to moisture loss.
- Heredity is a factor in skin dryness (fair-skinned women often have the problem). Poor diet (or diet low in fats), tension, health problems (such as hormone imbalance), and the air around you may also be factors. Dryness is usually more noticeable in winter than in summer.
- A great deal of skin dryness is the result of overuse of soap and water and of overexposure to sun and wind.

Care for dry skin. Avoid use of soap and water on the face; if you *must* wash your face, use superfatted soap or "soapless soap" and still keep face washing to a minimum.
- Avoid vigorous scrubbing that removes dry flaky surface skin and exposes "new" skin to moisture loss.
- Cream-cleanse the face for three minutes night and morning, using a rich cleanser.
- Use a skin freshener formulated for dry skin, and follow freshening with a night cream or day-use moisturizer.
- Avoid drying beauty masks; if you use a stimulating mask, make the treatment infrequent. You may use lubricating cream as a facial mask while you soak in the tub. A half-hour treatment is often as good as an overnight treatment. Follow with a light night cream.
- By day, wear a moisturizing emollient, or lubricating cream, under your cream or liquid foundation.
- To protect lips, wear lip gloss over your lipstick.
- Keep skin of eye and throat continuously protected with complexion oil.
- Avoid overexposure to sun and wind by use of creams and protective headgear, such as sun hat, scarf, or parka hood.
- Avoid "arid air." Be sure that home heating and air-conditioning provide adequate humidity.

IS YOUR SKIN OILY?

How to recognize oily skin. Pores are enlarged, particularly about the nose, and there are occasional skin blemishes.
- There is a tendency to perspire freely.
- Skin has morning "shine" due to oil accumulation during sleep.
- Shine appears often during the day as skin oils come through makeup.
- Skin may feel uncomfortably sticky or "dirty."

What causes oily skin? The skin oils are the natural lubricants and protectors of the skin. Persons with dark complexions—brunet skins—often have a normally rich supply of oils, a slightly less-fine texture and larger pores than the fair-skinned, and a tendency to perspire freely. Such skin has a good supply of pigment (the brunet coloring) so that tan comes easily, and the skin suffers less from exposure. Warm climate and warm weather increase oiliness. The fair-skinned also suffer excess oiliness, but usually in a "combination skin."
- Excess oiliness often accompanies physical changes of adolescence and sometimes reappears during the menopause. Oiliness can be increased by a diet overly rich in sweets and fats and by general poor health. There may also be a "lazy skin" condition in which the fat-producing glands release oil too readily—in a glob or droplet rather than in a steady lubricating flow. Emotional disturbance and excitement can increase both sweat and oil production; so can vigorous exercise.
- Oiliness is often apparent in the scalp condition as well as in the facial skin. Treatment helps "to dry up the oil" by improving both general health and surface skin care.

Care for oily skin. Use a cleansing cream to remove makeup but be sure all cream is quickly removed from the skin. Follow creaming with a soap-and-water washing or a detergent-lotion cleansing.
- Clean the skin three times a day—including a soaping or use of cleansing lotion.
- After washing, tone the skin with skin freshener; use an astringent on the middle face, where pores are often enlarged.
- A once-a-week facial is helpful to remove pore deposits and to prevent the pores' becoming plugged and permanently enlarged and to avoid skin eruptions. Use a detergent mask.
- At night use a deep-pore cleanser followed by astringent.
- Change makeup at midday and evening, but between changes do not repowder to remove shine. Repowdering only cakes makeup and clogs pores; instead, blot the shiny areas with tissue or a moist sponge.
- If you have dry areas—usually round the eyes and on the throat—avoid touching these areas with masks or astringents.

"COMBINATION" SKIN

How to recognize combination skin. The middle parts of the face—forehead, nose, and chin—usually show shine, enlarged pores, sometimes skin blemishes. These areas are oily.
- The area behind the ears may develop pimples and blackheads. This area is often oily.
- The sides of the face may show dry flaky skin.
- Skin round the eyes and on the throat is often dry, feels tight, and may show tiny lines of crepiness.
- The outer surface of the skin may seem dry, but whiteheads and pimples sometimes appear, indicating a skin that is basically oily with an outer surface that is dry and tight.

What causes combination skin? Combination skin may result from faulty skin care. If the surface is overdried by sun exposure, soap-and-water washing, or arid air, the natural (and perhaps normal) oil supply gets locked in the pores and cannot surface. The result is more surface dryness and more plugging of pores—whiteheads, enlarged pores, and skin coarseness.

In combination skin, the skin of eye and throat, which has few sweat and fat glands, is usually dry. While the middle face is being treated for excessive oiliness, these dry areas may be temporarily neglected. Because dryness is a surface problem and oiliness goes deeper, it is usually preferable to treat the oily areas till they are cleared, keeping treatment lotions and masks away from eyes and throat. After oiliness is arrested, dry areas may be treated with emollients.

Care for combination skin. From age 20 on a woman should keep a light cream on the eye skin night and day; this is the first area to become dry.

❧ Throat skin should also be treated with a moisturizing lotion by day, with complexion oil as a night conditioner.

❧ Treat oily areas as oily skin, washing with soap and water three times daily; rinse well. Follow washing with toning lotion. Have a mask treatment weekly to keep pores free of plugs.

❧ Cream the eye and the throat skin before you apply stimulant masks to the rest of the face.

IS YOUR SKIN "TROUBLED"?

How to recognize troubled skin. Acne—skin eruptions and blackheads and whiteheads—is characteristic.

❧ Otherwise the skin often has the shine, enlarged pores, and the other symptoms of oily skin.

❧ Troubled skin may, however, be sensitive and easily chapped and may feel dry and itchy.

What causes skin blemishes? Skin dryness appears on the surface layer, but oiliness (with blemishes) arises in the underlayers, where oil and sweat glands are imbedded. In acne the pores of the skin become plugged with fat deposits and these plugs appear as whiteheads (plugs below the top skin layer and not open to the air) or blackheads (pore plugs that are exposed to air at the tip; contact with air oxidizes the sebum, or fat, and creates the characteristic black speck). Sometimes these plugged pores become infected below the skin surface; a redness, or inflammation, appears; and eventually, due to the accumulation of white blood corpuscles that have rushed to destroy the invading bacteria, pus forms—and we have a "pimple."

Medical findings lean toward *internal* physical factors in acne, but the result appears on the skin surface, and the surface must be cared for so that there will be no acne scars. Chronic and extensive acne should be treated by a physician; only a dermatologist or trained facial cosmetician can safely clear sebum deposits so the skin will not be damaged.

Care for troubled skin. Clean the skin frequently—at least three times a day.

❧ Remove makeup with cleansing lotion and be sure that every vestige is removed.

❧ Follow with a soap-and-water washing and rinse well so there is no soap residue. Soap is drying and may tighten the outer layer of skin and thus encourage oil accumulation within the pores, resulting in whiteheads and pimples.

❧ Bedtime cleansing should open the pores and flush them. Follow soap-and-water washing and rinsing with warm-towel applications—or make a tent for your head under a towel and hold your face over a steaming basin or facial sauna for five minutes—till perspiration flows freely.

❧ After steaming, go gently over the middle of the face with cotton balls—one in each hand—stretching (not squeezing) the skin so that any sebum deposits that are ready to be released will emerge. (Do not force blackheads and leave pimples and whiteheads alone.) Remove released sebum with a cotton ball saturated with antiseptic lotion. If you do this with each bedtime washing, you will keep the skin condition much improved.

❧ Follow with a deep-pore cleanser or a detergent mask. Rinse with cool water.

❧ Tighten pore openings with astringent.

❧ During the day use a light makeup base to discourage pore plugs.

❧ Medicated treatment creams and medicated makeup should be used only upon the recommendation of your physician.

❧ Although ultraviolet-light treatment is sometimes used in acne, oversunning on your own should not be attempted. Skin may appear healthier and seem free of blemishes during the season of sun, but often the skin is damaged by overtanning. The outer layers become dry and thickened, concealing enlarged pores and pore plugs. As summer ends and the tan fades, there is often a fresh outbreak of these hidden pimples and blackheads.

IS YOUR SKIN "AGING"?

How to recognize aging skin. Look at your skin in a magnifying mirror. Aging skin has a fretwork of tiny lines and circles round the skin hairs that indicate loss of "fullness" in the underlying layers.

❧ There often is sallowness that indicates blood is not circulating freely close to the skin surface.

❧ The skin lacks elasticity—is slow to spring back into place when pinched or indented.

❧ There may be brownish spots, or accumulation of pigment, on some skin areas.

❧ Sometimes there is excessive itching and cracking.

❧ The skin feels stiff rather than soft.

❧ Dryness is noticeable; skin is tissue-thin and may appear "glassy."

❧ Crepiness appears around the eyes and upper lids and also on the throat.

❧ Sometimes facial hair becomes more noticeable.

What causes skin aging? Dryness in aging skin may be a matter both of surface-moisture loss and of lowered moisture content in the underlayers of the skin. The fat-producing glands become smaller as we age, and supporting skin cells retain less moisture and lose their fullness. Almost the only factor in skin "aging" that medicine attributes to *actual* aging is this excessive dryness that results from fall of estrogen production after menopause and sometimes as menopause approaches. With this estrogen decline comes a lessening of circulation to the skin; the pink glow disappears as a result of poorer circulation and diminished activity of the tiny skin capillaries.

Because "aging" is often noticeable chiefly in skin of face and hands—the areas we constantly expose—medical opinion now leans to the belief that "aging" is chiefly "weathering." Certain rays of the sun seem to produce unfavorable changes in skin that make it look "old."

Abuse of the skin through poor handling may also lead to wrinkles and lines; simple gravity pull on facial muscles can eventually lead to sag; and use of facial muscles in both smiles and frowns can cause the face to take on certain familiar aging lines.

Care for aging skin. If skin is excessively dry, see your doctor; estrogen therapy (if there is a deficiency) may help your skin and may also help you to avoid other health problems.

❧ Make use of refined-lanolin or lipide preparations that relieve tightness and soothe the skin.

❧ Injuries from overexposure to sunlight cannot be reversed, but you can protect your skin from further damage by using a sun-screen preparation when out of doors and by getting as little exposure as possible.

❧ Cream-cleanse the face to remove makeup and soil and to cut down on soap-and-water washing.

❧ Avoid heavy creams and masks; your skin will benefit from light moisturizers and light lubricants or emollients. Heavy creams may cause further drag on delicate tissues.

❧ Improve skin circulation by lying down frequently during the day with feet up, head lower than the hips.

❧ Keep your general health at its best with balanced diet, plenty of rest, fresh air, and activity.

❧ Use a moisturizer emollient under makeup by day and as a night cream.

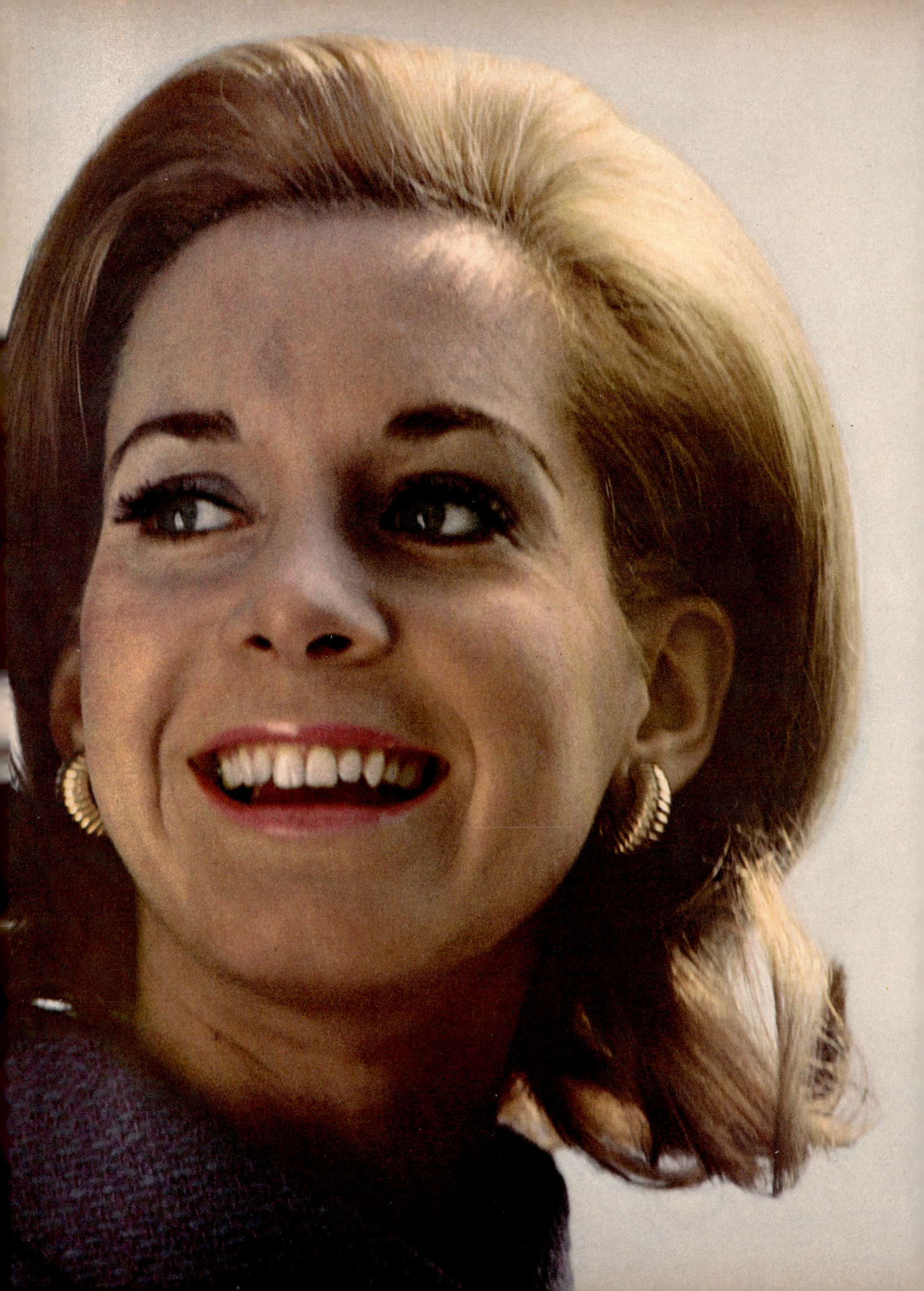

"Normalize" Your Complexion

Today it is agreed that two factors greatly affect skin beauty. One is inner—your health and feminine functioning. One is outer—the environment in which you live. What, then, can you do about the weather? Or air pollution? As far as your skin is concerned, you *can* do something. You can give it the care and protection it needs to stay moist. For moisture—the moisture in the skin cells and the moisture that is held against the skin by a moisture cream or lotion—is today considered the wonder-worker in skin beauty. If you can keep this atmosphere of your skin dewy and protect your skin from exposure to drying elements (sun, wind, soot, chemicals and parched indoor air), you help to ward off signs of age. Start your skin-renewing program by analyzing the kind of skin you have. The simplest way to test your skin for dry, normal, and oily areas is by use of sheets of blotting tissue (or the small sheets designed for cleaning eyeglass lenses) to reveal the oil pickup from the skin. In the morning—before you have washed your face but with any night cream thoroughly removed—press a tissue lightly to the skin, first to the outside of the cheeks and then to the throat and to the sides of the forehead. These areas are often dry; if they are, they will not mark the tissue or will mark it only lightly. Next, blot the middle of the forehead, the nose, the middle of the chin. These are often rich in oil, and, if they are oily, will leave a noticeable mark on the tissue. Normal skin will mark the tissue lightly; dry skin will leave little or no stain; oily skin, a noticeable mark.

IS YOUR SKIN NORMAL?

How to recognize normal skin. The skin feels smooth and soft and slightly dewy.
- In a magnifying mirror the skin texture appears smooth with no perceptible enlarged pores.
- The skin shows a pink glow—"good color"—from adequate blood circulation.
- Perspiration is neither excessive nor scant.
- Skin oils are imperceptible—the skin appears luminous but not shiny.
- The surface is clear with no blackheads, whiteheads, or pimples.
- The skin is elastic—it springs back readily when pinched or depressed.
- Skin hairs are fine and almost invisible.

What is normal skin? Normal skin reflects good health and a favorable heredity. It can protect itself from the outside and feed and cleanse itself from the inside. The skin produces enough water from its sweat glands to cool the surface and to balance the skin chemistry and also to distribute over the skin the fats produced by the oil glands; these fats soften and lubricate the skin.
- Normal skin is self-renewing; the outer layer is constantly being shed, and a new top layer is constantly appearing.
- The skin has a downy coating of "invisible" hairs that perhaps serve to exercise the sweat and sebaceous (oil) glands. It also has its own sun screen (pigment that develops as light rays penetrate the skin) that rises to the surface and, by filtering out unwelcome light, protects lower levels from damage.

Care for normal skin. Because we like to feel clean, we wash often. But we remove a great deal of the skin's protective coat each time we wash. With normal skin it is wise simply to rinse the face in the morning and to give face, neck, and ears their soap-and-water wash at bedtime. The skin thus has time to restore its normal balance during sleep.
- Use makeup removal creams—two coats—to remove makeup.
- Wash with soap and water, if you choose.
- Use a stimulating freshener to keep pore openings normal.
- Avoid overuse of treatments or beauty masks.
- After age 20 use a moisturizer on eye skin; on the throat skin as well after age 30.
- Protect skin against weathering with a creamy foundation or with a sun-screen preparation whenever exposed to much sunlight.

HOW TO TONE THE SKIN

After cleansing, the skin should be "toned" to remove the vestiges of cleanser, to stimulate the skin, and to close the pores slightly.

✤ For a dry skin, use a skin freshener that is formulated for dry skin.

✤ For normal skin, a normal-skin freshener.

✤ For oily skin, an oily-skin freshener followed by an astringent to dry up the oil and to further tighten the pore openings.

Pat the freshener on with a cotton square moving upward and outward along facial lines and with a rotary motion on the middle of the face—nose, chin, and forehead.

Skin stimulation. Slapping the skin lightly with a cotton square after you have applied skin freshener acts as a gentle stimulant to the skin. You may also use light "piano-playing" movements of the fingers over the face. Once or twice a week you may, however, want to use a beauty mask as a skin stimulant.

Mask treatment. Beauty masks are sometimes cleansing, drawing the oil and grime deposits out of the skin and helping to peel off the surface layer of dead skin cells. Usually the masks are intended to be "stimulating" by encouraging the local flow of capillary blood. Masks are also firming and tightening, clearing away at least temporarily the tiny fretwork of lines and making the skin glow.

✤ Sometimes these masks are "drying" and are a boon to a woman with oily skin.

✤ A woman whose skin is dry should use a lubricating mask as her beauty pickup.

✤ Masks come in the form of a "clay" pack or a cream or as a light liquid or as a jelly. "Packs" harden on the face; the face muscles should be relaxed and immobile while these masks dry (usual drying time is 10 to 15 minutes) and they are best applied while you lie in the tub. These masks are both stimulating (bringing increased circulation to the face skin) and detergent (cleaning pore surfaces).

✤ Quick pickup masks in liquid or gel form have little or no detergent action; they bring increased circulation to the facial skin and also "tighten" the skin to erase tiny lines.

✤ Beauty masks should not be used if tiny broken blood vessels are visible in the skin and should not be used frequently by any woman, for the repeated stimulant action of bringing increased blood flow to the skin capillaries may overstrain tiny blood vessels and lead to breakage.

✤ Any mask should be used only after the skin has been thoroughly cleaned by other methods. Follow the mask treatment with use of skin freshener and, if skin is dry, with an emollient, or lubricating cream.

Beauty pickup. Here is a quick 10-minute pickup beauty treatment that you may find useful before a party or as a part of your weekly beauty routine:

✤ Fill the bathtub with warm water and sprinkle in a fragrant skin-soothing bath oil.

✤ Clean the face before entering the tub.

✤ In the tub apply a stimulating or lubricating mask and lie back, letting the mask work while you soak.

✤ While still in the tub, remove the mask with cool water.

✤ When you leave the tub, apply skin freshener and then a conditioner.

CONDITIONING TREATMENT

Skin conditioning depends on skin type, and the treatment chosen should be right for a particular skin.

✤ Greatest need of dry skin is for protection against loss of water through evaporation. Creams that lubricate, soften, and protect the skin against moisture loss are called *emollients*. Sometimes a "moisturizer" or other treatment factor is incorporated in the emollient, but the cream itself, through its lubricating action, helps keep the skin dewy.

✤ For the oily skin, which needs no added lubricant, a nonoily vanishing cream or a freshening lotion can be used for skin conditioning; in excessively oily areas, an astringent is enough.

✤ When skin is troubled, the conditioner is often a medicated cream or lotion that is worn under the makeup or as a night cream. Medicated creams should be used only with your physician's approval.

✤ For sensitive skin there are hypoallergenic conditioners useful to women who are sensitive to some common cream ingredients. Most creams and cosmetics today exclude general irritants. It is also true that a person can be allergic to *anything,* and sometimes even to hypoallergenic preparations.

✤ Special eye-and-throat creams should be included in the conditioning treatment. Complexion oils, because of their lightness, are desirable for use in the eye area.

Conditioners can effectively bolster the natural beauty dew—the skin's own protective coating that keeps it fine-textured, supple, and soft. Today's more specialized creams are credited with going even further—with activating the skin into better condition. The circulation of blood in the lower tissues is increased; the skin acts to use oxygen better and to discharge wastes more effectively; more internal moisture reaches the "underskin," and the tissue is better able to hold this moisture. Result—a firmer, younger-appearing complexion.

Nourishing creams. These creams are not actually "absorbed." Instead, the cream spreads over the skin surface and fills in the tiny crevices, coating the skin surface. Some drugs are, however, believed to be susceptible to absorption, and this is the reason creams containing "active" ingredients should be used with discrimination. Hormones, for example, are believed to work through the top layers of the skin surface to act on the cells of the lower layers. There also are indications that skin may utilize vitamins A and D, possibly E.

Moisturizers. Skin can be dry because cell water content is low or because the skin lacks oils to protect against moisture loss. "Moisturizers" help the skin to retain a normal amount of water and can have either an internal or an external effect.

✤ In *external* moisturizing the oils in the cream form a coating over the skin, preventing the loss of moisture through evaporation from the skin into the air; the surface skin is thus kept soft.

✤ The *internal* moisturizing effect takes place in the underlayers (the true skin) where the cells are activated to make better use of body moisture; this results in plumping the tissue and in filling out tiny lines on the surface.

Skin activators. Estrogenic hormones, used in cosmetics for the aging skin, were among the first "moisturizers" with a below-the-surface effect.

✤ *Vitamin A* is believed to combat scaliness, drying, and chapping typical of older skin, and *Vitamin D* (usually the two are used together) seems to aid the action of vitamin A and may also hasten healing.

✤ A cream will, however, usually have a variety of ingredients: *Energizers* that make the skin receptive to the moisturizing ingredient; *carriers* to bring the moisture into the skin layers; *humectants* to hold water in the skin; *lanolin, vegetable and mineral oils, fats,* and *waxes* to soften and smooth the skin surface, slough away dead cells, and form a protective coat. *Scents, emulsifiers,* and *water* itself—are also part of skin creams.

How much cream should be used? Use as little or as much cream as directed, balancing these instructions, of course, to the size of your face. (Some faces and throats have more square inches of skin area than others.) Many treatment creams are equally as effective if left on for two hours as if left on overnight. In other conditions, such as excess dryness, the skin needs to be creamed day and night. Today's creams are light in texture, "disappear" quickly, and are not unpleasant for overnight use.

❧ Use your cream regularly and according to the instructions on jar or bottle. Choose the cream according to your individual needs, skin problems, and degree of aging, not according to the price or the looks of the package. A 20-year-old woman should not choose a cream designed for aging skin, but a woman between 25 and 30 may find that her skin has begun to show signs of withering. Choose from a cosmetic line that you know is reliable and whose advertising and labeling claims are commensurate with a good reputation. Above all give the cream you choose a fair try—at least six weeks of regular use to see how your skin responds.

Natural cosmetics. Cosmetic use of fruits, vegetables, honey, herbs and other natural products goes back to Cleopatra—and is probably as old as the first man and woman? Does it have any scientific support? Yes. Lemon, for example, is known to be a mild skin bleach and helps to restore the slight normal acidity of the skin after use of "alkaline" soaps. With some natural products it is the acidity (citrus fruits, tomatoes), in some the astringent qualities (herbs, cucumber), in others oils (coconut, banana, avocado), or the proteins and perhaps the hormones (as in egg yolk or honey) that soften or soothe the skin. Even in this day of sophisticated cosmetic chemists, lemons, herbs, and a variety of other plant products such as witch hazel and vegetable oils go into commercial cosmetics. Vitamins A, D and E in creams or ointments also have current dermatological uses.

Today you can buy strawberry creams, cucumber creams, lemon cosmetics, balsam hair conditioners, avocado creams and a variety of fruit, egg, and honey cosmetics as commercial preparations. Or you can buy a lotion in which to mix your own fruits and vegetables for your favorite natural creams. Some mixtures should be refrigerated to retain their color and freshness. Prepare in small amounts.

But you can go still further back to nature by using natural products directly on your skin as masks and astringents. Besides those already mentioned, some of the popular natural masks are mashed bananas, coconut milk, cow's milk, yogurt, oatmeal (mixed with milk), strawberries, apples, tea, carrot juice, rice water, grapes, cornmeal, tomatoes, yeast, rose water, pineapple juice, grapefruit, herbal extracts.

Keep all natural masks and juices away from the eyes (they are not dangerous but may make eyes sting). If you are allergic to any fruits and vegetables or other natural product mentioned here, consult your physician about using the treatment on your skin.

SKIN PROBLEMS

Most skin problems are health problems, but they become cosmetic problems, too, when they affect our look and our attitudes toward ourselves.

Acne. Most people experience a skin outbreak at some time or other, and acne is common among teenagers, in whom it is more nearly the rule than the exception as a part of growing up. Many women continue to experience a recurrence of acne around the menstrual period. Often women who take the Pill find their acne clears up; others experience their first acne outbreaks on the Pill. The contraceptive Pill is, however, often prescribed as a treatment for acne. The most serious form of acne, chronic pustular acne, is usually persistent and hard to clear and may last long after adolescence. It should be treated by a physician, who has both internal aids—antibiotics, hormone treatment, diet—and external means—light treatments, medications, removal of pore deposits—to help bring it under control. To control severe acne, treatment must be consistent, with regular visits to a physician and sticking to the prescribed acne-control personal hygiene measures. Often, too, the use of cosmetics is discouraged. Some facial salons, notably the Georgette Klinger Salons in New York and Beverly Hills, have also been very successful in helping with acne skin problems. Again, regular consistent treatment has brought the good results.

Scars. Plastic surgery can often correct serious scarring, but not always. Some people tend to form keloids (raised flesh) when wounds heal, and this tendency persists when surgical correction is tried. Uncorrectable scars can sometimes be covered by makeup. When fresh scars are forming, stay out of the sun. The healing skin is producing melanin, the skin coloring, or pigment, and sunlight speeds this formation. If the healing skin is exposed to sunlight, the scar may be permanently darkened.

Birthmarks. These can sometimes be surgically removed or hidden with tattooing or can be concealed with covering makeup. In some cases, though, they cannot be treated or successfully concealed and have to be lived with.

Skin problems of pregnancy. Usually, thanks to the high production of the feminine hormone estrogen during pregnancy, the skin condition will improve. Some women though, develop brown splotches, particularly around mouth and eyes. These usually disappear after the baby is born, or the physician can treat them.

❧ Stretch marks on the body can sometimes be avoided by keeping the abdominal skin well lubricated; if they form, nothing as yet has been found that can get rid of them.

Skin problems on the Pill. The contraceptive Pill often improves the complexion and is sometimes used as a treatment for acne condition, but in some women acne apparently is produced by the Pill, and going off it can correct the problem. Brown splotches that sometimes appear on the skin when the Pill is being used can be removed by dermabrasion, or face planing.

Brown spots. Other brown spots appear as a result of using certain perfumes on the skin and then exposing the skin to sunlight. They are very slow to fade. It is wise not to use perfume or toilet water on the skin when you are sunbathing. Brown spots that appear on the hands with age should be called to your physician's attention. They can sometimes be bleached with special bleach creams.

Moles. Everyone has a certain number of moles, and most are harmless and cosmetically innocuous. Disfiguring or annoying moles should be removed; this can be done by electric needle or by plastic surgery. In any event, moles should be examined by a physician, especially if there is any change in size or color.

Pierced ears. Skin around the opening in pierced ears frequently becomes red and irritated. This may be due to allergy or to infection. For health reasons, piercing should be done by a physician, but jewelers who pierce ears also are adept at it and will advise you on how to prevent infection.

HOW TO STROKE WRINKLES AWAY
BY JESSICA CRANE

Did you know you are partly responsible for the speed at which you age? And that you can check your tendency to rapid—or even moderately rapid—aging?

Those who see their skin wrinkling before age warrants deep wrinkles will often place the blame upon inheritance, sensitive skin, worries, and frustration. But none of these is so much at fault as your own insensitive handling of your face.

Starting in childhood, too much touching of your face and neck can be harmful and will eventually lead to a loosening and displacement of facial tissue. It is always possible to recognize the face that has been damaged by touching and pulling—the skin has lost much of its elasticity, there is a lack of firmness, the under-eye area is loose and baggy, the chin and contour of the face pose a distressing problem.

You can effect improvement even at this point. The first rule: Hands off!

Even if you have mild facial problems, you may be unconsciously overtouching your face. Ask yourself these simple questions right now:

- Do you ever move the layer of your skin from its bony surface—for example, resting your face in your hands?
- Do you ever tug your face up and down?
- Do you towel your face, massage it, or apply makeup with anything but a gossamer touch?

If the answer to any of these questions is yes, you have a problem.

Let us rehash some biological facts: Each layer of the skin can be broken down into other distinct layers. (The outer layer, or epidermis, alone is made up of five semilayers—and all five are easily visible when viewed under a microscope.)

Together, these layers are intimately associated with the nerves, blood vessels, sweat glands, sensory apparatus, cells, muscles, sebaceous glands, and pressure apparatus for touch. All of these are woven together, adhering fast to the underlying cutaneous tissue and the bony structure of your face. Yet, all of them together are so thin that they can be held and pinched by the forefinger and thumb.

The question, then, is this: *How gently must you treat your face?*

Are you familiar with the musical word "pianissimo," meaning "very soft"? Think, then, of the pianist coaxing the softest tone from his piano—delicate, sensitive, and yet sensuous. Think of the gentle touch of the softest velvet brush, just skimming the skin surface. Just such a gossamer touch is our *Stroking Touch,* which is the kind we suggest using for your face. (If you are a parent, it is the touch you should guide your children to use, for toweling, cleansing, or applying makeup.)

Another vital point: The skin under your eyes is very sensitive. Applying makeup to this area must become a veritable art. During application, think of it as "breathing on" makeup.

The exercises that follow will restrain those who, by their own admission, are likely to be heavy-handed. Others can benefit, too. At the very least, you should compare your own touch to the sensation you will receive when making the following touch tests.

Finger numbering.

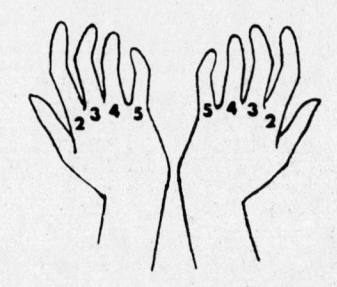

Art of touch. In the Touch Exercises, we will use fingers 2, 3, 4, and 5. Later on, when you practice stroking, you will use only fingers 3, 4, and 5. Thumbs are not used. Keep them out of the way, resting lightly under your palms. When finger 2 is indicated for any exercise, use the second finger of both hands. Do the same for fingers 3, 4 and 5. Curve your fingers just as a pianist does. It is important that the cushions of your fingers (and not your nails) rest lightly on your face.

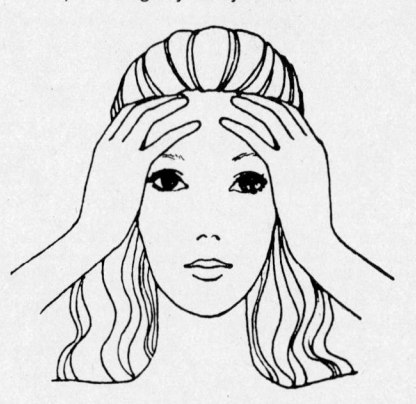

- Begin by placing fingers 2, 3, 4, 5 of both hands on your forehead below hairline. Position No. 1. Do this so lightly that you feel no pressure or contact at all.

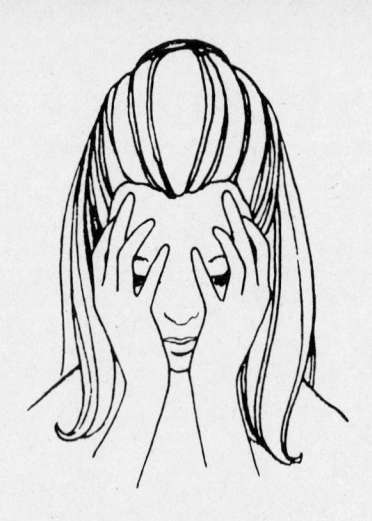

Touch Procedure No. 1. Move finger 2 of both hands up and back. Feel no pressure. Now move finger 3 of both hands up and back. Feel no pressure. Follow with finger 4, of both hands, then finger 5—up and back. Feel no pressure.

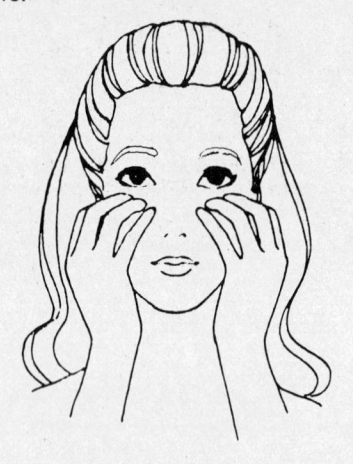

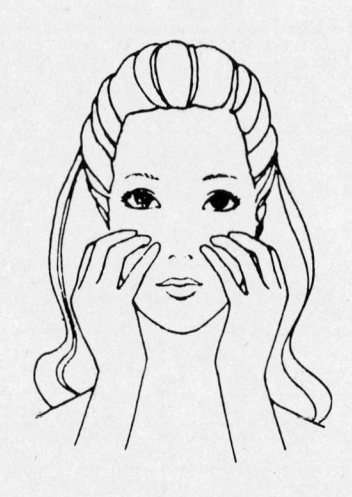

- Place fingers 2, 3, 4, 5 on cheekbones. Repeat Touch Procedure No. 1.

- Move down one inch on cheekbones. Repeat Touch Procedure No. 1.

🌿 Place fingers 2, 3, 4, 5 on contour area of chin. Repeat Touch Procedure No. 1.

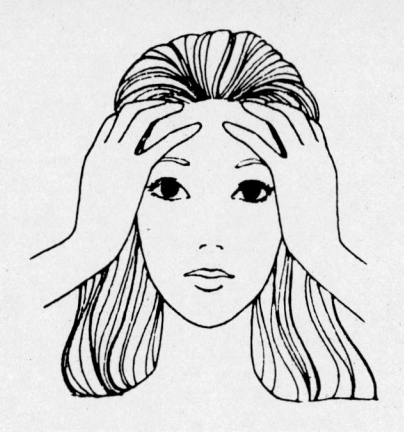

🌿 Return fingers 2, 3, 4, 5 of both hands to forehead close to hairline. Move fingers of both hands together in Touch Procedure No. 2.

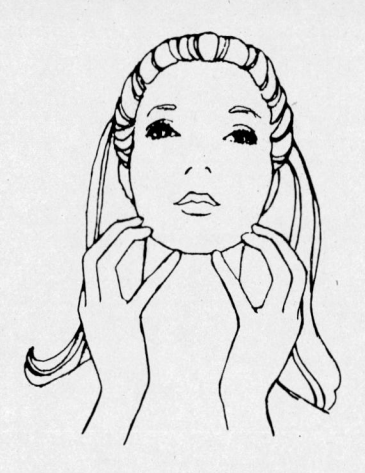

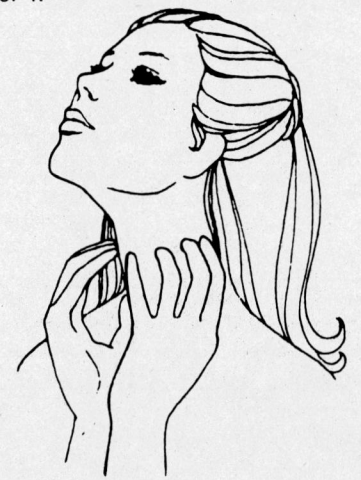

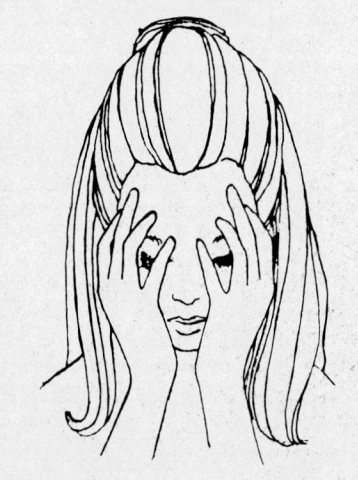

🌿 Place fingers 2, 3, 4, 5 on neck. Repeat Touch Procedure No. 1.

🌿 Move fingers one inch lower and repeat Touch Procedure No. 2.
🌿 Repeat—cheekbones, chin and neck (as earlier) with Touch Procedure No. 2.

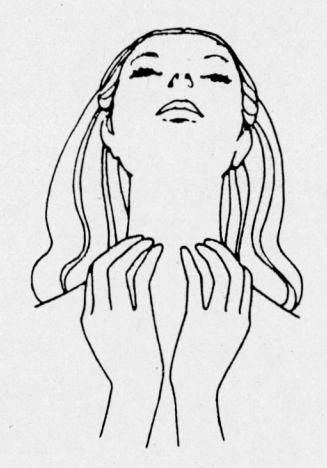

🌿 Move fingers down one inch and repeat Touch Procedure No. 1.

Touch Procedure No. 2. Move—all together—fingers 2, 3, 4, 5 of both hands up and back. Covering an area of about an inch. Feel no pressure; little contact.

Your stroking strategy. Stroking is the most delicate kind of massage, carried out in a soothing rhythm, consistent and relaxed. It is based upon the touch exercises. Your goals in stroking strategy are three:

🌿 To relax completely the muscles of facial expression, called the mimetic muscles. You accomplish this artfully, muscle by muscle.

🌿 To help erase from your face all extraneous expressions but one—young, smooth serenity. (Extraneous expressions mean those that you *want* to dispense with: Worry, dismay, tension, anxiety, hopelessness, and agitation. It is these expressions, collected over a lifetime, that prematurely trace lines on the face.)

🌿 To banish most of the distressing facial lines caused by these aging facial tensions.

Now, you may be asking: *"If stroking is so gentle and delicate, how can it possibly eliminate facial problems such as lines?"*

To answer, it is only the lightest finger approach, and the most consistent one, that relaxes tensed-up, rigid, and inflexible lines. Once they are relaxed, the lines seem to fade away from your face by themselves.

How often do you stroke? Stroke as soon as you open your eyes each morning—just for a minute or so. It's a delightful, positive way to start the day.

How much do you stroke? The accompanying chart will advise you how many minutes each day to devote to stroking. It is based on the average requirements of various age groups.

DAILY AMOUNT OF STROKING TIME
(in minutes)

Condition of face and neck	25 to 30	30 to 35	35 to 40	40 to 45	45 to 50	50 to 55	55 to 60	60 to 70	70 to 80
Poor	8	10 to 12	12	12	15	18	20	25	30
Fair	6	8	8	10	12	15	18	20	25
Good	4	6	6	8	10	13	15	18	22
Excellent	2	5	5	6	8	10	12	15	18

Let us take a few examples that show you how to use the chart on the preceding page to best advantage:

🌺 If, for example, you are in the 30- to 35-year-old group yet are singularly untouched facially, lean toward the stroking requirement for the age group below you. In other words, you need stroke only two minutes a day. If there is any question, however, stroke a few minutes longer each day.

🌺 If you are in the 40- to 45-year-old group but your face has deteriorated severely, put in a little extra time every day. Do as much as the next age group —say, 15 minutes a day. You may, of course, divide these stroking sessions up into, for example, three sessions a day of five minutes each.

🌺 By the same token, stroke the amount of time listed for an older group if you wish speedier results—more effectiveness—no matter what your age.

Here are your stroking patterns. Use them at least two minutes every day.

Stroking patterns. (Minimum of 10 strokes a day.)

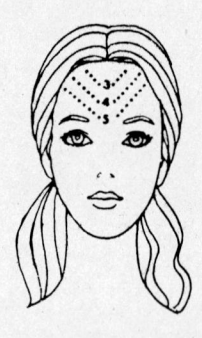

🌺 Use fingers 3, 4, 5 of each hand. Stroke letter V.

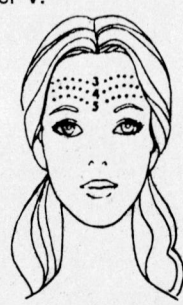

🌺 Use fingers 3, 4, 5. Stroke letter M.

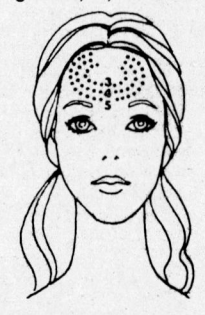

🌺 Fingers 3, 4, 5. Stroke letter C.

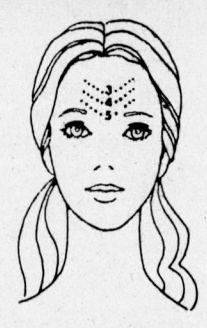

🌺 Fingers 3, 4, 5. Brush-stroke—in one-half-inch short strokes—small letter v.

The Basic "Woo" position. The following motions all require the face to be in "augmented" posture, or Basic "Woo" position. Here is how you achieve it:

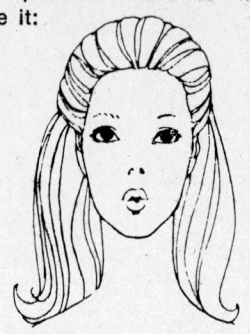

🌺 Relax your lips into a semiwhistle position.

🌺 Keeping your lips pursed, pull your chin down; you'll find this leaves your mouth open slightly. If you try to speak in this position, the sound you utter will arise deep in your throat, very much like the syllable *"woo!"* Hence, its name. (Of course, you need not make the sound "woo" every time you take the Basic "Woo" position.)

The Basic "Woo" position may be used as an exercise itself:

🌺 Take the Basic "Woo" position. Think *up*—and think *out*—think *up*—think *out*—push *up* and push *out*.

🌺 Hold this position to the count of five; then, very slowly, relax your face. When you do this exercise correctly, your face will feel tired after you have repeated it a few times. Therefore, practice for only a few minutes and then rest for awhile.

Basic "Woo" is a very important facial posture. It helps avoid the loss of facial structure that often comes with time. It also is a strenghening posture. People with unexercised faces should work gradually with this position. So, be sure *not to overdo*.

The tiny pucker lines you see above your mouth when it is in Basic "Woo" need not disturb you. They are an indication of weak muscles around your mouth and will be considerably or altogether eliminated by practice of exercises for the mouth. These lines can be reduced only by *concentrated relaxing* of the mouth into Basic "Woo" position. Do not purse lips tightly. When the Basic "Woo" is done correctly, with the mouth *relaxed* into the posture, the lines do not appear.

Because the Basic "Woo" position may seem tiring at first, do only three of these stroking exercises each day for the first week. (Do the first three exercises the first day. Then second three the second day, and so on.) After the first week, your face will get used to this position, you will find it more comfortable, and you may then do all the exercises every day.

Stroking exercises. For these exercises the face is in Basic "Woo" position:

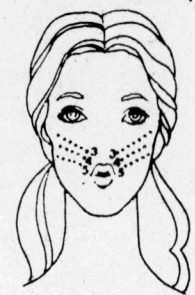

🌺 Fingers 3, 4, 5. Stroke V (up only).

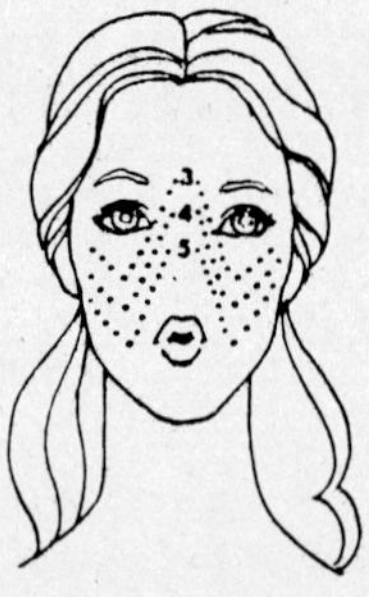

🌺 Fingers 3, 4, 5. Stroke letter W.

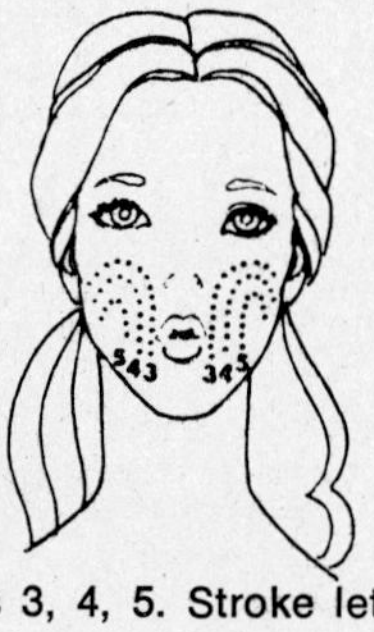

🌺 Fingers 3, 4, 5. Stroke letter M.

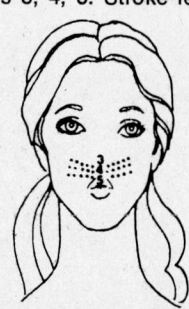

🌺 Fingers 3, 4, 5. Brush-stroke the upper lip in one-half-inch short strokes—small letter v.

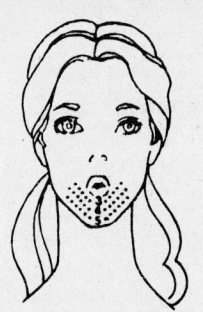

🌸 Fingers 3, 4, 5. Stroke letter V.

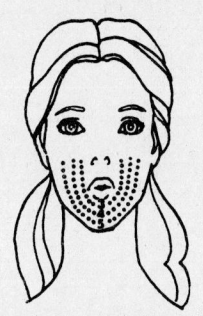

🌸 Fingers 3, 4, 5. Stroke letter U.

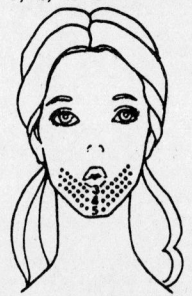

🌸 Fingers 3, 4, 5. Brush-stroke letter V.

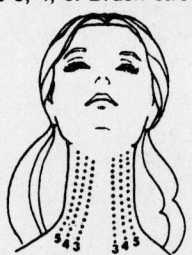

🌸 Right hand, fingers 3, 4, 5. Stroke letter I, left side of neck. Left hand, fingers 3, 4, 5. Stroke letter I, right side of neck.

"Structured" cream technique. One face cream is not enough to lubricate the skin correctly. Use three for this creaming technique. Cream No. 1 (base layer) should be of a heavier consistency than Cream No. 2 (the middle layer), with Cream No. 3 an oil.

🌸 Expose neck and throat. Cover your hair or pull it back from your forehead.

🌸 Take Cream No. 1 (the base layer) with your second finger and apply about a teaspoonful of it in a pattern of small dots to face and neck.

🌸 Repeat the same technique with Cream No. 2 (the middle layer).

🌸 Pour a quarter teaspoonful of Oil No. 3 into each palm.

🌸 Take the Basic "Woo" position and use the hand position shown here.

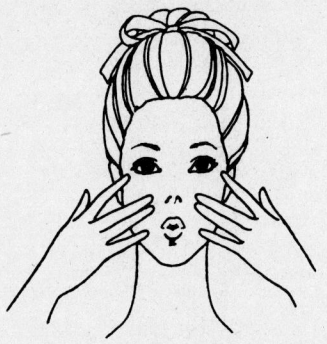

🌸 Then slowly stroke, first using fingers 3, 4, and 5 of both hands, in this pattern:

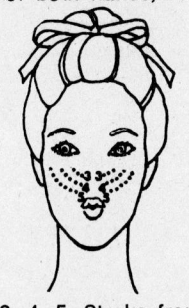

🌸 Fingers 3, 4, 5. Stroke from nostrils toward ears five times.

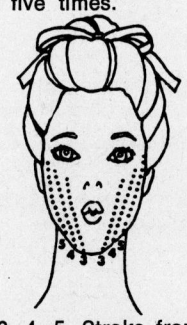

🌸 Fingers 3, 4, 5. Stroke from chin to temple five times.

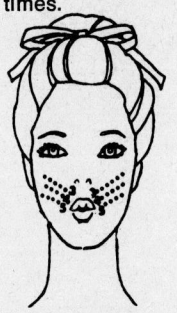

🌸 Fingers 3 and 4. Brush-stroke upper lip five times.

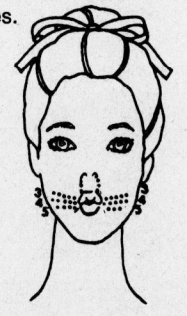

🌸 Fingers 3 and 4. Brush-stroke mouth corners five times.

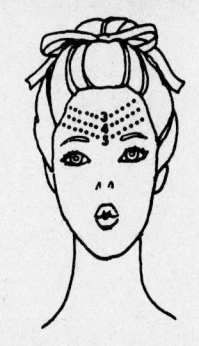

🌸 Fingers 3, 4, 5. Stroke forehead—letters V, W, M—five times each.

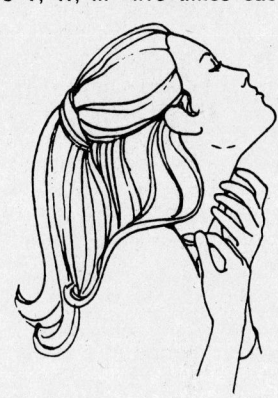

🌸 Lean head back, place lower lip over the upper lip. Use fingers 3, 4, 5. With left hand pressing the left collarbone, stroke upward with the right hand on throat five times; reverse hands, and with the right hand pressing the right collarbone, stroke upward on the throat with the left hand five times.

No stroking of area under eyes. Here, you merely dot creams on—at least one-quarter inch away from your eyelids.

Creams should be left on for a minimum of 15 minutes. Dry, normal-dry, or mature skin will profit from using the technique at least three times a week.

Any cream left on your hands should be applied to the throat in this way: While the left hand is firmly pressing the left collarbone, the right hand will stroke upward, a minimum of five times. Hands then alternate, right hand pressing down on the right collarbone, the left hand stroking upward, a minimum of five times.

With tissue, pat away the cream gently: Unfold a tissue and place it over the face. Pat gently to remove excess cream; repeat with fresh tissue. Unfold another fresh tissue and touch lightly to the corners of the eye, the nostrils, and the sides of mouth to remove excess cream at these points.

An ideal conclusion for the structured cream treatment is an ice-water treatment, followed by just a touch of Cream No. 2 beneath your eyes. Result—a glowing face!

THE TOTAL LOOK OF BEAUTY

"Beauty is an attitude," says Pablo Manzoni, creative director for Elizabeth Arden. "It consists of confidence, charm and being attractive by feeling attractive.

🌿 Beauty is individuality, and so it makes sense to be honest about yourself. Take the courage to sit in front of a mirror and play up the qualities of a good feature; emphasize what you like most, disregarding what you like least.

🌿 Get away from any inferiority complex about your looks. Stop saying: 'I hate my nose' or 'my chin, my hair'—or whatever. I believe no beautiful woman today is without a little facial fault—but one remembers her for other reasons. Because she looks at you directly. She listens when you speak. She has something interesting to say. She smiles freely. She is self-confident.

🌿 When a makeup artist looks at a face, he thinks only of what he likes about it—and goes on from there. I never feel that I have to correct a face—or use shading and highlighting to change it. I only try to bring out what is interesting.

🌿 You begin with a face, your own. Hair—and the way you wear it—can do much to improve the shape of your face. But, like makeup, it should not do away with the distinctive features that are all your own and individualize you.

🌿 And you needn't try to achieve one look that is right for you all the time. It won't be. You have many facets, different moods. At times you are romantic, at times glamorous, at times simple. There is no standard.

🌿 The psychology of beauty is really being able to feel good about yourself. When you wear something new, you instantly become more stimulated and alive. When you put on a makeup you like, you respond like a new person. You open out more and live for a while in a new dimension. Perfume also gives you this sense of being whole and beautiful. Wear it on your body so the scent keeps rising and gives *you* pleasure.

🌿 Perfume, makeup, clothes—they are all a way of expressing yourself.

🌿 Whatever you do for yourself contributes to your sense of well-being and gives you confidence. Then others are stimulated by your own assurance that

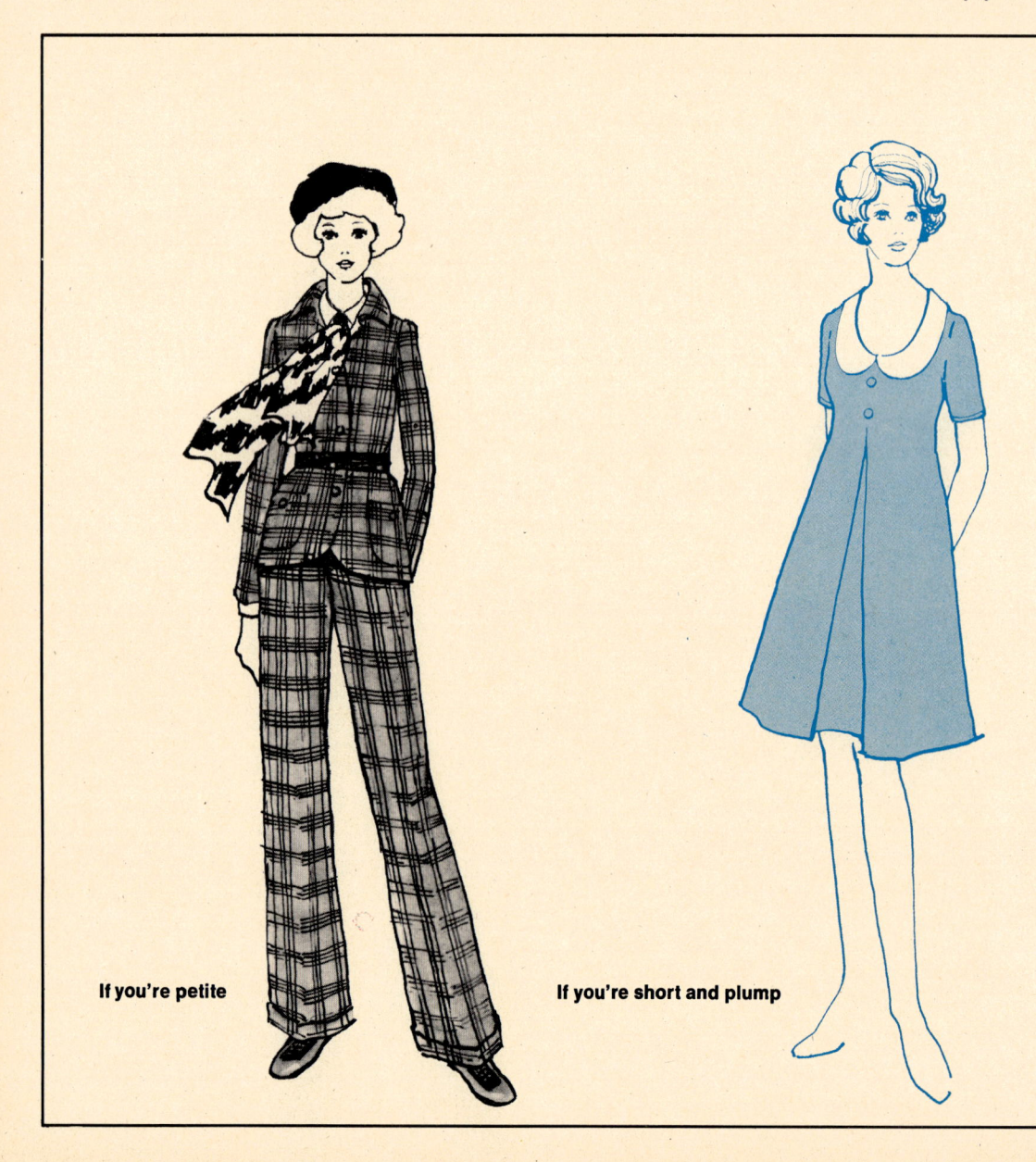

If you're petite

If you're short and plump

you are attractive. They admire you.

"Luckily, this is a time when there's an open choice about what you wear: Heels can be high or low, chunky, slim or wedges; skirts mini, maxi or to the knee; pants and shorts—wear either/or; put your waist where you want it— empire or belted high, low or in the middle. Belts can be wide or stringy, or you can borrow one of your husband's flashy ties for a sash. Even the elegant "little" dress and glamour evening gown are back. You needn't come out as a carbon copy of anyone. Instead, pick what's becoming to you and fits your life-style. Does this make putting yourself together easier? Or harder? If you've been dressing like everyone else, you now need to make discoveries about your individuality. First step is to get rid of any anxieties about being *too* anything—too short, too tall, too thick in the middle. You are *you* and now have the chance to make the most of your individual looks. The idea is to create your own image—a picture of yourself, your own look. Sometimes all that is needed to turn a look into a great look is a little change—in eyeglass frames, a tendril of hair at the ear, a scarf or a jewel. Apply good taste and good sense and emphasize the part of your body that is most important to you. There may be little you can do to change your face or your shape but much you can do to improve them.

If you're petite. Keep things in proportion; nothing too big. No puffy sleeves, flaring collars or oversized handbags. A favored look for the small, well-proportioned woman is that of the little boy—tailored, neat, with little buttons. You'll look great in tailored pants suits, little shorts, a short skirt with a slash. Keep shoes, boots slim.

If you're short and plump. Avoid loud colors and very tailored clothes, instead look warm and cuddly. And be careful not to load on too much—chunky shoes, for example, could be too much. If you wear necklaces or chain belts, wear *fewer* than a tall girl would. No busy hairdo with a bouffant skirt.

If you're tall. Take advantage of styles that only you can wear. The chubby jacket or shawl (popular again) looks best on a tall, thin figure, especially with a clingy, crepe, pencil-slim long skirt below. It gives the impression of a flower on a stem—slim below and full at the top. You can also carry off the flappy trenchcoat, long full hair, big sleeves. Don't slump. High-fashion looks are designed for a girl like you.

Heavy thighs. Forget about Bermuda shorts, little pants, short-short skirts.

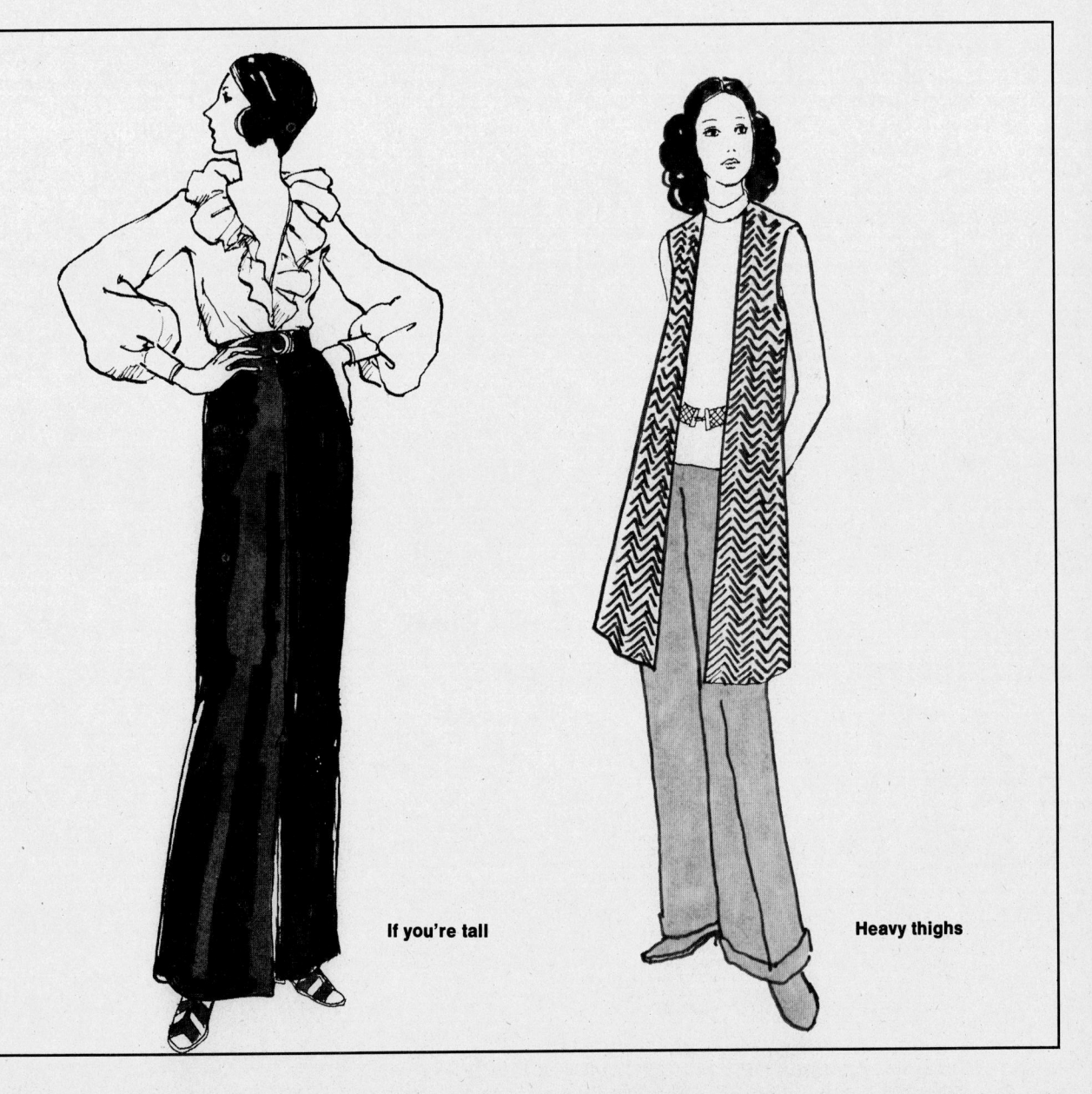

If you're tall

Heavy thighs

Knickers are good. So are pants with a long tunic top. Wraparound skirts of a fabric with some body are also good. Avoid clingy material.

Heavy legs and ankles. Camouflage them with boots, pants suits, midi skirts. Wide shoulders and wide belts help bring any heaviness below into balance.

Thick waist. A high waistline with the skirt falling straight down or with a slight flare will be becoming. As an alternative, belt your dresses low on the hips. A battle (Eisenhower) jacket over a straight dress or a dress with an A-shape skirt also camouflages a thick waist.

Oversized breasts. Wraparound blouses are a fine style; they don't make the breasts appear smaller but rather more in proportion—and they are comfortable. Avoid anything too tight (unless you want to emphasize fullness), high collars, gathers at neckline. Sleeves, especially full sleeves, help balance the bosom, so avoid sleeveless tops. A deep oval neckline is becoming. You can also wear a high waist with gatherings beneath the breasts over a trapeze skirt that falls with fullness or flare at the hemline.

Small bosom. An empire waist that is fitted close beneath the breasts makes average-sized breasts appear fuller. But it's better, if you are small-breasted, to capitalize on the flat-chested look that many of today's fashions are designed for. You can wear the skinny tank tops in clingy materials, sleeveless outfits, a long-waisted '20s-style dress with a low belt and bottom ruffle. Don't let public opinion get you down; the small-breasted woman *can* have glamour.

Short neck. Show all the neck you can. Pile hair up on the top of the head, wear necklines that are low in back as well as in front, or T-shirt necklines. Avoid high collars, turtlenecks, long, low-falling hair, neck scarves, neckbands, chokers, anything that makes you look hunched up. Slightly capped sleeves are helpful in creating balance.

Long neck. A neck can never be too long; it's a beauty asset and shouldn't be considered a problem. It allows you to wear a variety of styles beautifully— a low chignon, turtlenecks, long hair, neckbands, long earrings. Consider yourself lucky.

❧ While camouflaging what you think of as a figure problem, call attention to whatever you have that is an asset; it may be long slim legs, a tiny waist, very white teeth, long fingers or pretty hands (emphasize with many amusing

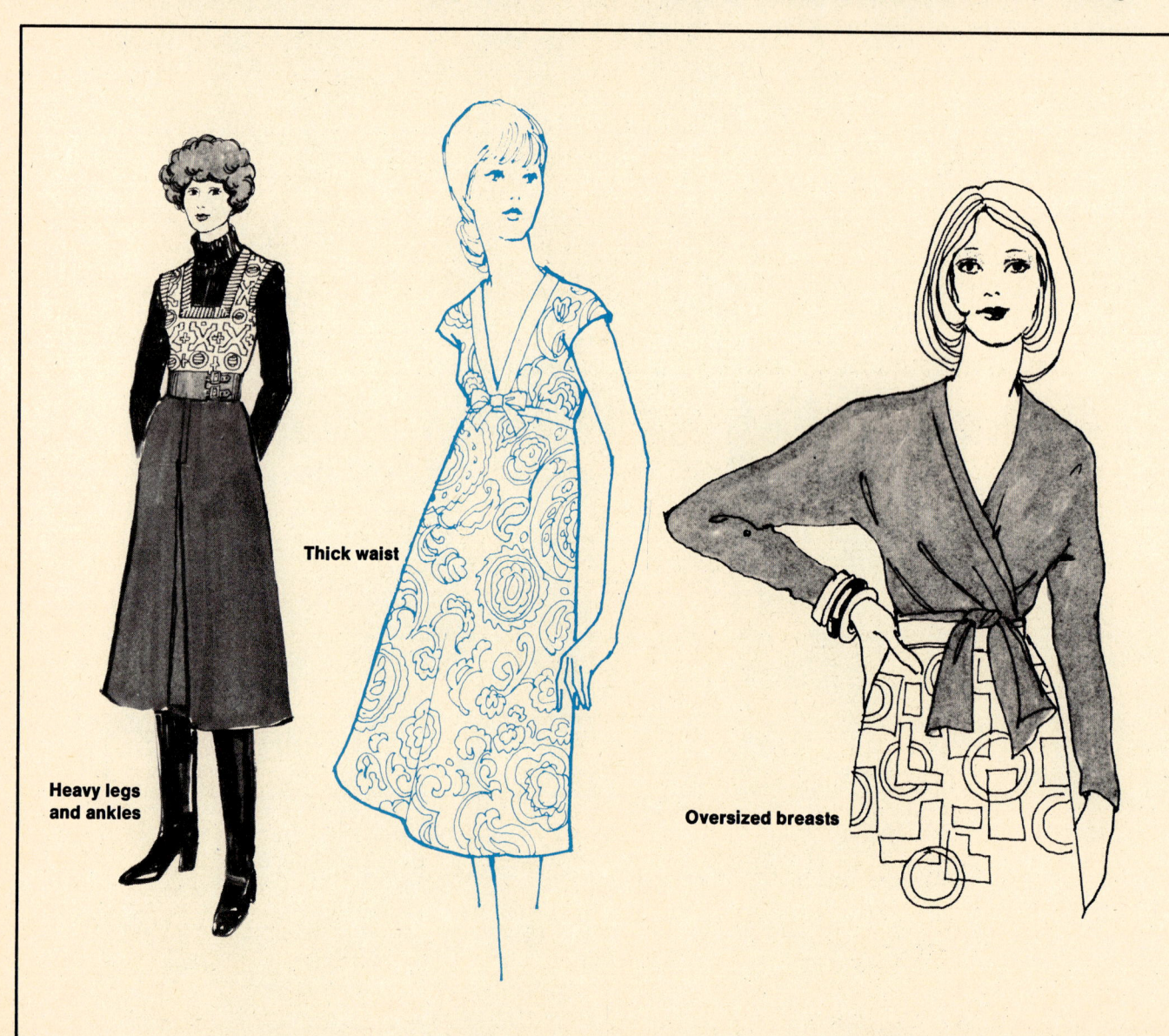

Heavy legs and ankles

Thick waist

Oversized breasts

rings), shapely hips, beautiful eyes. Keep in mind your total look."

SLIM-AND-TRIM EYE-FOOLERS

We are likely to think of our own head as being smaller than it is in proportion to the body. Because of the way we see ourselves, it is easy to unbalance the silhouette with a hairdo or hat that is too big for the figure it crowns. We often also fail to realize how large our hands appear to others. Watch these factors when you try to fool another's eye:

🌸 Keep hat, hair style, handbag, glove length, jewelry, heel height, and collars in proportion to the figure as a whole. Don't look at just one part of yourself—the head for a hat, the feet for a pair of shoes—when you buy or when you dress. See yourself as a whole—full length in a mirror and from *all* angles.

🌸 Wear hair high at back to stretch the neck visually. In a cap hair style, comb the bottom hair down and toward the ear at each side to hug the nape and to follow the curve of the head.

🌸 Dark foundation on the throat helps the face to stand out and "slims" the throat. Carry the foundation to the base of the throat and fan out toward the neckline. If a pale V under the chin is creating the appearance of a double chin, cover this area with a dark shade of foundation and use light foundation along the jaw line.

🌸 In your dress, fit the natural waistline and the shoulders and have the hemline and heel height in the correct length; then your figure will balance.

🌸 Keep any color note to one area—scarf, shoes, hat, *or* belt—and if you are short, keep the color note high, at throat or shoulder or on your head. Don't break up the silhouette with many patches of color.

🌸 Stick to one "eye catcher" in other ways, too. Don't overload yourself with jewelry, scarves, bows, and flowers.

🌸 Avoid both bunchiness and overtightness in any area you wish to slim. The princess line in a dress is most slimming; bulk *anywhere* will add bulk to that part of the silhouette.

🌸 Dark, neutral, and solid colors are slimming; light colors, bright colors, and prints add bulk.

🌸 Sleeve length can save your silhouette. For slimness, choose a sleeveless dress, a short cap sleeve, or a long fitted sleeve. If arms are heavy, wear a three-quarter or below-the-elbow sleeve. Avoid a sleeve that cuts the upper arm in half.

🌸 Shorty gloves are slimming and should be chosen by the little woman to wear with sleeveless or cap-sleeve dresses; with three-quarter or elbow-length sleeves, the glove should reach

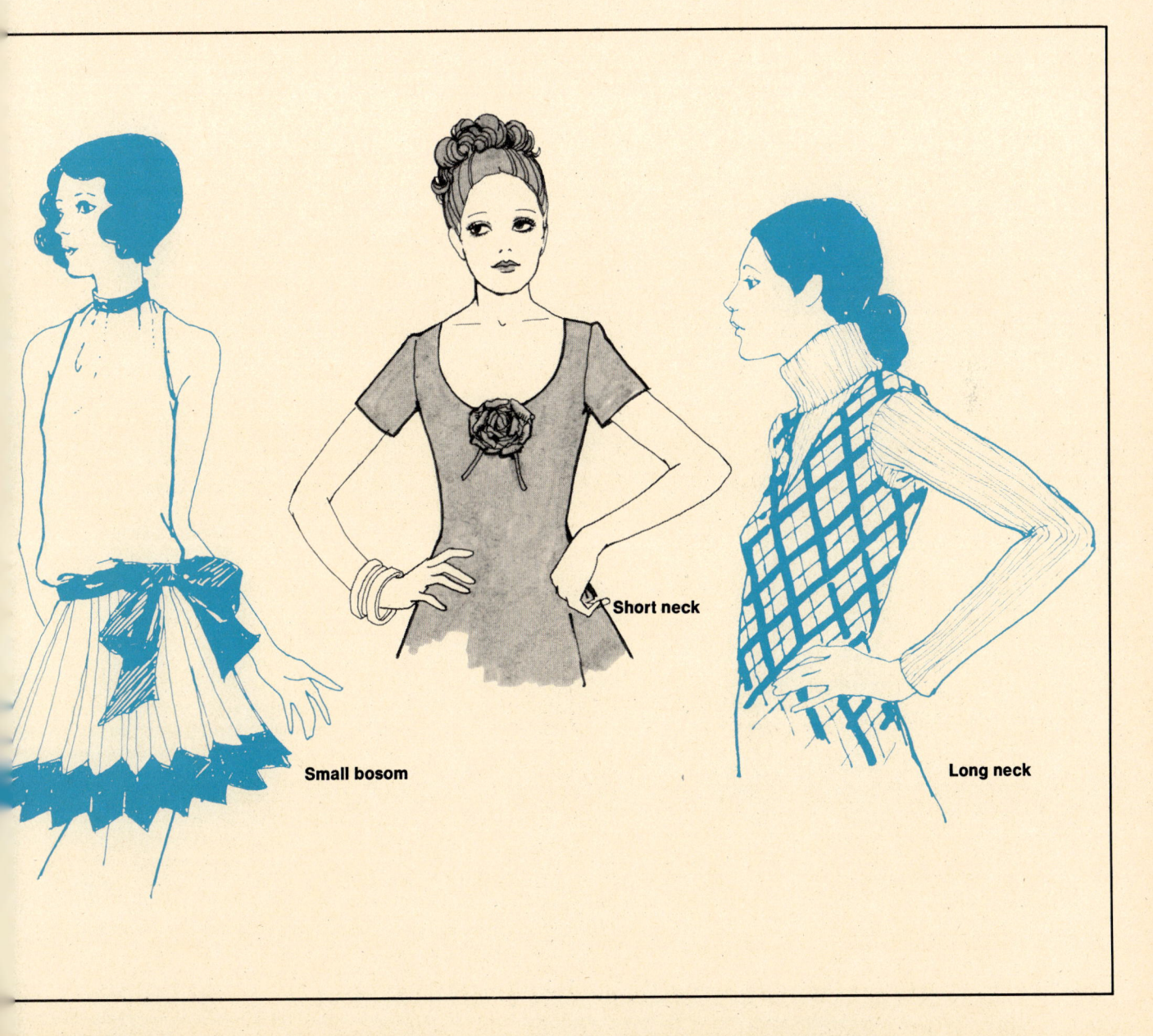

Small bosom

Short neck

Long neck

the hem of the sleeve. Gauntlet-type gloves should be worn only by the tall woman. White and bright-color gloves exaggerate hand size; if hands are large, wear gloves to match the costume color.

✄ Skirts should be in the length that is currently fashionable. There is always a becoming fashion length for your figure size.

✄ Strap shoes make the legs seem shorter; a slim pump in the same color as your stockings will make the legs seem longer.

✄ The portrait neckline, the V-neck front *and* back, and the scoop neckline are slimming. The cowl neckline and high collar make the neck and throat appear shorter. If neck is short, avoid choker necklaces and expose the ears to slim and lengthen the throat. The long bob and the low chignon are becoming only when throat is long.

✄ Stand with a long line forward to make the slimmest impression; carry the rib cage up, the shoulders down, and shoulder blades spread, and try to touch the ceiling with the back of the head.

✄ Keep legs close together with one foot slightly ahead of the other and one hip and one shoulder slightly forward to have this long-line look.

TAKE YOUR MEASURE

Because we all are built differently, it is hard to say what is "ideal" and it is often hard to decide even what is "average." So find your own "ideal" by analyzing your figure and comparing it to the "average" or to the "ideal."

Are you below or above average height?

✄ If you are 5′1½″ or under, you are considered *short.*

✄ If you are 5′1½″ to 5′3″, you are *moderately short.*

✄ If you are 5′3″ to 5′5″, you are *average.*

✄ If you are 5′5″ to 5′6½″, you are *moderately tall.*

✄ If you are 5′7″ or over, you may call yourself a *tall* girl.

Consider proportion. You also have to consider *where* you are long or short. Are you long through the waist? The lower legs? The back? The thighs? The neck? Or are you short in any of these areas? Or are you fairly well proportioned throughout?

Women's fashions are made according to certain basic "bodies" that take into account this difference in proportion of the female figure.

✄ The short-waisted figure is called a "junior" and is built according to these proportions for an average. size-11 figure:

Height without shoes 5′4″-5′5″
Bust 33½″
Waist 25½″
Hip 35½″
Length of waist in back 15¾″

✄ The regular "misses" figure is longer waisted and has these proportions for a size-12 figure:

Height 5′5″-5′6″
Bust 34″
Waist 26½″
Hip 36″
Length of waist in back 16¼″

✄ The short-waisted fuller "woman's figure" is labeled "half-size" and has these proportions for a size-16½ figure:

Height 5′2″-5′3″
Bust 39″
Waist 33″
Hip 41″
Length of waist in back 15¾″

✄ The regular "woman's figure" is again fuller but longer-waisted. For a size-40 figure:

Height 5′5″-5′6″
Bust 44″
Waist 37″
Hip 46″
Length of waist in back 17⅜″

These are realistic sizes for "average" women, but ideally our measurements are a little different. It is good to strive for something like the following:

✄ The waist 4 to 4½ times the wrist measurement, with the bust and hips 10 inches larger than the waist.

✄ The ankle 1¼ times the wrist measurement and the calf 2¼ times the wrist measurement.

WHAT'S YOUR FIGURE TYPE?

The "ideal" feminine shape is an ellipse —an elongated oval. Just as hairdo and mouth and eye makeup balance the face to approximate the "ideal" oval, so the figure can be balanced toward this "ideal" ellipse. In actuality women are, of course, of many shapes and sizes, many heights and body builds; fashion also wanders all over in its choice of silhouette for any particular year and season. So whatever your basic shape, you will at sometime or other (if you are the right weight) have the figure type that is in vogue. And from the cycle of fashion silhouettes you can be guided to the style that will (again, if you are of the right weight for it) flatter your figure type.

The rounds. Round and pear-shape figures tend toward curves and toward putting on fat rather than muscle. Women with such body shape sometimes lack "bounce," and inactivity may add to their weight problem.

✄ Both figures look best when the natural waistline is fitted and the skirt is easy across the hips. Skirt should be long and full enough to cover the top of the knees when you sit. A cinched-in waist gives you shape.

Round—This figure is usually average or below-average (under 5′5″) in height and small boned; the "round" woman may take pride in her tiny feet and wrists, and her waist often is tiny, too. If not, it *should be.* Work on the waist-whittling exercises to give yourself littleness here. Fashion's version of the *round* silhouette is the short dirndl skirt and puff-sleeve peasant blouse, and a round hairdo.

Pear-shape—Short-waisted and measuring two or more inches larger at the hips than at the bust, this figure is usually long through the thighs and lower legs. Because this figure "runs to hippiness," fat easily accumulates in the buttocks and thighs. Walk as much as you can and sit as little as possible to keep the hips slimmed. Fashion approximates the pear-shape in the small slope-shouldered fitted bodice and ballerina skirt, slicked-back pony-tail hairdo or high topknot, and slim flat slippers.

The ovals. Both the small oval figure and the more elongated elliptical figure are well balanced in height and width. Bust and hips measure about the same, with the waist 10 inches smaller; the waist is fairly long (about 16½ inches from nape to waist at the back for a 5′5″ height). Both figures are compact, firm-muscled; the smaller and shorter oval is curvier and may become plump, though during youth overweight is usually not a problem. Both types are fairly active and have a good supply of energy. The smaller oval is the "ideal" little-woman figure; the ellipse is taller (5′5″ or over) and wears "misses" fashions becomingly.

✄ Both ovals and ellipses should work on figure-firming exercises; though these women rarely have a weight problem in youth, pounds can sometimes creep up unexpectedly after 35.

Oval—Small-boned or with a medium frame and below-average or average in height, the oval is the smaller, more "feminine" version of today's "ideal" figure. In fashion the oval is represented by rounded shoulders and slim bodice, easy waist, and peg skirt; the oval cap or medium-full hair style goes with it.

Ellipse—The taller ellipse is well made,

well muscled and of average or medium-tall height with a medium frame. The overblouse with slightly rounded shoulders, the slim skirt, and a hairdo that tends toward the bouffant are fashion indicators of this classic figure.

The squares. The square and oblong types are likely to have large bones, to be energetic, and to run to muscle rather than to fat. Both figures look well in tailored clothes; both need diet control so as not to become "beefy" and both should avoid overdevelopment of muscles while firming them. In fashion, strive toward a "tailored" look and for simplicity in accessories.

Square—Usually of average or below-average height, this figure tends to be heavy at the waist; exercise for waist slenderness. Watch out, too, for heavy foods in the diet. We have the square shape in fashion when we wear the boxy jacket with squared shoulders and a short straight skirt. Shoes are usually square-toed with this fashion phase; handbags are tailored; and the hairdo tends toward a low pompadour or a short pageboy bob.

Oblong—Often slim and well-muscled (but sometimes flat-chested) and usually above average height, this figure may have a problem of underweight. But oblongs can be heavies, too, and care should be taken not to weigh an ounce more than is "ideal." In fashion, the oblong is represented by the A-line skirt with easy jacket and straight (but not wide) shoulders, the full coat, and the portrait neckline.

The slims. The triangle and the stringbean figure types are usually tall and naturally slender. Both should watch posture so as not to slump or to slouch. Both should take care to keep hem length, hat, shoes, and handbags in proportion to the figure. Both have the satisfaction of looking well in most fashions.

The triangle—Here shoulders are broad and hips are slim. In fashion this figure is created by wide (often padded-out) shoulders and the hip-length fitted jacket with a slim skirt. Waistline is often easy. Hair is usually worn fairly full and below ear length.

The stringbean—Usually tall and often underweight, this is the fashion-model figure. Care should be taken to become posture-perfect and to acquire body grace. In fashion this figure is seen in the shift and the sheath. Hair style, whether long or short, is usually close to the head. Only the stringbean should dare to wear styles that are bunchy round the middle; she can also comfortably wear a high waistline.

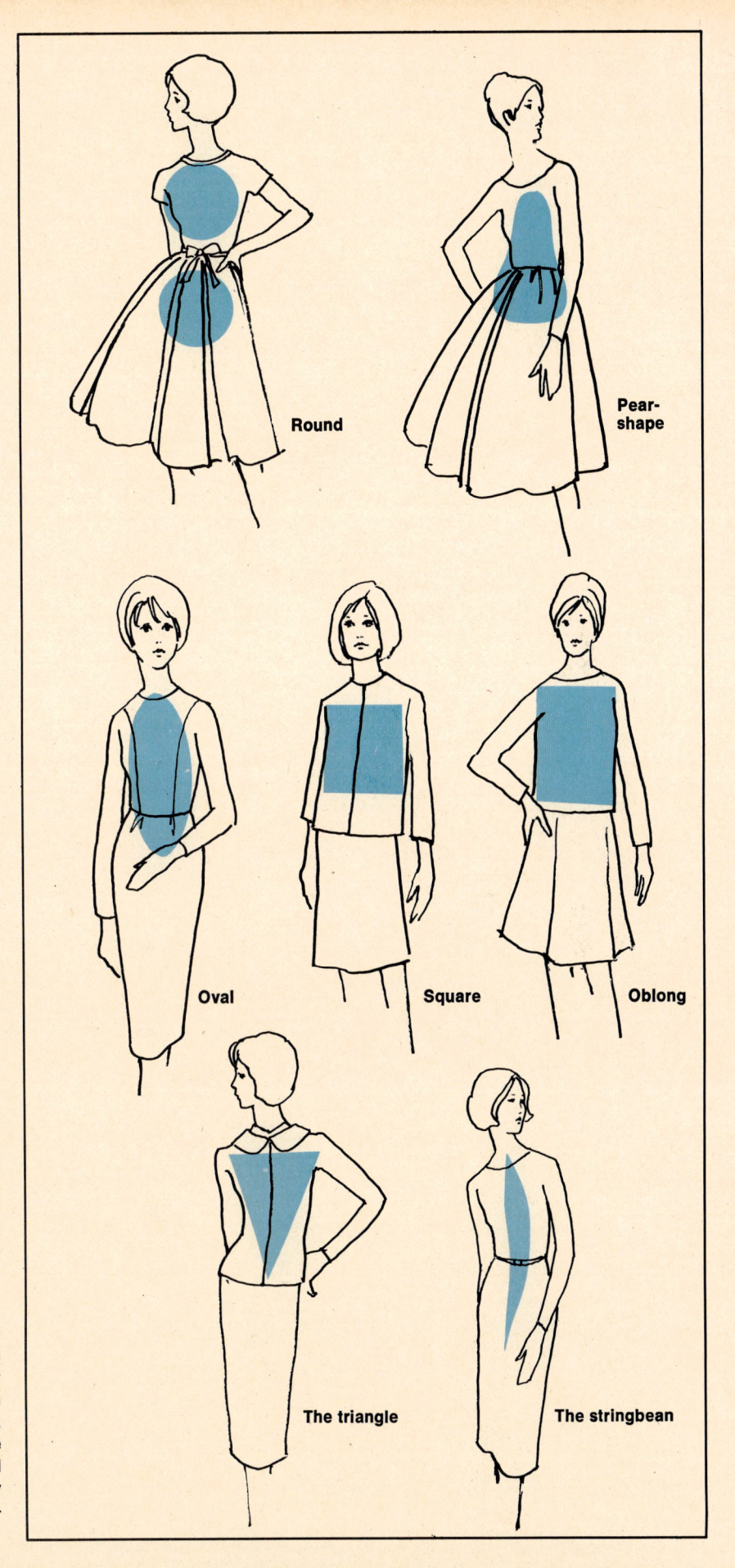

HOW TO LOOK PRETTIER IN A PICTURE

Perhaps the most important secret of beauty before the little black box is the ability to feel relaxed—whether you are posing or taken by surprise. You will feel more at ease if you know what to do with your arms, your legs, and your head. Then your face will almost take care of itself.

Snapshots. Relaxation is the key to a natural look in snapshots: A sitting or kneeling position often feels more relaxed than a standing pose. When you can't sit, lean against a tree, a fence, or a low wall. Make use of hand action as often as you can. Adjust your hat or gloves, touch some flowers—props of any kind are a help in relaxing your hands.

✤ Focus your attention on an object or person alongside or behind the photographer, but do not stare fixedly at one point. If you must be photographed in bright sunlight, keep your eyes shut till the picture is about to be snapped and then open your eyes at the photographer's cue.

✤ Get into the mood of the picture: If you are to be photographed against a landscape, ask the photographer if he wants you or the view. If he wants you simply as a foreground figure, look toward the view, not toward the camera. Be sure that you stand at an angle to the camera; avoid direct views, front or back.

✤ If you are pictured against a low wall or a car or other large object, rest on it or half sit on it and lean forward from the waist, keeping the head up, the chin lifted; this helps lift your figure out of the background.

✤ If you are photographed against an interesting and active background, again ask the cameraman whether he wants you or the setting. If he wants the setting, you might better stay out of the photo. If you are to be in it, work out a natural action that makes you a part of the activity. Don't simply stand by and look on.

✤ Choose the right clothes for your setting. A tourist's outfit, becoming as it may be, often looks out of place against quaint backgrounds or places of historical interest or even of scenic grandeur. Sometimes it is better to stay out of the picture than to appear as a sore thumb.

Scenery. If the camera is catching you and local color, join the scene by working out a natural action that helps you become part of the setting attractively. Do it charmingly—don't clown.

✤ Sitting helps you relax. A side view, with torso straight and chest high, is kind to the figure. Keep your head well up so your face catches the light. Hands clasped on the knees minimize leg faults. You need not always turn toward the camera. (If you do, look a little to one side of the cameraman.)

✤ Relate to any object you're photographed with. An interesting door? You will be slimmed if you stand partly behind it. Flowers? Get your face close to them, even sniff them—but don't pull back to gaze at them.

✤ When you stand beside a large object, keep the figure at a slight angle to the camera; a hand on the forward hip minimizes hip size. A place to lean makes for relaxation—a key to looking pretty in a picture. When photographed against a building or a high wall, don't stand close to it or lean

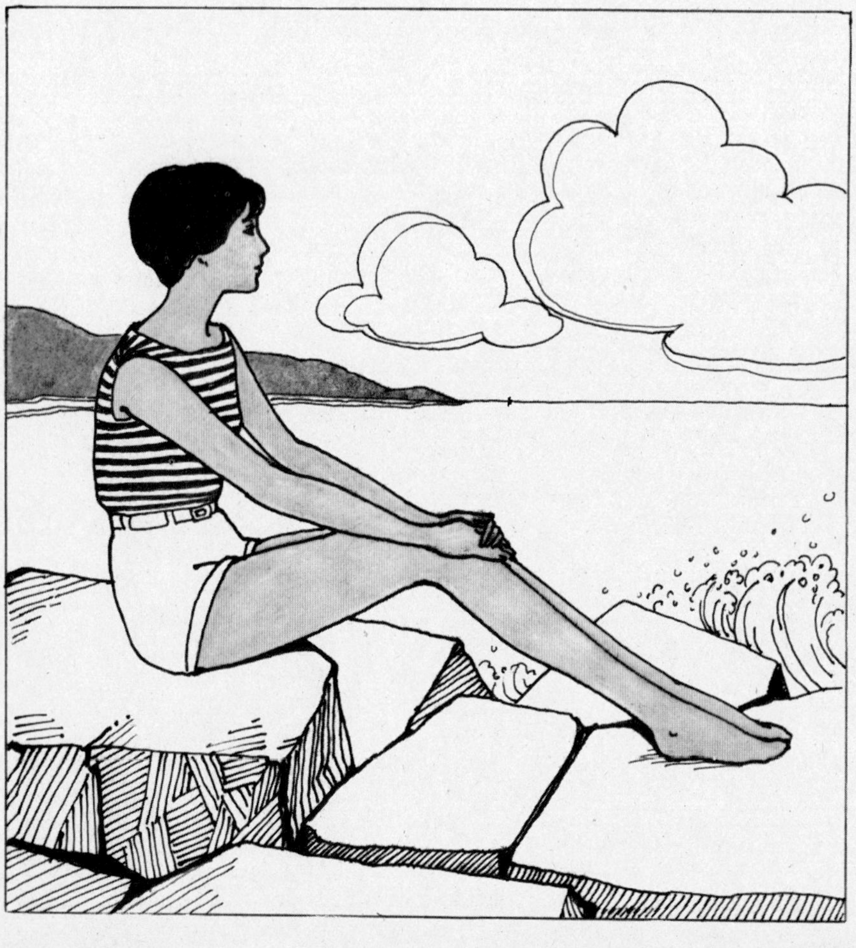

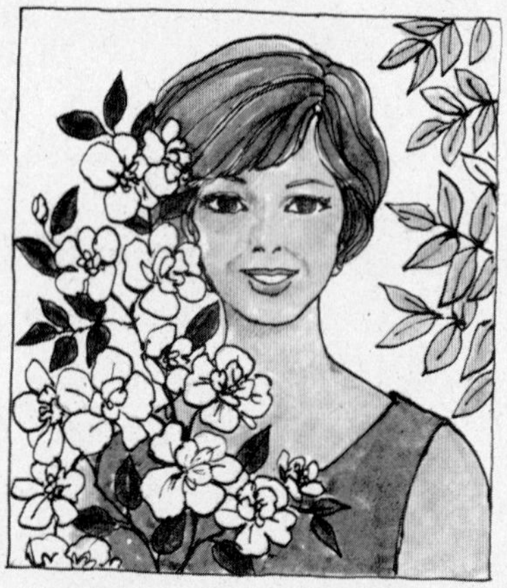

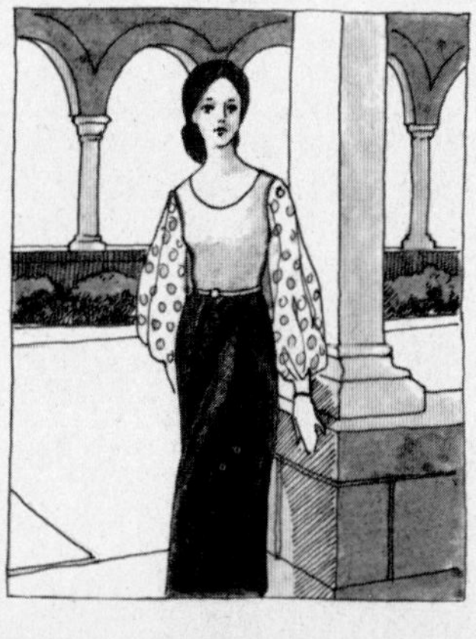

against it; to be a few feet in front of it is more flattering. The head bent back gives the face good light.

🌸 An interesting setting? Look toward the camera (but not directly into the lens), not at the scenery, and let the setting become your backdrop. Among columns, stand close to one, knees relaxed, one foot forward, taking care not to let the other hip jut—and relax.

Closeups. For a pretty face in a closeup or even at longer range, try these tricks: Seek back light—that is, have the back of your head toward the sun so you needn't squint and so your face won't crack up with lights and shadows. If you smile, keep it gentle to avoid lines in the face. Glasses or sunglasses are better off the face. Like backlighting, a wide-brim hat puts the face in shade. Be sure that the brim shades the whole face and doesn't cut it into halves of light and shadow.

Action shots. All beach photos need not be in swimsuits. If you have a figure problem, wear a becoming cover-up; a hat shades the face from harsh sand-and-sea light.

🌸 Standing with one foot in front of the other gives a long appealing leg line.

🌸 If you are photographed in a swimsuit while lying down, keep the torso a quarter turn away from the camera. Bring the top knee over the other and the top foot back; dropping one arm behind you prevents your looking all arms and legs.

🌸 Are you caught in action? Try not to overlap the figure of any companion, but don't separate completely. A side view defines your action; clothing that swings creates a feeling of movement.

🌸 Hand action is helpful in relaxing you for a photo. If you are to be photographed with a car, it is better to be inside, framed by the window, than to stand outside. Touch chin or hat for casual action. Your hair will stay back if you face into the wind and use your sunglasses as a hair holder.

Portraits. Posture practice helps you look slim and at ease before the camera: Keep the midriff slim by lifting the chest slightly and flattening and spreading the shoulder blades. Keep elbows and knees slightly bent, the elbows out a little from the sides of the body so that light shows between waist and arm, and the waist outline is defined. Keep the head up, the neck long at back, and tilt the top of the head away from the camera.

🌸 Standing, keep the torso at an angle to the camera so that one shoulder and one hip are somewhat back. Bring one knee forward a little over the other, one foot a little ahead of the other, and at a 45° angle to the other. When you sit, cross your legs below the knee or at the ankles, keeping the knees and feet close together. Legs that are crossed directly at the knee look heavier than they really are.

🌸 Hands should be held in profile to the camera, with the fingers curled slightly and the thumbs tucked into the palms. If you shake your hands before the picture is taken and then curl the fingers gently, your hands will help put you at ease.

🌸 Don't force a smile or smile too broadly. Instead, moisten the lips lightly with the tongue just before the picture is taken and then smile gently so that you look pleasant but have no deep lines beside the mouth and your eyes are not lost in your smile.

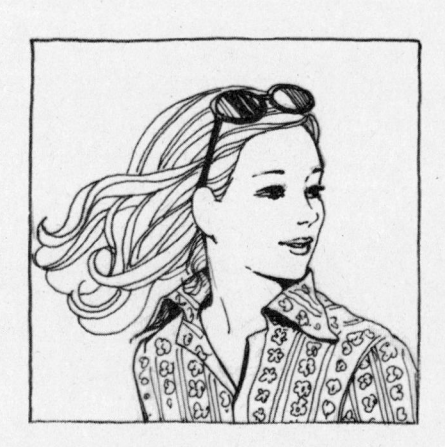

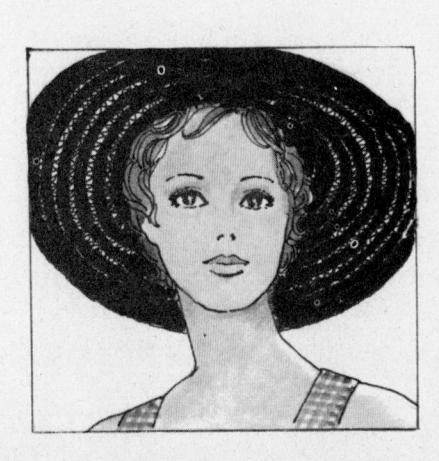

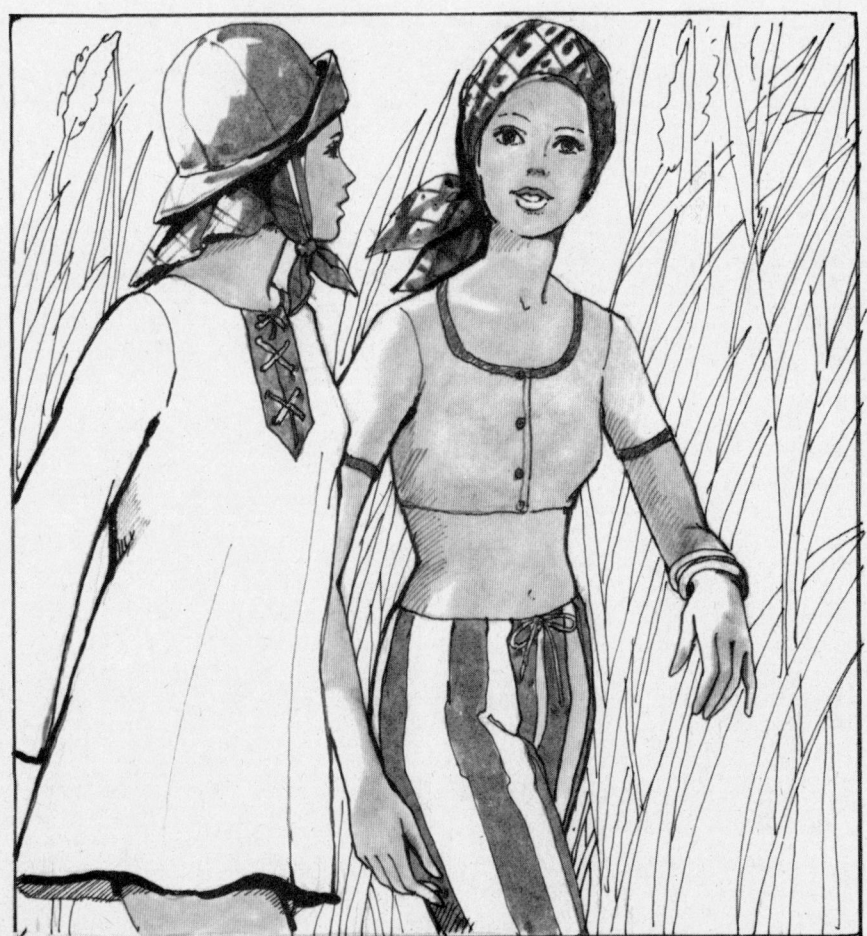

BEAUTY FOR THE WORKING WIFE

If you have a home and a family and a job besides, a lot is expected of you —and you are expecting a lot of yourself. Good appearance builds the impression that you manage things well, and others accept the fact that you do. This can make things easier all around. How do you find time for your personal upkeep?

Simplify your wardrobe. Keeping clothes in good repair is a short cut to grooming ease. A few outfits, each in working order, keep you better dressed than a closetful of clothes that fall short of perfection. The guideline is to put no item away unless—and until—it's ready to wear again. If a dress needs repair or a trip to the cleaner, if a ripped stocking should be tossed out, the time to act is when the garment is taken off.

✤ As for handbags—don't use yours as a catchall. Keep the contents to a minimum—everything you need, but *only* what you need.

Have a well-made face. For skin care and makeup, learn to limit your choice. Your skin-care needs are cleanser, toner, and lubricating cream. Your makeup needs, too, are limited: Two makeup bases, one loose powder, two lipsticks or lipstick and gloss, eye-shadow kit, eye liner, rouge, blusher, a brow make-up in a shade near your natural brow color—that does it.

✤ Keep your start-the-day makeup in a small case or tray that will be handy and ready to use. Carry your to-work makeup in a case or bag that fits into your handbag. You need only a lipstick, mascara wand and a pressed-powder compact. Other take-along grooming aids are comb and purse-size fragrance dispenser.

✤ Do a complete makeup at day's start—practice will make you speedy. A damp cloth pressed over the finished makeup acts as a fixative. You need not then change makeup during the day. An occasional patting of pressed powder and a lipstick touch-up will keep your face fresh-looking. If skin is oily, excess oil can be removed with special tissues.

A good hair style is a must. Get a good basic haircut and a simple styling that a few curlers or a spraying will refresh between sets. Save on shampoo-and-set time this way:

✤ Shampoo under the shower, taking care that hair is well-rinsed. This means that water pressure should be reduced so the underneath hair as well as top layers get a full water run-through. Keep a steel-wool pad over the drain so that shed hair doesn't stop the plumbing.

✤ Dry the hair before setting. Use a warm-air blower or remove the hood from your hair drier and use the hose as a blower.

✤ For a really speedy set, dry the hair thoroughly and then set on hot rollers.

✤ A small hairpiece or a wig more than pays its way.

Keep hands well-groomed. Gloves are your best hand protectors. This means rubber gloves for dishwashing and other "wet work." But also wear cotton gloves to protect hands and nails while you dust, vacuum, make beds, and simply pick up. These are tasks that otherwise wreck a manicure. Rub hands lavishly with hand cream or lotion before you put your work gloves on and you will get an extra beauty treatment. In winter, dress gloves protect hand skin from chapping and also keep the hands clean —so wear them, don't just carry them.

✤ And remember to keep a dispenser of hand cream or lotion at every water faucet—and to use it, a little bit at a time so that it rubs in quickly.

✤ A once-a-week manicure is a must. If polish won't stay pretty for a full week, then you must plan for a midweek polish change. Or, if you can't cope with colored polish, buff a glow onto your nails. Or use clear liquid polish.

Take care of your feet. Comfortable feet make life simple. If you have a stand-up job, give feet and legs regular rest. Changing shoes at midday and after work helps; sitting or lying down from time to time with feet higher than hips is a kindness to feet and legs. Regular visits to a foot doctor relieve serious foot problems. Well-fitted shoes and stockings are a kindness you deserve.

✤ And treat yourself to a once-a-week pedicure. This means a good long soak for the feet, smoothing rough areas (use a pumice stone—you can get one in any drugstore), and buffing toenails as well as a neat straight nail clip.

✤ Put shaped toe plasters or moleskin on rubbed or tender areas. For a special treat, rub the feet with hand or body lotion and slip on soft cotton socks; keep feet thus soothed for an hour or two—even overnight. Foot powder or spray on the feet and inside the shoes gives daytime comfort.

Underarms need attention. Today most women are aware of underarm problems and use an antiperspirant as routinely as they brush their teeth. Underarm hair should be removed as often as is necessary to keep underarms free of shadow. Shaving underarms takes only half a minute, so you can shave daily as a part of your bath routine. Softened by bath water, hair comes off quickly.

Showers, yes, but baths too. The shower is a quick easy way to move ahead with morning grooming. Don't neglect it as a timesaver, but don't completely abandon the luxury of a tub bath. A 20-minute soak in a warm fragrant tub saves time, too—if it relaxes mind and body, gets you off to a good night's sleep, or perks you up so that daily tasks seem easier.

✤ After your morning shower, dry the skin carefully and then pat or spray on bath powder; girdle and stockings slip on easily over powdered skin.

Learn to relax. Relaxation is a timesaver because it renews your energy. Lying down with feet higher than the head is relaxing; a warm tub bath is restful— and so, surprisingly, is exercise. A noon-hour walk, a before-dinner romp with the children, and other changes of pace help you feel rested and renewed.

LOOKING PRETTY AT 40-PLUS

There's really very little difference in what an over-40 woman does about her looks from what a woman in her 20s should be doing. The problem is that over-40 women start to do aging things. They begin to feel that some hair styles are too young for them. (Maybe straight, loose waist-length hair is, but most salon styles for medium-length to short hair can be worn at any age.) They begin to do the wrong things to their skin—to use heavier makeup, heavier creams. Or they won't adopt new ideas, such as false lashes. The ideal age for any woman is "age indefinite." If you keep your figure, are healthy, active, self-assured, you needn't worry about what's "too young for you."

Most of the suggestions we make here apply just as much to women in their 20s and 30s as to the 40-plussers. The most important thing after 40 is to stop thinking of your age and to start thinking of what makes you look your best. Stop trying to project an image of "who you would like to be" and start to like "who you are." Put the accent on your charm, and you won't have to try to hide anything—you just make the most of the what you have. No one will wonder how old you are—they'll just say: "Doesn't she look great?"

Skin care. Some people at any age have excessively dry skin that needs constant protection. If you're one of these, your doctor will tell you what to do. Otherwise, if you have "normally" dry skin (we say "normally," because the majority of women over 30 have some dryness), don't suffocate your skin with heavy creams. You do need to use an emollient at night—but not *all* night. Put it on after you have cleaned your face, let it stay on for 15 minutes, then remove it. This is enough to lubricate the skin—while you sleep, your skin will have a chance "to breathe."

🌿 A moisturizer is not a lubricant. This cosmetic is intended for daytime use under makeup—to smooth down the surface cells and to lock in your own natural moisture. Put your moisturizer on clean skin, and let it set for 10 minutes before you apply your foundation. If you don't wait this long, the foundation will sink into the pores with the moisturizer and "pollute" your skin.

Makeup. Don't use a heavy, concealing makeup just because you think you're older. You need just the opposite—a sheer, thin, transparent liquid makeup that merely tints the skin. This is makeup that is promoted for youthful complexions, but you need this light makeup as much as the young do. More than ever, as you grow older, you should avoid makeup that looks stagy.

🌿 Don't try to hide wrinkles. Covering makeup that you *think* hides flaws and wrinkles merely fills them up and makes them more noticeable. Let your skin shine through. If for any reason you want to use a concealing makeup—to change your skin tone or because you're used to it—apply it lightly and remove the excess. If you need to cover a tiny flaw, use a delicate bit of cover makeup in that particular area only.

🌿 Under-eye shadows need not be coated with a lot of eye whitener to be concealed. It is better to blend them into the general skin tone by using a foundation about two shades darker than your skin tone on the whole face. This makes the under-eye shadows less noticeable.

🌿 Contouring is not usually necessary, even with a full face. Complicated trickery only makes you look older. Use your blusher toward the outside of your face so that your features shine out of a glow of warmth and your bone structure and eyes will be beautified. This is more complimentary to your face than contouring at any age.

🌿 No, you probably don't need to make up your throat. Bring the makeup over the jaw-line and chin, and then fade it out into the under-jaw shadows. Makeup only emphasizes the wrinkles and lines and, perhaps, the sagging of the throat; natural skin reflection onto the face from chest skin is also becoming.

🌿 Old-style powders filled and caked; today's translucents give a delicate softness to the skin that keeps down shine without filling the pores. Powder down the middle of the face—forehead, sides of nose, upper lip, chin—for today's elegant look. Do not repeatedly repowder to keep makeup alive during the day. This can give a heavy look. Instead, splash the face with handfuls of water over the makeup; pat dry, and your makeup will be refreshed—and will last.

Eyebrows. At any age the eyes are the center of interest and communication—where your personality shines through. Most important is the shape of the eyebrows. For today's fashion, the brows should be fairly thin, light and beautifully shaped. The contour should be arched and lifted—like the edge of a bird's wing. A beautifully shaped eyebrow opens the space around the eye and makes the whole face look more beautifully formed. Don't draw your brows in a hard line or make them too heavy; they should look soft and clean. Old-fashioned brow shapes suggest age.

Eyes. Eyes can be emphasized by your use of shadows. Yes, line the eyes—but in a soft, slightly smudged line in the upper and lower lashes. Do your eyes in a monochromatic color scheme—for example, line with dark green, put green shadow on the upper lid to the crease, brown-green under the brow, blending the shades into each other. The secret is the darkest at the lashline, the lightest below the brow, and the medium shade in between.

🌿 Yes—you should wear false lashes (unless your own lashes are long and thick and can be extended by mascara). As we age, our lashes often become thinner and faded. The use of well-chosen false lashes offsets this aging effect and brings the eyes up for attention. You have to choose the right ones for your eyes—perhaps avoiding the extra-heavy "moth wing" lashes. Thin, spiky false lashes or shaggy flexible lashes can be very becoming.

Eyeglasses. Even if you wear contact lenses, you probably use eyeglasses sometimes, too (to find your contacts). And, of course, you wear sunglasses. Plastic lenses are not only protective (won't shatter) but they also are lightweight and make eyeglasses more comfortable to wear. In addition, they reduce the weight on the nose piece, so you are less likely to get indentations where the glasses rest. Choosing frames that are an asset to your appearance is more important than ever after 40. Study smart-looking women you see wearing glasses on TV or in magazines and newspapers for good ideas. Change your frames often to keep them in line with fashion (at least whenever you change lenses). Some fashion frames cannot be fitted with corrective lenses or, at least, not with bifocals. However, you can still find good-looking frames that will put happy emphasis on your eyes, where it belongs.

🌿 If you need visual aid in doing your eyes, helpful devices are available—stick-on magnifiers for mirrors and enlarging mirror "glasses" on extended frames.

Mouth. Keep your lip color light now—but change with the fashion. Use the color underneath—the gloss on top. If you need to reshape the mouth, use a brush. Make a well-defined line. Apply lip color lightly so it does not seep into tiny lines around the mouth.

Facial flaws. Some facial flaws become more noticeable as we get older—moles, for one. Your physician will advise you about removing them. Discolored brownish spots on the face, even tiny lines, can now be removed by dermabrasion—face-planing (this can be done by a plastic surgeon or by a dermatologist)—or even by chemical "peeling" (this should be done by a qualified physician). Dental care is particularly important at any age—restoration of lost teeth keeps your face in better shape; toothcapping or other restoration work can enhance the appearance of your mouth. No woman of any age should have to repress her smile because her teeth look bad. Facial hair—it sometimes develops on the upper lip after menopause—can be removed by wax or facial depilatory creams or professional electrolysis.

Figure. Repeated weight loss or gain can add up to sagging facial skin, double chin and other woes. Find the weight you can maintain and stick with it, instead of putting on and taking off and making yourself not only miserable but less attractive. By the time a woman is 40, she should have a well-formed personality and should have learned that it is better to use less than more—in her eating, her dressing, her makeup.

Hair. Fluff and soft curls are now fashionable; they soften and flatter the older face. Hair that is healthy and clean, well-cut and well-set enhances anyone. Color? Whether you go gray gracefully or color your hair is your own personal choice. Going to a lighter shade than your natural color is the key after 40. Avoid reds, but try warm brown, warm light brown or ash blond to flatter your skin tone.

USE YOUR BODY GRACEFULLY

Good posture and graceful body movements help to keep you well-groomed. When you stand well, clothing fits well; graceful and efficient movements help you avoid disarray. Here, from the John Robert Powers Charm School, New York, are suggestions to help you move gracefully.

Walking. When you walk, feet should move parallel to each other, never crossing over to "toe a line."

🌿 With each step, lead with the thigh, keeping knees slightly flexed so they act as shock absorbers.

🌿 Shoulders should be relaxed so that arms will swing easily, the palms of the hands facing the skirt, fingertips just brushing the sides of the skirt.

Stairs. Keep the back straight and the head up when you go up and down.

🌿 Going up, place entire foot on each step, pushing and lifting with thigh muscles.

🌿 Going down, sight each step as you approach it. Keep weight on back leg till other toe is firmly placed on step below.

Standing. Make front view slim and tall by turning the body slightly.

🌿 The forward foot should be pointed straight ahead, the back foot placed at a 45° angle just behind the front foot.

🌿 Weight should be divided equally so back hip does not slide out.

🌿 To stand restfully for long periods, keep knees slightly flexed, never locked.

Sitting. You will appear graceful if you approach a chair from an angle and,

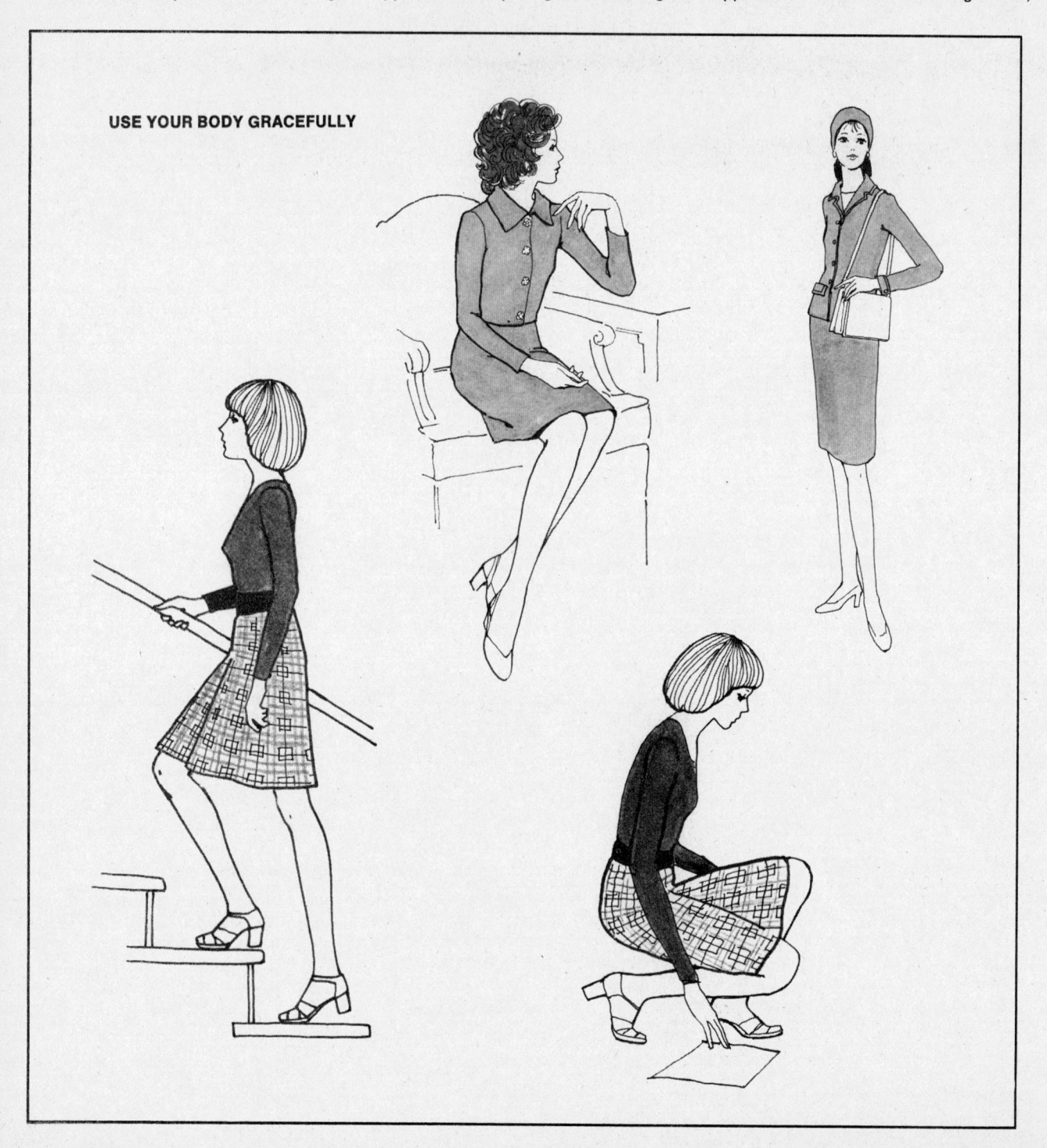

before sitting, pause in the basic standing position described above. This places the body at an angle to the chair.
- Sit on buttocks, not on thighs, but keep the body at an angle to present an S-curve to anyone facing you.
- This means the shoulders are shifted slightly to one side and the head is slightly tilted away from the angle of the shoulders.
- The knees are turned to the same side as the shoulders, and legs are swept to the other side, with the toe of the back foot resting on the ankle of the front foot.
- Do not cross legs at knees; cross them at the ankles, if at all.
- Hands may be cupped in lap—or one elbow or hand may be placed on the armrest, the other left on lap. Never place both elbows or both hands on armrests at the same time.

Automobiles. To get into a car gracefully, stand first in good-posture position beside the open door. Place near foot on car floor, slide hips onto the seat, pull in head and shoulders, and then bring other foot into the car after you.
- To get out, swing door open; place outer foot on curb, slide out head and shoulders, and, straightening to standing position, bring out lower torso; the other foot comes out last.

Picking things up. Any object to be picked up from the floor should be approached so that you stand beside it, one hand directly over the object, one foot slightly ahead of the other foot for balance.
- As you pick up the object, bend deeply at the knees, keeping the buttocks tucked under and the back straight.
- Return to standing position in good body alignment.

Carrying accessories. Carry handbags, umbrellas, and other accessories on the left arm (unless you are left-handed) so that the right hand will be free.
- A strap handbag is carried on the left arm, with the arm at waist height, and the slim end of the bag forward.
- A clutch handbag is carried in the left hand.
- Do not carry handbags, packages, newspapers, or magazines tucked under an arm.
- Wear gloves to keep the hands clean; don't carry the gloves to keep *them* clean. If you do carry gloves, fold glove fingers and hold these in the palm of the hand; the glove cuffs should be placed neatly one atop the other and folded together over the outer side of the hand.
- When putting gloves on in public, hold the hand upward, palm in, and pull the glove down over the hand.

Hand grace. When you have *nothing* to do with your hands, let them do nothing:
- Let one hand rest easily on a chair arm; let the other rest in your lap, palm up, fingers slightly curled.
- Or clasp the hands lightly and let them both rest palms up in your lap.
- Or place one hand over the other and hold them slightly to one side, resting, palms down, on the upper thigh.
- The hand appears most graceful in profile, so learn to keep your hands at a slight angle to the viewer.
- Hold the index finger slightly extended, the other fingers gently curled, and the thumb curled just within the palm.
- When walking with a man, hold *his* arm, tucking your hand into the bend of his elbow. He should not hold your arm or propel you along by the elbow.

Arm grace. Outline the waist: When standing or walking, hold the elbows down but slightly out from the waist so the waist outline will be distinct; the arms will appear graceful, and the figure will appear slimmer.
- When standing, it is graceful to fold the arms across the chest or to clasp the hands behind you, but again, keep elbows down and slightly away from the side of the body.
- Shoulders should be down and level if arms are to swing gracefully; if one shoulder droops, the entire figure loses its grace.
- Avoid carrying heavy packages, schoolbooks, or the baby always on one arm; one-side-man-ship can throw the shoulders, arms, and spine out of line.

Breast beauty. If the upper part of the body is properly carried, the breasts will have a better contour.
- Keep the shoulder blades down and slightly spread.
- Keep the ribs up.
- Hold the abdomen in for a long slim line below the breasts.
- The breast is mostly fatty tissue and has little muscle; it depends upon the skin and the muscles underneath the breasts for support.
- A good bra helps keep the breasts in line; there is less breast movement to break down fatty tissue and less chance for gravity pull to stretch the breast skin. The support of the bra allows fatty tissue to build up; and also makes clothes fit better.
- The bra should support the breasts from below and from the sides and should not flatten the breast at the front.
- If breasts are heavy (and during pregnancy and nursing), a bra can be worn loosely fastened while you sleep to prevent stretching and pulling when you toss and turn.
- To put on a bra correctly, slip the straps over the arms and then bend forward at the waist. Position the breasts comfortably in the bra cups and then fasten the bra at back. Straighten and position shoulder straps.

Leg problems. Any leg structural faults can be minimized by standing gracefully, by wearing skirts or shorts of a length that is flattering, by wearing simple shoes. Developing the leg muscles will help disguise bone faults—bicycling, swimming, brisk walking help.
Heavy legs—Exercise—walking, swimming, or bicycling—will help reduce leg fat. If legs are over-muscled, simple heel stretches and toe pointing will improve their lines.
Thin legs—The same exercises that help reduce heavy legs help thin ones develop shape.
Flabby thighs—Check your work chair. If it is too long and too wide you may be sitting on your thighs instead of upon your buttocks. The spreading and flattening of thighs by the body's weight will over a long period of time result in looseness and flabbiness of the thighs. A good work chair and regular exercises will help.
- Avoid wearing tight girdles or depending upon a girdle to hold your abdomen flat. Too much support for hips and thighs encourages flabbiness and building up of fat in these areas.
Prominent veins—Blood is pooling in the veins and is distending them. Get off your feet as often as you can. Five-minute leg rests every two hours—feet elevated so they are higher than the hips—can be helpful.
Leg fatigue—Try a quick-change leg bath. Put legs under the bathtub faucet or the shower and turn on water as hot as you can stand it for two minutes; change to cold water for two minutes; change back to hot and again to cold. Five minutes of this hot-cold treatment refreshes legs.
Sore muscles—Knead out soreness with leg massage:
- Lie on back; bring knees to chest and using the whole palm of both hands, stroke legs upward from ankles to above the knees.
- Then, with both hands, grasp first the calf muscles and then the thigh muscles of one leg at a time, using a kneading motion to work over the entire leg, pressing the muscles firmly.
- Stroke the entire leg with the palms.
- Repeat on other leg.

MISS CRAIG'S INSTANT-THINNING PLAN FOR ABDOMEN AND WAIST
BY MARJORIE CRAIG

As surely as there are instant coffee and instant tea, there is an instant way to make rolls of fatty inches disappear from the abdomen and waist. This instant method does not require dieting, and the result is not an optical illusion. It is a simple matter of correcting the way you stand. Bad posture can add from one to five inches to your girth that dieting alone can never get rid of.

To get in condition, one must systematically exercise muscles in all parts of the body, However, one can give the appearance of being 10 pounds thinner simply by correcting bad posture. Almost everyone can stand in correct posture in an instant—for an instant. The big trick is to learn to hold yourself straight and tall, naturally, for longer than an instant. To do so, you will need to strengthen muscles so they can form a natural girdle that will hold in those inches around your midsection.

To discover if you need posture work, take this simple two-part test:

✤ Stand the way you normally do, and while in this position, take the measurement of your waistline.

✤ Now lift your shoulders, pulling them back as you pull your stomach in, and while standing in this corrected position, again measure your waistline.

If you find that your measurements become smaller by an inch or more the second time you measure, incorrect posture is causing you to look thicker and fatter than you really are. The time has come for you to lie down on the floor and begin to strengthen your posture muscles. Do three simple exercises and right before your eyes—almost in an instant—your figure will show improvement.

Experience has shown that posture-correcting exercises can be started most easily on the floor. In this way the inexperienced exerciser is not struggling against the pull of gravity. In a sense, gravity will be helping you to get the maximum results with the minimum amount of strain and struggle.

EXERCISE 1.

Basic position—Lie on your back on the floor. Bend your knees. Place feet together on the floor close to hips. Keep knees slightly apart. Place arms on floor close to your sides.

Action—Push your waist back. This means: With a rolling hip movement, pull your pelvis back so that the small of your back touches the floor.

✤ Keeping waist back, pull your ribs up. This means: Pull your ribs up away from your hipbones so that you get the greatest distance possible between ribs and hipbones without lifting your spine.

✤ Keeping waist back and ribs up, pull your ears up. This means: Feel as if someone is holding the top of your ears and thus stretching your neck away from your shoulders while you keep your chin at a right angle to your neck.

✤ Holding waist back, ribs up, ears up, pull your shoulders back and down. This means: Keep your shoulders as flat on the floor as you can, and at the same time pull them down toward your feet; feel as if your arms were being pulled by the tip of your elbows.

✤ Hold your body in this corrected position for the count of 10. Relax. Say and do this five times: Waist back. Ribs up. Ears up. Shoulders back and down. Hold. Count to 10. Relax.

When you can do Exercise 1 with ease, add Exercise 2.

EXERCISE 2.

Basic position—Stand with back and head against the wall—heels 8 to 10 inches out from wall, feet 4 to 6 inches apart and parallel, toes pointing straight ahead. Have arms at your sides, elbows pressed against wall.

Action—Bend knees, keeping feet in set position; slide down the wall to the place where you can easily push the small of your back firmly against the wall. Raise rib cage up away from hips. Pull ears up, away from shoulders. Push shoulders back and down. Hold. Count to 10. Relax.

✤ Slowly slide your back up the wall to the point where you can still keep the back of your head and your spine at the waistline pressed against the wall.

✤ In this position, repeat five times.

When you can do Exercise 2 with knees only slightly bent, you are ready to add Exercise 3 to your routine.

EXERCISE 3.

Starting position—Stand against the wall—heels 4 inches out from the wall, feet 4 inches apart and parallel, toes pointing straight ahead. Have arms at your sides, elbows bent and pressed against wall.

Action—Bend knees slightly. Separate knees further without moving feet. Push waist back against the wall. Raise rib cage away from hips. Pull ears up away from shoulders. Push shoulders back and down.

✤ Holding your body in this corrected posture position, walk away from wall. Keep knees relaxed, hips "tucked" under. Holding this position, walk back and forth across the room 10 times. Keep arms relaxed and loose as you walk.

Continue to do these exercises until correct posture comes naturally.

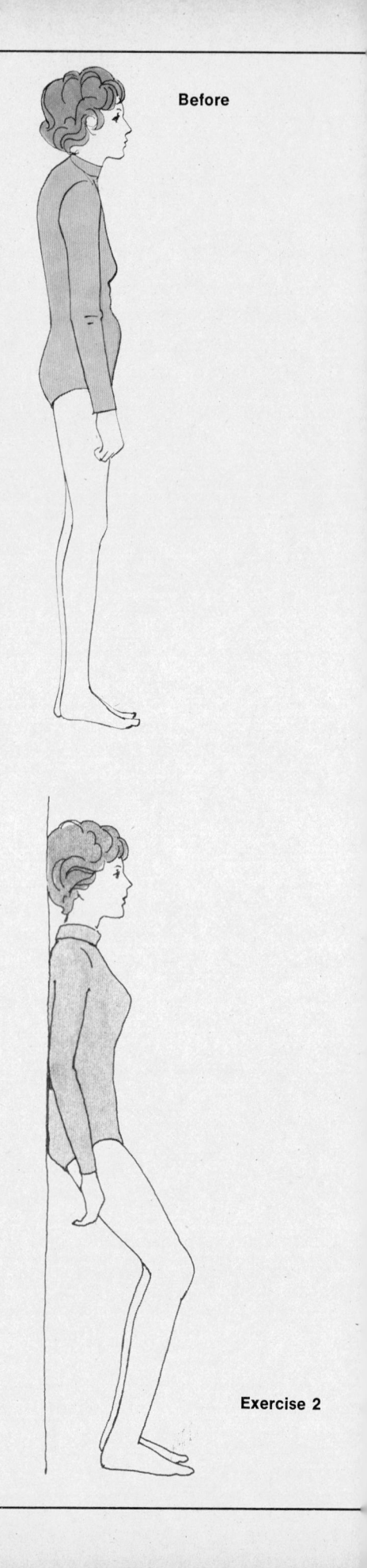

Before

Exercise 2

After

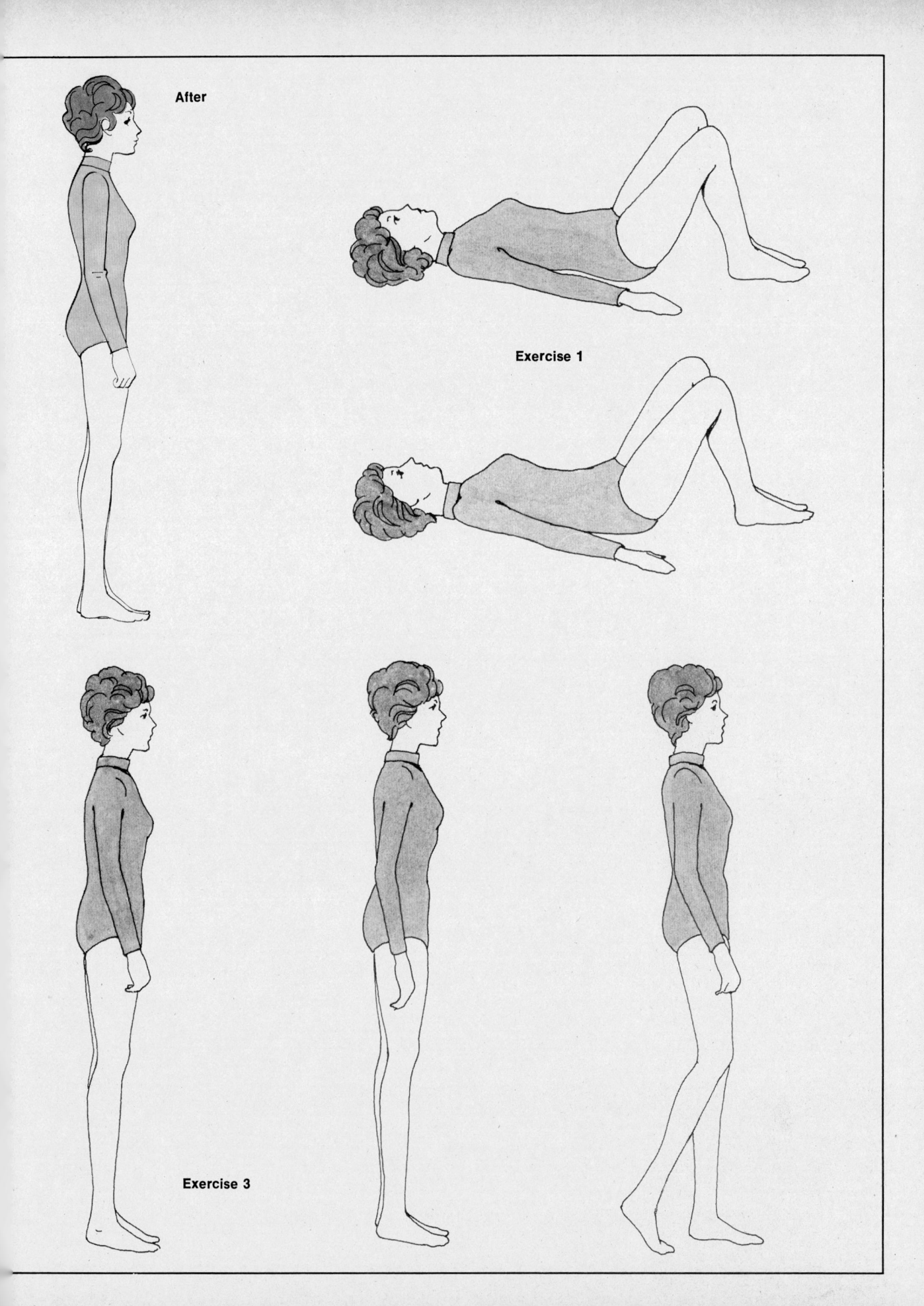

Exercise 1

Exercise 3

GROOMING AIDS

You will need a well-organized closet and the determination never to put clothes away unless they are ready to be worn again.

❧ A rear-vision mirror so you'll know what evil lurks behind you in the form of hanging hemlines, hair on collar.

❧ A well-stocked sewing kit—needles and thread and straight pins (safety pins for emergencies only). Repairs often take only a minute or two.

❧ A kit of grooming musts—manicure and pedicure needs, a shaver or depilatory, deodorant and antiperspirant, and tooth-care, and hair-care needs.

❧ Brushes—powder brush, shoebrush, clothesbrush, toothbrushes, hairbrush, nailbrush.

❧ An appointment book.

❧ A dressing table with a good light so that you see yourself clearly and apply makeup neatly so that others are aware only of a prettier you.

Well-groomed personality.

❧ Keep appointments on time.
❧ Do not linger on the telephone.
❧ Do not rush. Allow enough time.
❧ Keep your manners, whatever the situation.
❧ Learn to deal with frustration.
❧ Be adjustable.
❧ Keep your voice pleasant and well modulated, but loud enough to be heard.

REFRESH WITH A BATH

Most women enjoy a tub bath—and even a shower devotee should center her weekly or twice-a-week grooming session on a good tubbing. Here you can use water softeners and other soothing bath preparations to make soap more effective and the bathroom fragrant. You can lie back and enjoy a relaxing soak that pampers both nerves and skin. And you can get many other benefits from a tubbing. Here are the five basic bath temperatures:

Cold bath—35°-60°
Cool bath—70°-80°
Neutral, or tepid, bath—92°
Warm bath—95°-105°
Hot bath—98°-120°

Bath helpers. Start with a clean tub. Water softeners, bath crystals (salts), and other bath preparations in the water help to avoid an afterbath ring. If you use powder cleanser in the tub, be sure to rinse the tub well so no irritating grit remains.

❧ Bath preparations—bubbles, oil, crystals, or some standard water softener—will add greatly to the bath's pleasure and its cleansing power. Any kind of bath preparation helps soften the water and makes it more soothing to the skin; soap lathers more lavishly in softened water. Bath preparations also give fragrance to the water and to the air of the bathroom and leave a subtle scent on the skin.

❧ Bathing water should ordinarily be a little warmer than tepid—about 98° to start—not so hot as to be enervating.

❧ Relaxing in the tub for five to 10 minutes before you start soaping eases tired muscles, relaxes taut nerves, loosens soil, perspiration, and body salts from the skin, and distends the pores so they will be more receptive to the cleansing action of the soap. If water cools too much during the soaking time, add some hot water to keep yourself warm. A tub pillow or a folded bath towel should be used as a headrest when you relax full-length in the tub.

Bath soap—Use a large bar for the tub, a smaller size for shower and basin. Soap in the same fragrance as your other bath preparations is a nicety, but the scent of soap lasts briefly, and you will find little soap fragrance left a short time after bathing. For the tub, a hard-milled rich-lathering soap is preferred (it won't quickly dissolve). A water softener will encourage suds and will leave no bathtub ring.

Bath crystals—These salts are both water-softening and fragrant. They should dissolve thoroughly in water, so place the crystals in the stoppered dry tub directly under the faucet and then turn the hot water on hard.

Bath bubbles—Powder or liquid, bubble bath softens and scents the water and creates a blanket of foam to soothe you while you soak. Soaping reduces the bubbles, so enjoy them before you start sudsing. Again, bubbling bath powders or liquids should be placed in a dry stoppered tub under the faucet and the water then turned on hard to build foam.

Bath oil—Bath oil is highly fragrant and leaves a slight film of oil on the skin— particularly helpful when skin is dry and likely to chap. You can usually find an oil in the scent of your preferred perfume, so use only a few drops sprinkled lightly in the filled tub. Some bath oils are designed for treatment of dry skin; these require a soak of 20 minutes or longer to be effective.

Bath powder—Afterbath dusting powder is used after drying to prevent chapping. Puff powder generously over the skin and into the body folds and creases and the armpits and between the toes. Sprinkle powder into bras, girdles, and stockings so these garments will go on smoothly and will not become damp and uncomfortable with perspiration. Bath powder is usually scented, but the fragrance is not long lasting.

Friction—Afterbath friction is a scented alcohol rub that helps tighten the pores after the bath; friction may also be used as a between-baths freshener—or for a sponge bath or a rubdown after exercise.

Bath accessories.

Large terry towels	Shower cap
Full-bodied wash- cloths	Large-size bar soap
Bath mat	Bath mitt
Nonskid mat for shower	Long-handled back brush
Bath spray	Nailbrush
Bath tray	Pumice stone
Headrest	Shaving kit or other depilatory
Water softener	
Headband	

BATHS THAT YOU CAN TAKE

Bedtime bath. A bath at bedtime should bring on relaxation and help you sleep better. Put clean linens on the bed and turn the bed down before you enter the tub.

❧ This is a warm bath—98°-105°.

❧ This time you suds *before* you relax. Make all movements leisurely, letting warm water continue to trickle into the tub as you soap.

❧ After your sudsing, relax for about 10 minutes.

❧ Rinse in warm water.

❧ After you leave the tub, gently blot the skin dry. Powder well so that skin will not chap.

Daytime relaxer. This is a neutral bath —92°. Use fragrance in the bath and have the tub half full when you get in.

❧ Cream eye skin, place witch-hazel-moistened cotton squares over the eyes, and rest the head on a bath pillow or a folded towel while you relax for 10 to 20 minutes.

❧ Let tepid water continue to run into the tub while you soak; the moving water is an added relaxant.

❧ After your soak, wash briskly and rinse with a spray of tepid water.

❧ Blot the skin gently dry. Powder.

Fatigue reliever. This is a hot bath— 98°-120°—and is good for general tiredness and sore muscles.

❧ Start with water at body temperature; soap first, letting hot water trickle into the tub while you wash so the bath gradually becomes hot.

❧ Soak for 10 to 15 minutes in the hot soapy water.

❧ Finish with a cool-water rinse.

❧ Blot dry and follow drying with a

rubdown, using body lotion or bath friction, kneading the muscles to release any remaining "knots."

Wake-up bath. Cool water—70°-80°—helps you to get awake in the morning.
✄ Start with a cool tub and gradually let cooler water run into the tub as you soap.
✄ Bathe briskly this time, skipping the soak. A soap-filled bath mitt helps quick sudsing.
✄ Use shower or spray to rinse.
✄ Dry briskly. Powder well.

Invigorating bath. This is the cold bath —35°-60°. Take it only if you enjoy the shock. This bath should last no more than five minutes—and it actually warms the body as it invigorates.
✄ Have the tub fairly full when you plunge into the water.
✄ Rub the skin vigorously all over while you are in the water.
✄ Dry briskly, powder well, and wrap up in a warm robe.

Warm-up bath. If you like a hot bath—98°-120°—to comfort you in winter, start with water at about body temperature and gradually let in hot water till it reaches hot-bath temperature.
✄ Suds but do not soak, for hot water can be enervating.
✄ After washing, splash the skin with cool water.
✄ Dry vigorously and powder well.

Cool-off bath. This is a neutral bath—92°—and is your real hot-weather refresher, keeping you cool longer than a cold shower.
✄ With water a little below body temperature and a woodsy or flower fragrance in the tub, soak for at least 20 minutes.
✄ Blot skin dry after the bath and use bath powder lavishly—puffing it on first and then smoothing it—so clothes will slip on without sticking. The skin will be cooled enough to keep you comfortable for four to six hours.
✄ Repeat this bath as often as you like on hot days; it is *not* enervating.

Skin soother. Allow an hour. This warm —98°-105°—bath is primarily a soak in water treated with a bath oil especially formulated to aid skin dryness.
✄ Start the tub at body temperature and let warmer water trickle in as you soak. The length of the soak is important for the treatment to be effective. This bath can be taken without soap if skin is sensitive, and no rinse is then needed.
✄ Blot the skin dry to avoid irritation and to leave a slight film of oil on the skin surface. Do *not* use bath powder.

After sunning. A neutral bath—92°—with a half pound of bicarbonate of soda or cornstarch dissolved in the tepid water will relieve soreness in minor cases of sunburn.
✄ Soak in tepid water for 20 to 30 minutes.
✄ Follow the bath with careful drying and a gentle application of body lotion or medicated cream.

SHOWER BATHS

The shower is quick—you need not wait for the tub to fill nor need you scrub away a ring after the bath. A shower also rinses soap away easily, and water-temperature changes are easy to make. You miss out, however, on the luxury of the long in-tub soak and the use of bath fragrances. Still, the shower has some special purposes that even confirmed tubbers may want to try. Here are shower-bath hints:
✄ Turn on water and adjust water temperature *before* you enter the shower. This protects against accidental scalding.
✄ Have a nonskid mat on the shower floor.
✄ Use a full-bodied washcloth with a small-size bar of soap that is easy to hang onto or use a soap-filled bath mitt for ready sudsing.
✄ A terry-lined shower cap will protect your hairdo.

Grooming shower. If it is not rushed, the shower can serve as the daily grooming bath. Take at least 10 minutes for a complete cleanup. Don't neglect areas that may be hidden by the shower cap —ears, back of ears, hairline.
✄ Water should be warm—98°-105°. Use a bath mitt or soap and a washcloth to suds each body part from head to toe; use a brush to scrub the back thoroughly.
✄ Finish with tepid water.
✄ Powder well and get into clean clothes.

Quick fresh-up. After exercise or as a late-in-the-day fresh-up or even as a bedtime soother, a shower can be a quick cleanser.
✄ Start with warm water, using a soap-filled bath mitt for quick sudsing.
✄ Finish with cool water.
✄ Dry briskly, powder well.

Fatigue reliever. The shower is ideal for the invigorating and fatigue-relieving alternately hot-and-cold bath.
✄ Turn water against the body part by part, alternating hot and cold water and vigorously rubbing the body part against which the water is striking.
✄ Switch from hot to cold and back to hot in three or more cycles. Be sure the water plays against feet and legs as well as the upper torso.
✄ Follow with an invigorating toweling and use of an afterbath lotion or friction.

Backache reliever. After your regular tub or shower or even as a between-baths treat, turn the shower on hard with the water very warm.
✄ Sit on the floor beneath the shower, resting your head upon your knees and letting the hot water beat down upon back and shoulders.
✄ Three minutes of this, and muscle tension is relaxed.

Afterswim shower. Follow your swim with a warm shower, using soap to remove chemicals, salts, and sun-screen preparation.
✄ Follow with a cool rinse.
✄ If you plan to sun-bathe after the swim, reapply sun-screen preparation before exposure.

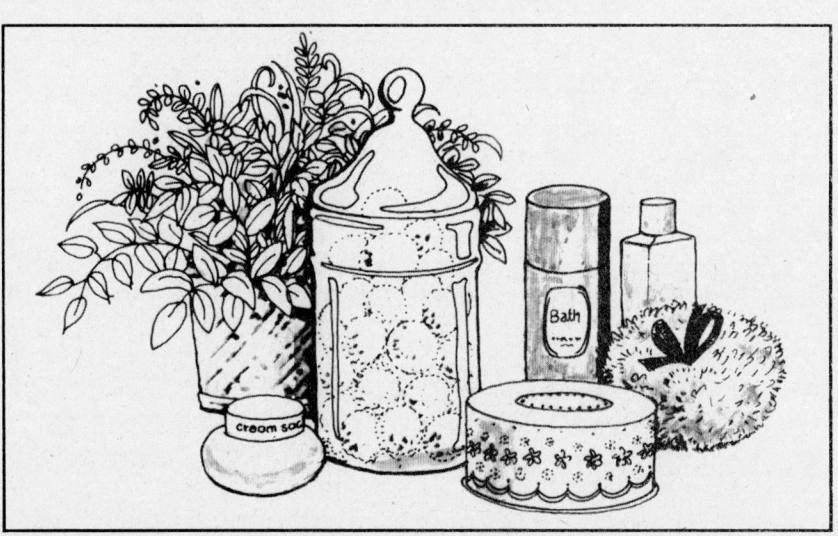

GUIDE TO GOOD GROOMING

To relax and to pamper yourself in mind and body, you will find there is nothing quite like the luxury of a tub bath. Quick and cleansing as a shower may be, you need a bath-oil bath to leave your skin soft, smooth, and clean, to leave *you* feeling lovely. A tub bath also prepares your skin for many of the other grooming musts. Foot calluses and rough skin are more easily rubbed away, toenails respond better to clipping, and cuticle around nails of toes and fingers can be erased gently and quickly after softening by a soak in the tub. Hair removal from legs and underarms becomes speedier, and gentler, if you shave when hair and skin are water-softened. This is the time, too, when stray hairs of the brows are least troublesome to pluck.

Grooming bath. A complete head-to-toe cleanup (besides your daily baths or showers) is in order once or twice a week. Set aside at least an hour (two is better) for a scrub down in the tub and all that goes with it.

- Shampoo and then roll up your hairdo or clip the hair into large curls in the shape of the setting. Cover with a net.
- If you use an electric shaver to remove body hair, do armpits and legs before entering tub.
- Clean the face and, depending on skin type, apply lubricating cream or a beauty mask.
- Place two large terry towels in a warm place so they will be ready to wrap in when you emerge from the tub. Draw your beauty tray near the tub and be sure all needed grooming aids are at hand.
- Make this a warm bath—98°-105°. Slip out of your robe and into the fragrant tub when it is about three-fourths full. Let a small flow of water run into the tub to keep the water warm while you soak.
- Place your head upon a folded towel or bath pillow, cream the eyes, place astringent pads over the eyes, and soak for 10 minutes.
- After your soak, exercise gently by stretching first one leg and then the other to push the foot against the end of the tub. Relax and repeat, making each leg as long as possible from hip to heel.
- Remove the facial mask or cream with the bath water. This is a good time to tweeze eyebrows because the softening effect of soap and water makes brow hairs easy to pluck; this is also the time to remove leg and underarm hair if you use a safety razor or a chemical depilatory.
- Wash from head to toe; push back cuticle of toenails and fingernails while you are in the tub so that you can complete your manicure once you emerge. Use a pumice stone on rough areas of feet and hands.
- Rinse in tepid water.
- When you leave the tub, dry thoroughly in a large warm towel, sponging or patting the skin dry.
- Follow with a lavish body rub with bath friction (scented afterbath rub) or body lotion. Powder the body creases and under the arms and between the toes to prevent chapping.

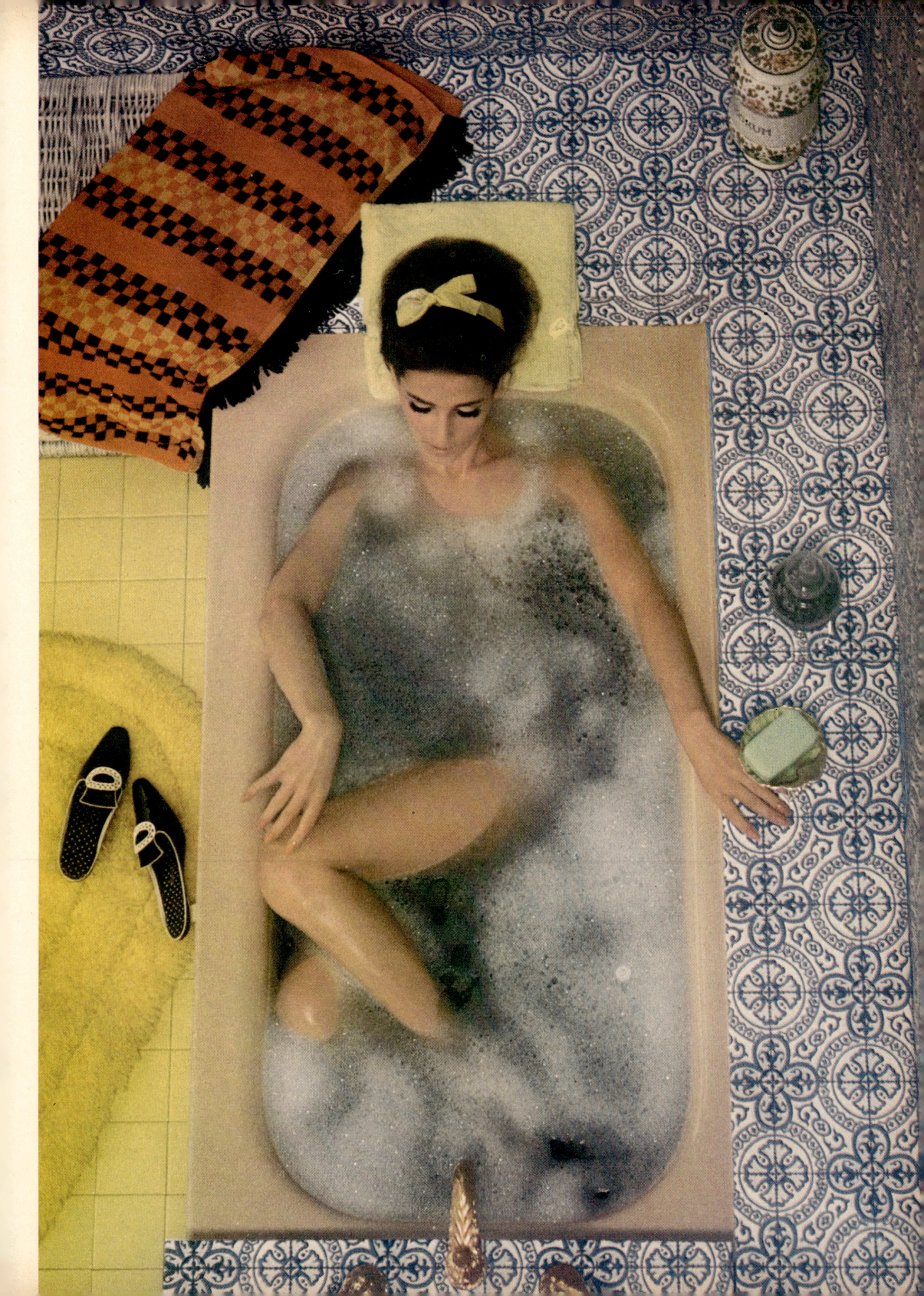

GROOMING AIDS

The skin spills out about two quarts of perspiration a day through its approximately three million sweat glands. This moisture cools the body by evaporation and also distributes skin oils and keeps up the natural balance of the skin. Most sweat is produced by the appocrine glands—and this sweat is normally odorless. In contact with the air and with germs on the clothes, an odor may, however, develop in time if skin and garments are not cleaned.

In both men and women (and somewhat more plentiful in women) are other sweat glands, called the eccrine glands, that go into action at some times of emotional excitement. The sweat from these glands does have a distinctive (but not necessarily unpleasant) odor. Menstruation also produces sweat odor in some women.

Deodorants. Frequent bathing is the best deodorant there is, but various preparations can also be used to mask or to prevent odors that may form between baths.

Deodorant powders—Antiseptic and absorbent deodorant powders can be used on the body-skin generally, between the toes, and in shoes and stockings, girdles and bras, even on hatbands and in gloves, to absorb perspiration. Patted in the armpit over the antiperspirant, deodorant powders help the heavy perspirer. There are special deodorant powders for use on menstrual pads.

Cream and spray deodorants—Scented to mask body odor, deodorant creams or sprays can be used as an accessory to the underarm antiperspirant and as as aid in masking menstrual odors or foot odors; or used anywhere where odor may form and an antiperspirant cannot be used. Some "deodorants" are also antiperspirants; the label should be examined to clarify this.

Deodorant colognes — Often called "summer colognes" these highly fragrant (usually citrus scented) toilet waters are used as a general body "splash" to cover body odors and to cool the skin.

Deodorant soaps — These antiseptic soaps reduce the possibility of odor by destroying or reducing the number of skin bacteria that otherwise would work on the perspiration to create a rancid smell. Bacteria are more often found on the clothes than on the skin, so clean garments will prove a necessity if "body odor" is to be avoided.

"Intimate" deodorants.—The vagina is normally self-cleansing and douching or use of an internal deodorant on a regular basis should not be necessary. Consult your physician about unusual discharge or odor. Deodorants for the perineal area may be needed—particularly during menstruation. These are available as sprays or powders.

Antiperspirants—The armpit is poorly ventilated and richly endowed with sweat glands; here moisture production should be stopped to prevent odor and damage to clothing. Antiperspirants—creams, sprays, lotions, powders, liquids—incorporate a chemical that acts upon the skin to stop perspiration temporarily. The effect lasts longer in some persons than in others. The best time to apply is in the morning; bathing does not undo the antiperspirant effect.

⚘ An antiperspirant is most effective when applied to clean dry hair-free skin, but usually it is unwise to apply the compound directly after shaving or use of a chemical depilatory. An antiperspirant may safely be applied directly after dry shaving.

⚘ The antiperspirant should dry before top garments are put on; when it is dry, an absorbent powder can be used for further protection.

⚘ Antiperspirants can safely be used on the palms of the hands as well as on the armpits; do not use on the face or feet or over the body generally. It is safe to stop perspiration in limited areas, but to stay alive, the body as a whole must perspire.

Hair removal. Bath-time is usually the best time for hair removal. There are several methods, all with some advantages and some disadvantages.

Wet shaving—The bath softens hair and skin and prepares hair for easy shaving, so the best time to use the razor is in the tub. At other times, use shave cream and warm water to create a lather.

⚘ On legs, move the razor upward against the direction of hair growth, stretching the skin in the other direction with the free hand. Use long smooth strokes.

⚘ For underarms, move razor downward against the direction of growth.

⚘ Do not use an antiperspirant directly after wet shaving; instead, shave at bedtime and apply the antiperspirant in the morning.

Dry shaving—For an electric shaver, skin and hair should be dry.

⚘ Powder the legs well and then move the shaver in long smooth strokes upward against direction of hair growth.

⚘ In armpits, powder for dryness and then shave with short firm strokes downward against direction hair grows.

⚘ Use a powder brush to remove loose hair and excess powder.

⚘ If there is no skin redness, you may safely use an antiperspirant directly before or after dry shaving.

Tweezing—Tweezing of eyebrows is best done in the bath—or just after face washing—when the skin and hair have been softened by soap and water. Pluck in the direction of hair growth and then apply an astringent. Do not tweeze hair from a mole; instead clip the hair close to the skin.

Chemical depilatories—Chemical hair removers may be used in the bath. A before-use patch test for any skin reaction is advisable. These depilatories are drying and one may develop a sensitivity to them. And do not use chemical hair removers if you have swollen or broken veins or if skin is broken or irritated.

⚘ With a wooden spatula apply the cream in a thin layer over the area to be treated. Allow the cream to remain on for the required length of time (usually five minutes) and then wash away the depilatory in the bath.

Abrasives—Pumice-stone abrasive, usually shaped to the area to be shaved, wears away the hair to skin level. Hair must be completely dry, so do not try this method after the bath.

⚘ Use a circular motion over the area to be treated and work only a small area at a time.

⚘ If skin becomes irritated, skip this over-rubbed area.

Waxing—Hair-removal waxes pull the hair out by the roots and so discourage regrowth. Do not use wax on the underarms and preferably have a salon treatment before you try a leg wax at home.

⚘ Wax should be warm enough to be fluid but not hot enough to burn.

⚘ Apply warm wax to the legs with a wooden spatula.

⚘ Once the area is coated, press a piece of surgical gauze into the wax. Use this gauze to pull off the wax as soon as it has hardened.

⚘ The wax must be yanked off sharply if the hair is to come out by the roots.

Mouth freshness. Your mouth should look and feel clean and attractive.

Mouthwash—If teeth are in good repair and well-cleaned, it isn't necessary to use an antiseptic mouthwash regularly. The mouth is self-balancing, and water rinsing is usually all that is needed after brushing. For comfort and a refreshed taste and to avoid bad breath, you may, however, choose to use a mouthwash solution; some persons feel poorly groomed unless they do.

Teeth—Teeth should be brushed after you eat anything. Take at least five minutes to brush the teeth and brush each area at least 10 strokes.

⚘ The teeth should be brushed away from the gums in the direction in which the teeth grow—up on the lower teeth, down on the upper teeth—and with a forward-and-back motion on chewing surfaces. Hold elbows down while you brush—this puts the hands in "working" position and makes the brushing easier and more effective.

❧ Use the dentifrice of your choice—or ask the advice of your dentist. If teeth stain readily, as a once-or-twice-a-week tooth whitener use a mixture of one part salt with two parts baking soda.

❧ After brushing, use dental floss for further cleaning. Cut off an 18-inch length of the floss, twist ends round the first two fingers of each hand, leaving a one-inch working length between the thumbs. Guide the dental floss between the teeth, working the floss back and forth to clean the area but not to injure the gum.

❧ A mouth irrigator helps keep spaces between the teeth clean, is particularly good for those with bridges.

❧ See your dentist as often as you need to—at least twice a year. And have any lost teeth replaced as soon as possible. If a tooth is missing and not replaced, other teeth may "wander." The replacement should have the same shape as the original tooth to best support its mates.

Eye care. Rest is the best relief for tired eyes, but temporary relief can be had by bathing the eyes with a mild eyewash or by using eye drops. If tiredness persists, see an eye doctor. The eyes need not be bathed regularly for hygienic reasons because the eyes themselves are their own best protectors against foreign objects and infections. You may, however, bathe the outside of the eyes freely with cold water—this is especially good on waking—and repeat frequently if there is tiredness or redness.

Eye pads—Use eye pads when sunbathing; use them as well while your facial mask dries and while you soak in the tub. Cotton squares moistened with a mild astringent, such as witch hazel, make excellent eye pads. Cream eye skin before applying.

Eye drops—Drops that "brighten" the eyes will clear temporary redness, but drops should not be used habitually.

FRAGRANCE

In your fragrance sequence of perfume, bath oil, toilet water, and sachet (and often in dusting powder and other cosmetics), the fragrance essence is the same but the "carrier" varies:

Perfume—This fragrance essence is diluted in a small amount of alcohol, which evaporates after application, leaving the aromatics to be diffused by body warmth.

Toilet water—This is essence diluted in a far larger quantity of alcohol and is intended as a base for the perfume.

Bath oil—Here the essence is carried in a skin-soothing oil; this is the most concentrated form of fragrance.

Cream or liquid sachet—Perfume essence in a cream carrier; cream sachet is applied directly to the skin, like perfume, and is sometimes preferred in hot weather because perspiration does not wash the cream away.

Powder sachet—This is powder with a high concentration of fragrance. You may use the powder directly on the skin but it is oftener used to scent clothing.

What is your perfume type? To help you to choose a perfume and to know what you are buying, perfumes have been classified into various types, depending on their essential ingredients. If you enjoy and wear a perfume of one group, you can usually wear another perfume of the same type. You may, however, be able to wear perfumes of several types. What type (or types) you enjoy depends upon the harmony between your skin oils and those of the perfume. It is this mixture of the perfume essence with your skin oils that creates the true fragrance.

Single floral—This has the fragrance of a single flower and many women and girls start with such a fragrance because it reminds them of a familiar and loved flower.

Floral bouquet—This group holds some of the most-loved "name" perfumes. The fragrance is predominantly floral but no single flower scent stands out.

Modern blend—These perfumes may be floral or woodsy but a predominant "top note" is characteristic. These perfumes are called "modern" because they include some new manmade aromatics.

Forest blend—These are the outdoor—mossy, woodsy, leafy—fragrances that are often definable by their clean fresh fragrance.

Oriental—These richly resinous fragrances are often described as "heavy" and are particularly long-lasting.

Fruity—These usually citrus-scented perfumes are often classed with modern blends.

Spicy—These are characterized by familiar spice fragrances—clove or cinnamon, for example—or by a spicy flower scent, such as carnation.

How to choose a perfume. Perfume should be tested directly upon your skin at a pulse spot, and enough time should be given to judge the scent truly.

❧ Apply the perfume to the clean wrist and then sniff to catch the top note.

❧ After two minutes, sniff again to discover how you like the developing fragrance.

❧ Wait 10 minutes—till the true scent has developed—and again sniff test to determine how you like the fully developed fragrance.

❧ Buy a small quantity and wear the perfume for a few days to learn what the scent is like to live with.

❧ The perfume should give you pleasure—a lift to your spirits—and should also be pleasant to others.

❧ Perfume should be pleasant to the scent but it also should be long-lasting on your skin. If the scent is right for you, the fragrance from one application will last about four hours.

How to use fragrance. Each of the items in your fragrance sequence has its own use and its own purposes.

❧ Sachet perfumes your clothes. Hang envelopes of sachet in your chosen fragrance in closets; place sachets among your underthings in bureau drawers; attach sachets to your clothes hangers and to your garment bags when you store your clothes; you may also place sachets among your bed linens.

❧ Bath oil perfumes the bath water and the skin. The scent is long-lasting but definably different in effect from perfume; so do not neglect to use perfume in addition to the bath oil.

❧ Toilet water forms the base for your perfume and is used for overall scenting—splash toilet water over your body or atomize the scent into your hair. Hair holds fragrance well because here the perspiration does not wash the oils away. Toilet water is not meant for use without perfume—the scent quickly disappears unless set off with perfume touches.

❧ Perfume is the "spot announcement" of your scent. Apply it to the pulse spots—throat, wrist, elbow, back of the knee—for a pervasive long-lasting fragrance. Or atomize perfume onto the throat and hair as a finishing touch to your dressing. Reapply perfume after about four hours. Perfume can be applied with fingertips, the stopper of the bottle, or with an atomizer (this is the way perfumers suggest it be applied).

Fragrance pointers. Test fragrance on a clear dry day when the scent comes through at its truest.

❧ Test on clean dry skin—and do not try to sample more than two or three perfumes at one time.

❧ Keep perfume in its own box, protected from light, air, heat and cold.

❧ Keep stopper tightly closed.

❧ Perfume does not keep indefinitely once the bottle has been opened; so use generously, not sparingly.

Nude Beauty

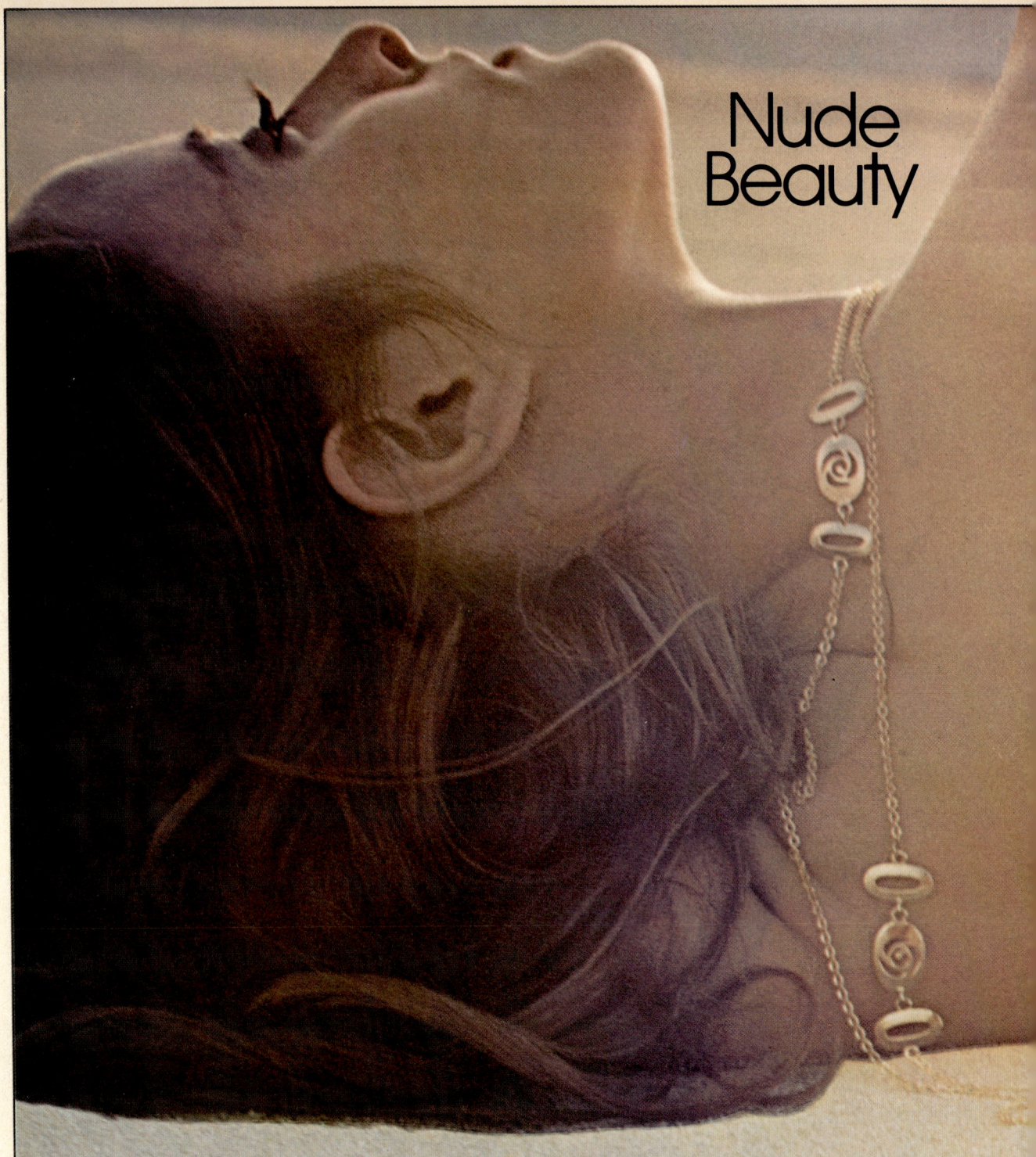

Just because your back is out of sight—and maybe out of reach—it often is skipped at body-pampering time. The middle of the back—between the shoulder blades—is an oily, high-perspiration, could-be blemish zone. Scrub well here with a long-handle brush when you bathe or shower. Dry areas are shoulder blades, the midriff, over the ribs. A friction lotion helps buff off flaky skin. Use a brush with buffing lotion on knees, elbows, feet.

❧ Well-buffed and creamed body skin tans smoothly. But keep sunning time short to avoid aging effects. Sunburn? Avoid it. Use a medicated cream to soothe even a little burn (dangerous area is around the edge of your swimsuit). Apply your burn preventer often. A brief word about cocoa butter: It sounds as if it would give you a beautiful brown shade—like that! But alone, though it softens the skin and keeps it "buttered," it doesn't screen out burning ra of the sun. Some cocoa-butter products have screening agent added. Check the label. Same i true of baby oil (great skin softener, but not a burn prevent

❧ Body hair? For leg hair, chemical depilatories or wax d the best job of stubble-proofing

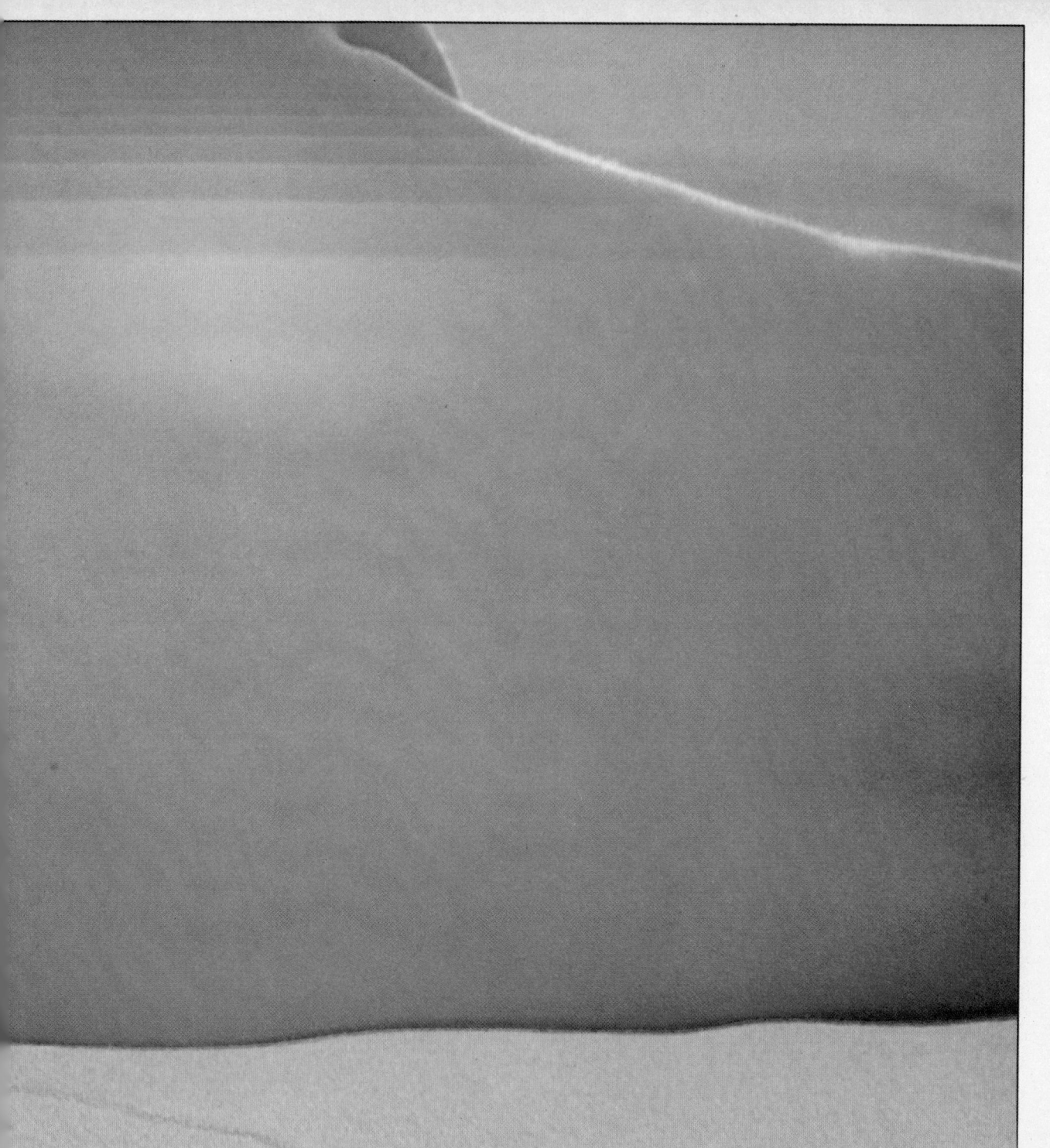

aution: Don't use wax on under-
rms—it can cause irritation.
having is often a satisfactory
ethod; an electric shaver leaves
ubble soft and avoids skin
crapes. Dust the skin first with
ath powder for an effective job.
ith your lady safety razor, use a
having cream for close cutting
 hair, fewer cuts on the skin.
eam skin after shaving, too,
 you have no raw spots.

☙ Should you tan your bosom all over? No. Body makeup evens the color if you are going braless and deep-plunge in your dress. Suit strap marks? These are a no-no (though body makeup will help here, too).

☙ Salt, pool chemicals, even perspiration—these can cause skin irritation. So can sand. Some so-called "sand rashes" may actually be due to particles of stinging sea creatures that wash ashore. Your soothing cream-coating helps protect the skin against these. Sometimes your skin can be irritated by protective products you use. Desist—or change. Or even see your doctor. Shower if you can after your swim to wash off salt and pool chemicals. Reapply your burn preventer or—before dressing—use body lotion.

PROFESSIONAL MANICURE TO DO AT HOME

Manicure needs.

Nail clipper	Polish remover
Cuticle clipper	Cuticle cream
Emery board	Cuticle remover
Cotton balls	Cuticle pusher
Orangewood stick	Nail-patch kit
	Solvent
Soft nailbrush	Polish base
Towel	Polish
Dish of warm water	Polish sealer

Shaping the nail. Remove the old polish and then, when nails are dry, shape the tips.

❧ If nail is broken or peeling or split, use a nail clipper. With a quick clean cut, clip the nail straight across to take off the split or broken part and to leave the tip in a squarish shape. Smooth the tip slightly with an emery board, but do not attempt to round the sides; let the nail at the sides grow out to about the length of the flesh at the fingertip and even after the nail reaches this length, continue to shape only the tip.

❧ If the nail is longer than fingertip length, gently smooth and shape the tip, but do not file into a point. A pointed nail breaks easily; kept slightly squared to start, the nail, as it grows, takes an oval shape.

❧ Use an emery board for shaping, not a metal file; a file puts too much pressure on the fragile nail tip and may cause it to shred.

❧ Place the emery board at a slight angle to the surface of the nail and brush the emery across the tip of the nail in one direction only. The movement should be light but firm so it will smooth but will not shatter the nail.

❧ Clip and shape nails only when they are absolutely dry; water softens the nail, and a soft nail will shred under filing.

Cuticle treatment. If the nail cuticle (skin around the nail) is carefully pushed back and any loose bits are nipped away, the nail will look longer after the polish is applied.

❧ Apply cuticle-massage cream lavishly to the cuticle and the fingertip and massage each nail for about one minute with this cream. This exercises the nail and helps to loosen dead skin.

❧ After massaging, cover the whole nail with massage cream and then put the fingertips into a dish of warm soapy water; soak them for at least 10 minutes. Do not skimp on this soaking time. Cuticle takes time to soften. When it is softened, the cuticle may be easily pushed away from the nail and will not crack or tear.

❧ After soaking, remove hand from water and dry each nail carefully.

❧ Next, apply cuticle-remover cream with a cotton-tipped orangewood stick. Use the cream lavishly so that cuticle, nail, and the space under the nail tip are saturated.

❧ Now, starting at the side of the nail, carefully lift the cuticle away from the nail with the stick. Do not bear down on the nail bed or scrape the surface of the nail. Instead, work around the edges, keeping close to the outer layer of dry skin and loosening the skin from the side, not from the top.

❧ When cuticle is loosened, take a nipper and gently clip any hangnails or bits of loose skin, but avoid clipping the entire cuticle.

❧ The nail must be clear of bits of loose skin if the enamel is to go on well; a gentle washing with a soft nailbrush will help clear away much of the loose skin. So will gentle massage.

❧ To massage the nail, wind a piece of towel around one or two fingers of the other hand and work the towel gently across the base of the nail in one direction only with a buffing motion.

Nail patching. A splint, or patch, over the nail tip helps keep it braced against damage and protects a broken nail as it grows out. Nail-patching takes some skill and some time to learn. But do not be concerned if your patches are a little lumpy at first. They are protecting the nail and this is the main thing. As you grow in skill, the patches will become smoother.

❧ To start, dampen a cotton ball with quick-acting polish remover and work the cotton over and around and under the nail to remove any cream.

❧ Tear off a piece of the paper that comes with the nail-patch fixative, or glue. Be sure to tear—don't cut—so the edge of the paper is uneven; the patch then holds better and does not peel off.

❧ Place the patch on your work surface and brush the top of the patch generously with the fixative.

❧ With the brush, lift the patch and position it on the nail with the uneven edge of the patch toward the base of the nail and leave enough of the other end extending to fold under the nail tip.

❧ Dip a cotton-tipped orangewood stick in a little solvent (polish thinner) and use the tip of the stick to fit the patch firmly to the nail and to overlap the nail tip and to fit smoothly into the sides and under the tip of the nail. The solvent also removes any excess glue.

Once the patch is on, it will last through two or more polish changes *if* you remove the polish carefully with a cotton ball dampened with polish remover.

Nail polish. Besides giving color and beauty to the nails, polish helps them to resist breakage and tearing, acting as a protective sheath.

❧ First, apply polish base—two coats if the nail has been patched. Let each coat dry completely before applying the next coat. If you do not allow enough drying time, the patch may separate from the nail.

❧ Apply two coats of nail enamel, again letting each coat dry thoroughly. Coat the nail from base to tip, beveling the tip by running the tip of the thumb of the other hand lightly along the edge of the nail.

❧ When enamel is dry (it is best to allow an hour's drying time for the second coat; wait at least 20 minutes), apply the sealer. First, run the brush lightly across the top of the nail to protect the tip, where there is most wear, and then coat the entire nail. Reapply sealer every day or two, always brushing first across the tip, and your polish job should look well till next week's manicure.

BETWEEN-MANICURE TIPS

Artificial nails. This fingertip magic is easy to come by. Take one set of artificial nails. Strip your own nails of polish and be sure cuticle around nail is pushed back and clean. Fasten artificial nails firmly with accompanying adhesive, allowing an hour or more for them to set. (Hair-drying time is a good occasion. Manufacturers suggest you put nails on at bedtime to give them several hours to adhere firmly. Okay—*if* you sleep alone and have no next-day housework!) Apply polish—two coats—the length of one nail in three smooth strokes.

Nail-hardeners. They really work. Follow package directions; some can safely coat the whole nail; others are only for the tips. Used faithfully, they can give your nails a hardness that resists workaday wear and tear. When a break or split does happen, a nail bonder painted across and then lengthwise on the break (both under and over the nail tip) is a quick repair.

Cuticle care. Between manicures, give cuticle a daily treatment with a cuticle brush and a push back with washcloth or towel after a hand-washing. Then regular creaming (hand cream or lotion by day, cuticle cream at bedtime) keeps the cuticle under control.

Nail shaping. File only when nails are bone-dry—never right after wet work, a bath, hand-washing; during your manicure, shape nails before soaking them.

Nail cleaning. To keep the underside of your nails clean, use a nailbrush during each hand-washing; run an orange-stick tip gently under the nail after you dry your hands; keep underside of nails creamed or soaped when you do rough work. Use nail white—cream or pencil—beneath the nail tip; if nail or skin is stained, a little hydrogen peroxide on a cotton swab will bleach it.

Enameling. Polish protects and beautifies the nail. The secret? For everyday, use a translucent polish—colored or clear. Between manicures, as long as polish is unchipped, apply a new coat each day—it dries quickly, takes only a minute. The build-up of polish strengthens the nail and gives it a jewel-like look.

HAND AND NAIL-CARE PROBLEMS

Breaking nails. If nails break easily due to household work, a triple-coat polish job will strengthen and protect them.
* Take care not to strike tips of nails against hard objects. When you reach into handbag or kitchen drawers, reach with the back of the hand, fingers curled, to protect nails.
* If nails split at the tips or peel, they may need a rest from liquid polish and remover. Use a buffer to exercise the nails and to give them gloss. Polish will go on more smoothly, too.

Freckles and liver spots. These can be bleached with use of a cosmetic preparation or they can be concealed by water-resistant cover makeup. If hands are protected from exposure to sunlight, freckles will fade; use a sun screen on your hands to avoid freckling.

Calluses. These are more easily prevented than removed. Soften calluses on the palm of the hand with hand cream or lotion, avoid the cause, and the callus will eventually peel off.
* To prevent calluses (they are a thickening of the thin palm skin in defense against rubbing), pad the handles of electric iron, mops, sweepers. Pad the palm of your work gloves as protection when you rake or hoe.

Warts. These are fairly common on fingers and hands. Small ones can be treated with a preparation your doctor will prescribe for you. Large ones can be burned off with an electric needle.

Nail biting. There are preparations you can paint on your nail tips to discourage your nibbling. There are nail hardeners, as well, to help nails resist damage.
* Try to make yourself conscious of your action whenever you start to bite your nails. Awareness of what you are doing can help you discourage the habit.
* Find a substitute. When hands are busy, with knitting or other handwork, you are less likely to nail-chew.

Stiffness. Simple exercises will help limber your fingers.
* Place fingertips of both hands together so that corresponding fingertips touch; press fingertips together to flatten the length of each finger against its mate without the palms touching.
* Arch wrists and rest fingertips on a flat surface. Then tap each finger separately upon the surface five to 10 times.

Swollen veins. Hold hands up, rather than let them dangle, and blood will not accumulate to distend the veins, and hands will not become reddened from an excess of capillary blood in the skin.
* Hold the hands at shoulder level; shake vigorously to aid the circulation.

Redness and roughness. Keep hands clean. After you have used household soap or detergent, rewash the hands with mild hand soap.
* Rinse hands carefully after you have had them in soapy water. Dry them whenever you take them out of water; dampness, especially when combined with cold and wind, encourages chapping.
* Avoid leaving the hands in water for long periods. In water, skin cells lose moisture; they don't absorb it.
* Avoid putting the hands into very hot water.

Hand protectors. Use proper kitchen tools to protect your hands. Don't use fingernails as pan scrapers, package openers, or for other tasks for which there are better tools. Use openers to budge hard-to-open jar lids so that hands are not strained. Save your hands from burns by having potholders handy at the range or grill.

Gloves. Wear dress gloves to keep hands clean, to protect hand skin when weather is cold and damp. And there are some household jobs for which only gloves can give protection to the hands:
* When hands are in contact with staining materials, paint, wax, oil, dust, caustics, and other irritants.
* When you handle steel-wool pads and other abrasives, even scouring powders.
* Whenever you put hands in water, if hand skin is sensitive to soaps, detergent, or other household cleanser.
* When you garden, do yard work, and polish the car.
* A little talcum powder sprinkled in rubber or plastic work gloves helps the glove slip on smoothly and absorbs some of the perspiration that can make wearing such gloves a discomfort. Lined gloves are comfortable, too.

Hand creams and lotions. These are more than a feminine indulgence; they answer a real need of the hand skin. In the hand, there is little natural skin oil and usually little fat cushion beneath the skin surface. Much of the natural oil can be removed by the soaps and detergents that cut grease from dishes, soil from clothes. In addition, the natural chemistry of the skin is slightly acid, and most cleansers are alkaline. Chemical balance, natural oil, and cell moisture are infection preventers as well as skin smoothers. Regular use of hand-skin conditioner—lotion or cream—can help to restore the natural skin balance. Keep conditioner at every sink.
* When you apply hand cream or lotion, use a generous amount, smoothing it on as if you were putting on a glove. Holding the hand up with fingers pointed upward, smooth the conditioner over the fingertips, down over the knuckles, over the back of the hand, and well over the wrist. Finish with a washing motion, rubbing both hands together till the conditioner is well worked into the skin.

ARM PROBLEMS

Flabby upper arms. They result from stretching of the arm skin through use, through loss of muscle tone, or perhaps from accumulation of fat. Arm-toning exercises can help.

Rough elbows. Lotion rubs will help. Make a cup of the palm of one hand and pour into it a teaspoonful of hand lotion. Rub the palm of this hand against the opposite elbow in a brisk rotary motion.

Hair on outer arm. Unless some glandular disturbance is causing hair growth (check with your doctor), overgrowth or darkness of hair on the outer arm is probably an inborn characteristic. If the hair is so conspicuous that it cannot be ignored, it may be removed with cream or wax depilatory. Shaving is *not* recommended; it leaves stubble or shadow to discomfort you. Electrolysis is a way to get rid of it permanently.

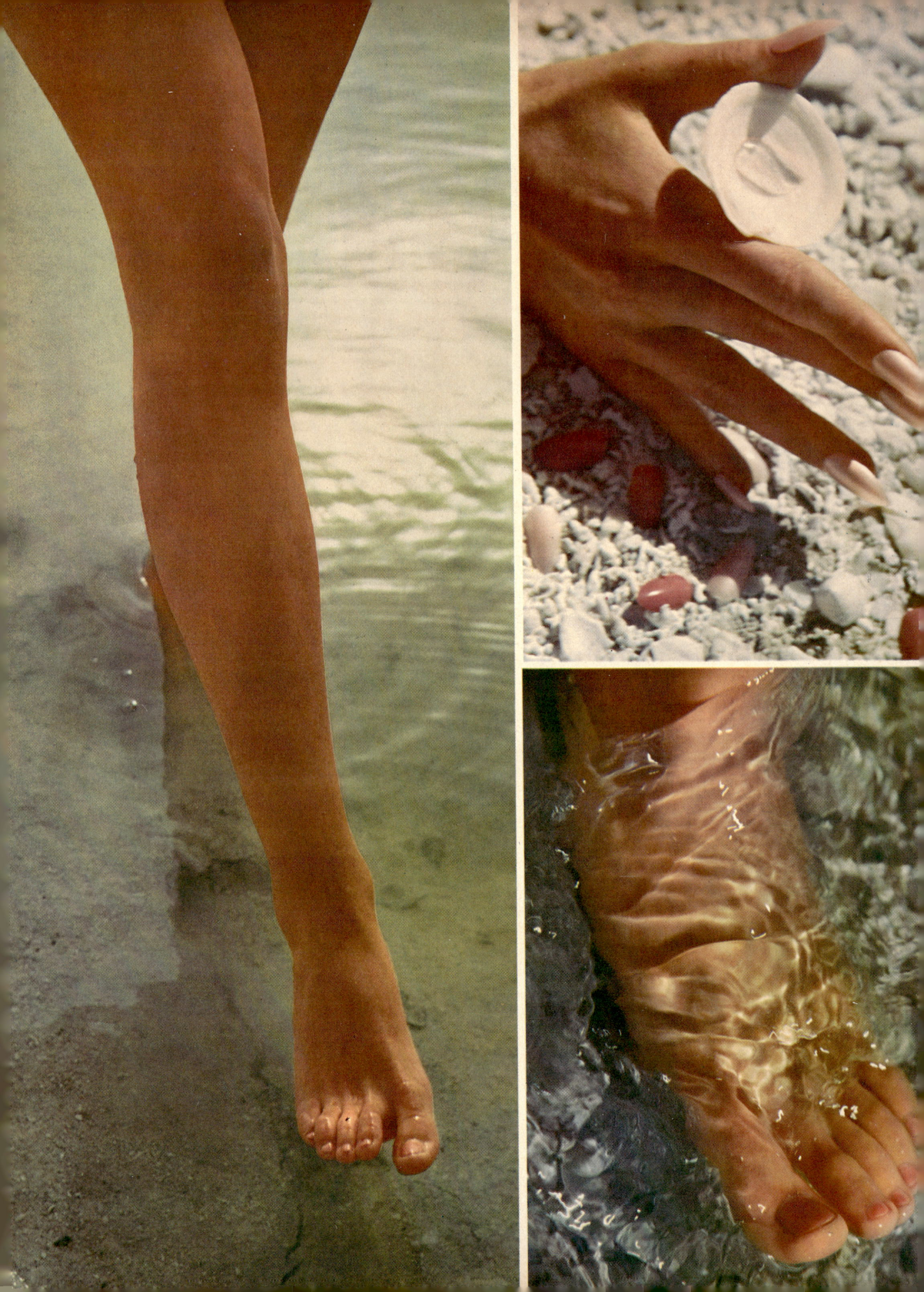

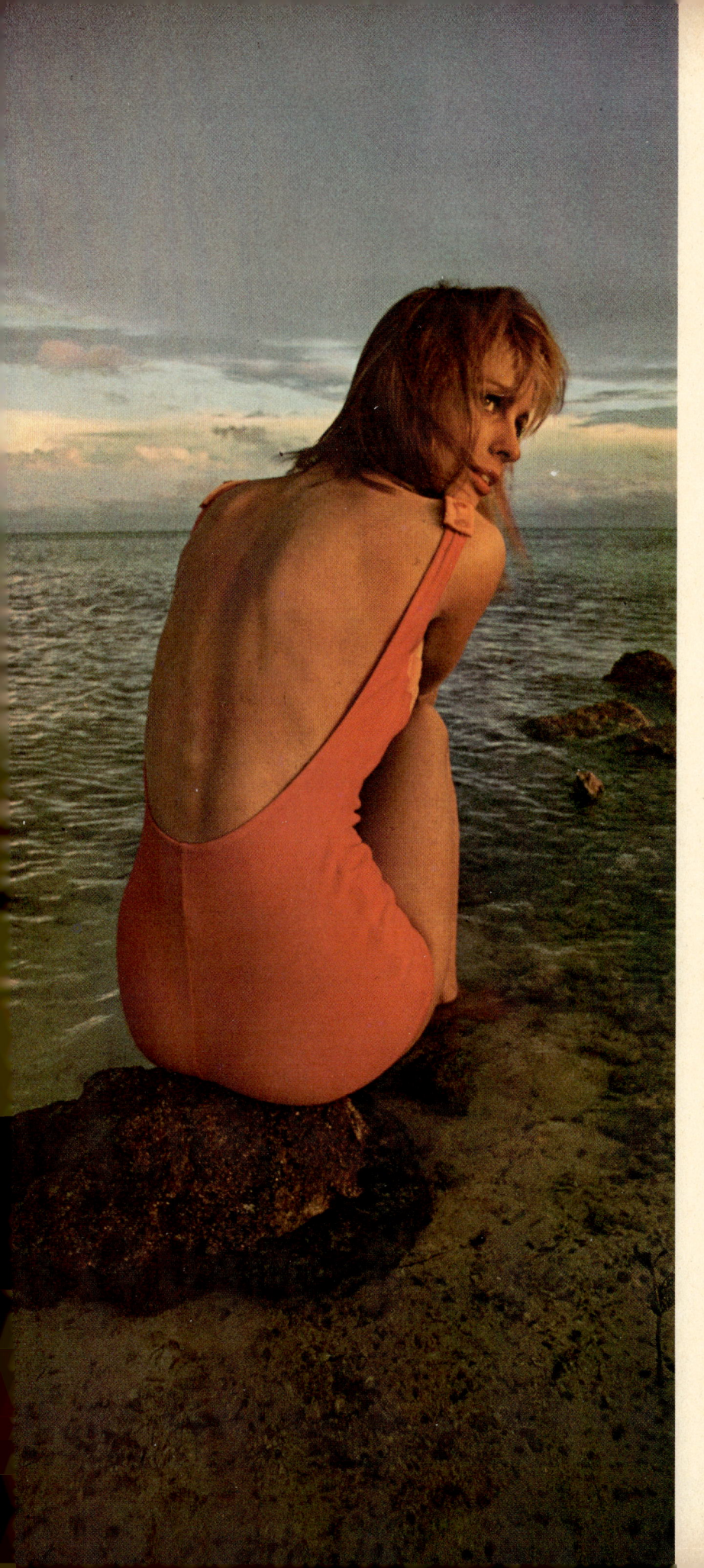

Instant Beauty Aids

Instant tan? With smoothly applied body makeup you can appear golden or toasty your first moment in the sun. Or use a tinted tanning preparation that simulates a tan while it protects the skin against burning.

Instant fingernails? They are easy to put on, once they have been shaped and fitted to your own fingernails. Shape at the base, not at the tip, using a long flexible emery board. Buy false nails in opaque or translucent color, or buy them clear and then apply your own nail polish.

Tinted leg makeup. Buffed to a soft sheen, this is a great summer beauty maker. It covers leg blemishes (such as visible veins) as it provides instant hose and instant tan. Bare legs—suntanned or made-up—should be meticulously free of hair. Chemical or wax hair removers leave the cleanest surface, but shaving the legs daily is faster.

Feet need beautifying? Corns and calluses are ugly and must go. For instant foot beauty, cut the toenail straight across at the tip; apply colored nail polish to the entire nail surface.

❦ You need two kinds of foot cream to beat dry foot skin. One to friction off the rough dead skin; another just to keep the dry spots moisturized. The sole, the edges of the foot, and the heels are dry-out spots. Make them your special field of care.

WHAT CARE FOR YOUR FEET?

How nice it is to be able to slip out of your shoes without being embarrassed by the condition of your feet! But foot care means comfort as well as beauty. Aching feet can be damaging to posture, health, temper, and facial lines—and may eventually disable you if you don't correct the cause. If you have foot problems, see a chiropodist or podiatrist—and be astonished at how much difference just one visit can make. Meanwhile, a little care, a little consideration—and some simple grooming—for your feet, ankles, and legs can make a tremendous difference in how all the rest of you feels.

Foot problems. Feet will not tire quickly if shoes and stockings are properly fitted—especially if they are long enough.

❧ Buy shoes late in the day when feet are expanded.

❧ Fit the larger foot and always stand when the foot is being measured.

❧ Both shoes and stockings should be one-half inch longer than the big toe to give room for expansion.

❧ After taking off shoes, grasp big toe and rotate it slowly. This also prevents calluses forming under the big-toe joint.

Swelling ankles—Rest feet as often as possible, keeping the feet elevated, preferably higher than the hips. At least, keep the knees higher than the hips by using a footrest at home and when traveling.

❧ Be sure that shoes and stockings are not so tight they will become unbearable if feet swell.

❧ See your physician if the trouble is chronic.

Broken veins—These may be concealed with use of water-resistant cover make-up.

Foot burn—Wear shoes with leather soles and uppers—leather is porous and helps to ventilate the feet.

❧ Change stockings at least twice a day.

❧ Sprinkle absorbent powder on feet and inside of shoes—or spray with foot spray—when you put them on and, if possible, renew each four hours.

Chapping—Use a body lotion or hand cream on the foot skin at bedtime and before putting on hose. Apply talcum powder to absorb moisture after the bath. Use chap cream on knees and ankles if these areas roughen.

Hard corns and calluses—These show areas where shoes rub, and well fitted shoes help the problem. Have existing corns and calluses removed by a foot doctor (a podiatrist or chiropodist).

❧ Cover rubbed areas with moleskin or callus pads to prevent calluses redeveloping.

❧ A pumice-stone rub after each bath can keep foot calluses down.

Soft corns—These appear between the toes and are a fungus infection, as is athlete's foot. Have your doctor prescribe treatment.

Ingrown toenails—These are usually caused by too-short shoes and improperly cut nails. A foot doctor can help.

❧ To avoid, cut toenails straight across (do not taper at the sides) and no shorter than the flesh of the toe.

❧ Wear shoes at least one-half inch longer than the foot.

Perspiring feet—Wear well-ventilated shoes and change shoes daily and stockings twice a day.

❧ Use an absorbent foot powder generously on feet and in shoes.

Foot relaxers. A 10-to-20-minute soak in warm water—add three tablespoons of baking soda for each quart of water—relaxes the feet. Dry feet well after the soak.

Massage—Particularly useful as a relaxer to homemakers is a tension-easing foot treatment from the Golden Door Beauty Spa. Called "happy feet," it helps to relax the entire body. Use warm scented oil or foot cream to soothe foot skin as you knead, knuckle, and wring the feet.

❧ Knead the bottom of the foot across the heel, arch, and ball and to the base of toe joints; continue kneading crosswise till the entire bottom has been massaged.

❧ Take one toe at a time and squeeze it between the fingers and then rotate it in both directions. Squeeze hard and pull away from foot as you rotate. Repeat with all toes.

❧ Put the fingers of one hand between the toes and place the other hand over the toes and squeeze.

❧ Pick up limp foot by grabbing one toe at a time, shaking, and then dropping it.

❧ Insert fingers between toes from sole side, using opposite hand; grasp bundle with free hand, and extend leg, squeezing with both hands. Release. Repeat three times.

❧ Grasp the ball and arch with opposite hand and wring foot like a wet towel. Leaving hand in place, take other hand and place on heel and wring. Repeat in each direction.

❧ Grasp foot with left hand, make the right hand into a fist, and work the knuckles over the entire top of the foot from above the ankle to the toes.

❧ Repeat entire process on the other foot.

Foot rest—Lie on back on bed or couch or on the floor facing a wall. Lift legs from hips so they make a 45° angle with your reclining spine and place feet firmly against the wall. Hold the position for about 10 minutes or for as long as is comfortable.

The pedicure. Pedicure needs are:

Nail clipper	Cotton-tipped stick
Metal file	
Cuticle pusher	Body lotion
Basin of soapy water	Towel
	Cuticle remover
Cotton balls and squares	Polish remover
	Polish base
Adhesive tape	Nail polish
Foot powder	Polish sealer

Foot bath—Start your pedicure after a bath or start with a 10-minute soak in warm soapy water.

❧ Go over any rough areas on the ball of the foot or at the heels with a pumice stone, rinsing the feet often as you work. Use a nailbrush on the toenails to remove loose cuticle.

Cuticle treatment—Dry the feet and then use a plastic cuticle pusher or a cotton-tipped stick to work away dead skin around the nails.

❧ Apply cuticle remover and work again around the nails with a cotton-tipped stick.

❧ Rinse toes in soapy water and then, to loosen cuticle, massage each nail with the corner of a towel.

❧ Dry feet well and then give the feet and legs, all the way up over the knees, a massage with rich body lotion.

❧ If any areas are callus-prone, soak a cotton square in body lotion and fix it over the rough spots with adhesive tape. Leave on overnight.

Nail care—Clip toenails straight across and no shorter than the length of the flesh of the toe. Smooth the tips with a metal file so that nail tip is somewhat beveled, but do not file down at sides. The squarish shape is comfortable and pretty.

❧ Place cotton balls between the toes to keep them separated while you apply polish.

❧ Apply base coat, two coats of enamel, and a seal coat.

❧ Use colored polish whenever feet are to be exposed, whether on the beach, in open shoes, or at home.

GOOD-GROOMING CHECKLIST

Grooming is all the careful top touches, plus fastidious concern about all that goes on underneath. If you feel clean, comfortable, and put together from top to toe, if you are pleasantly fragrant and attractively made up, you are helped to feel poised, organized and competent.

Here are some ways to keep your appearance in control.

Protect your vitality. Start good grooming with the inner you. This means a nutritive diet, regular meals, and adequate hours of sleep to keep up your energy. It is hard to feel (and to be) well-groomed when you are tired. Eat an adequate breakfast and skimp (if you're calorie-counting) on evening nibbling. Get enough sleep so that you feel rested. You may need as few as six hours or as many as 10—but if you get less sleep than you need, you won't feel up to daily tasks.

Work at figure control. Good grooming is easiest when you are the best weight for your height and frame. If you are of normal weight, your clothes fit well and you feel comfortable in them. So be sure your figure matches the proportions of the dress size you consider desirable for you. A regular exercise program, plus calorie-counting, can bring your figure under control. Exercise helps too, in bettering your posture and in smoothing your body lines and increasing energy.

Budget your time. It is hard to be well-turned-out if you have had to rush to get ready. Time has to be put aside for grooming as for everything else. If you keep up with the attentions your body needs, it is easier to dress on a minimum time budget. Learn to make fairly accurate time allowances: "If I must be there at four o'clock, I must leave here at 3:45. So I will start putting on my clothes at 3:30; I start doing my hair at 3:15 and my make-up at three. If I start my shower at 2:45, I'll be sure to make it." This kind of backtracking on your schedule works more effectively than saying: "I have to be there at four. It takes me about an hour to get ready, so I guess I can start at three."

Take care of your clothes. Clothes should be well-fitted and well-cared-for. A hem line that sags at sides or back or is even half-an-inch too long spoils the look of you as a whole person. Heel height in your shoes matters too; the relation between heel height and skirt length is an important grooming keynote. Be sure that all slide fasteners are locked, that hooks and snap fasteners are closed, that any snags and catches are taken care of. Important to good grooming is a well-organized closet so that clothes come out ready to wear; your sewing box should be handy and well-supplied. A full-length mirror is a must—items that look all right separately sometimes look all wrong when you wear them together. Check your look front, back, and from both sides.

Care for your accessories. Your feet should be comfortable and well-cared-for so that you can walk and stand gracefully. Have shoes well-brushed or polished, the heel lift in good condition. Do your stockings fit snugly? Check their leg length as well as foot size when you buy. Your handbag is smartest when it is inconspicuous and comfortable to carry. To look well-groomed with a strap handbag, carry it on your arm or over your shoulder so that the slim end is forward. Keep the contents of your handbag neat so that if you should drop it, you need not despair. Fitting it with correct accessories helps. Include an appointment book and address book with a strap or slide closing, a makeup case, wallet and coin holder, a tissue case.

🍃 Gloves should be worn, not carried; they are less likely to be lost, and they keep your hands clean as well as warm. (You need not remove your gloves to shake hands.)

🍃 Umbrellas with a strap are easy to carry—and less likely to be forgotten. When not in use, keep your umbrella tightly rolled and fitted into its case.

Be neat underneath. Undergarments should be invisible except to give a well-molded line to your body and to make your clothes fit you better. A body stocking is a great figure smoother; even if you need more contouring than it gives, it works well when combined with girdle and bra. Underwear should be fresh daily—and this goes for stockings too. Hosiery wears better when washed and rested between wearings.

Have a neat head. Schedule your hair care so that your hair looks pretty most of the time. If there are days when it simply isn't right, have a wig or other cover-up that helps you look well-groomed. If you choose a scarf as a cover-up, tie it prettily so that it will look part of your design, not a makeshift.

🍃 A good haircut is basic—and if your hair is short, three weeks is about the right time between trims. Don't try to make any hair setting last a full week. Five days is the most you can expect—and you may as well face the fact. Shampoo your hair as often as you like so that it is always clean and shiny. If hair is short and needs to be fluffy, it isn't unreasonable to shampoo often so that your hair doesn't appear stiff.

🍃 If you use a tint or a bleach and toner to achieve your hair color, you need retouches every three to four weeks. When shampooing between touch-ups, use a conditioner after the shampoo to keep your hair glossy and manageable and in good condition.

🍃 Time your permanents too for an always-becoming hair style. You'll need a new permanent every three to four months on an average, but some women need one every two months. It depends on your hair and the type of wave you have.

🍃 Brush your hair to keep it manageable, but don't overbrush. And take care in brushing not to strike the scalp with the brush bristles.

Keep your complexion clear. This means that the skin looks clean, that it is softened with cream, that it has glow but not shine, and that any blemishes are made inconspicuous. Use the cleanser that does things for your skin. Oily skin needs frequent daily cleansings; dry skin needs weatherproofing with a round-the-clock moisturizer. Eye and throat skin need special care, for these areas are the first to show discoloration and a parched surface. Skin blemishes should be treated with both medication and a cover cream so that such imperfections will be virtually unnoticeable.

Keep your hands looking cared-for. Hands need constant care if they are to look well-groomed. Too many hazards to hand skin are encountered in the home to allow us to be casual about creaming the hand skin, about wearing protective gloves for work that demands them, and about keeping the nails protected as much as possible. If you use a nail hardener, you will find your nails grow a little and are less likely to tear and to chip. Polish is protective, too. If you want your polish to last a day or two, apply three coats, letting each coat dry before applying the next. For the nicest-looking nails, remove polish daily—if you have the time—and apply a single fresh coat.

Be pleasantly fragrant. Use toilet water as a base for your perfume—spray it all over you and then touch your perfume to your pulse spots. You will probably need a deodorant and an antiperspirant too. An antiperspirant stops perspiration (most women need to apply it under the arms daily). A deodorant merely covers or deters perspiration odor. A deodorant can be applied generally over the body; use it as often as you consider necessary to keep yourself inoffensive.

FIGURE BEAUTY

You are ideal in weight if you are nicely but thinly padded, if you curve in and out at the right spots. For lucky you we offer a sensible program of exercise to keep your figure trim and beautifully aligned plus a diet plan that will save you from someday waking up and saying, "Oh, dear me! I'm fat!" If you are underweight, you probably feel you have no shape at all. For you, good news! The same exercises that firm the muscles of normal-weight women and trim the curves of the fatty, help you to develop a shape of your own while you beef up your diet to give you those needed pounds. If you're overweight, you have to cut calories—and exercise. See our 1,000-calorie diet plan and start on our figure-firming exercises. Lazy? You can begin with yoga exercises you do in a chair and move along to our four-week yoga slimming plan. Feeling strong? Step ahead to Bonnie Prudden's four-week shape-up with spot-reducing exercises—these really use energy, deliver diet spunk.

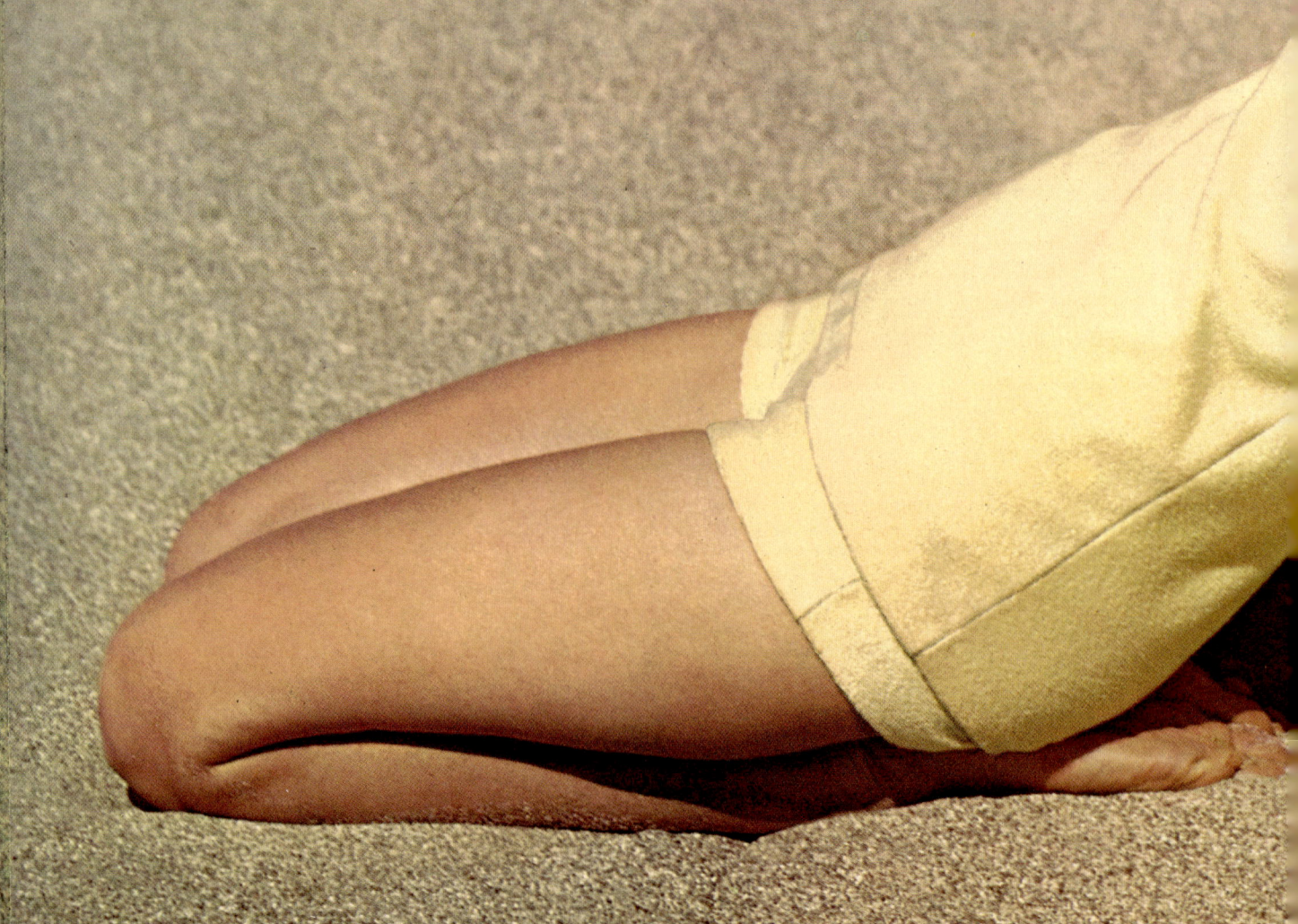

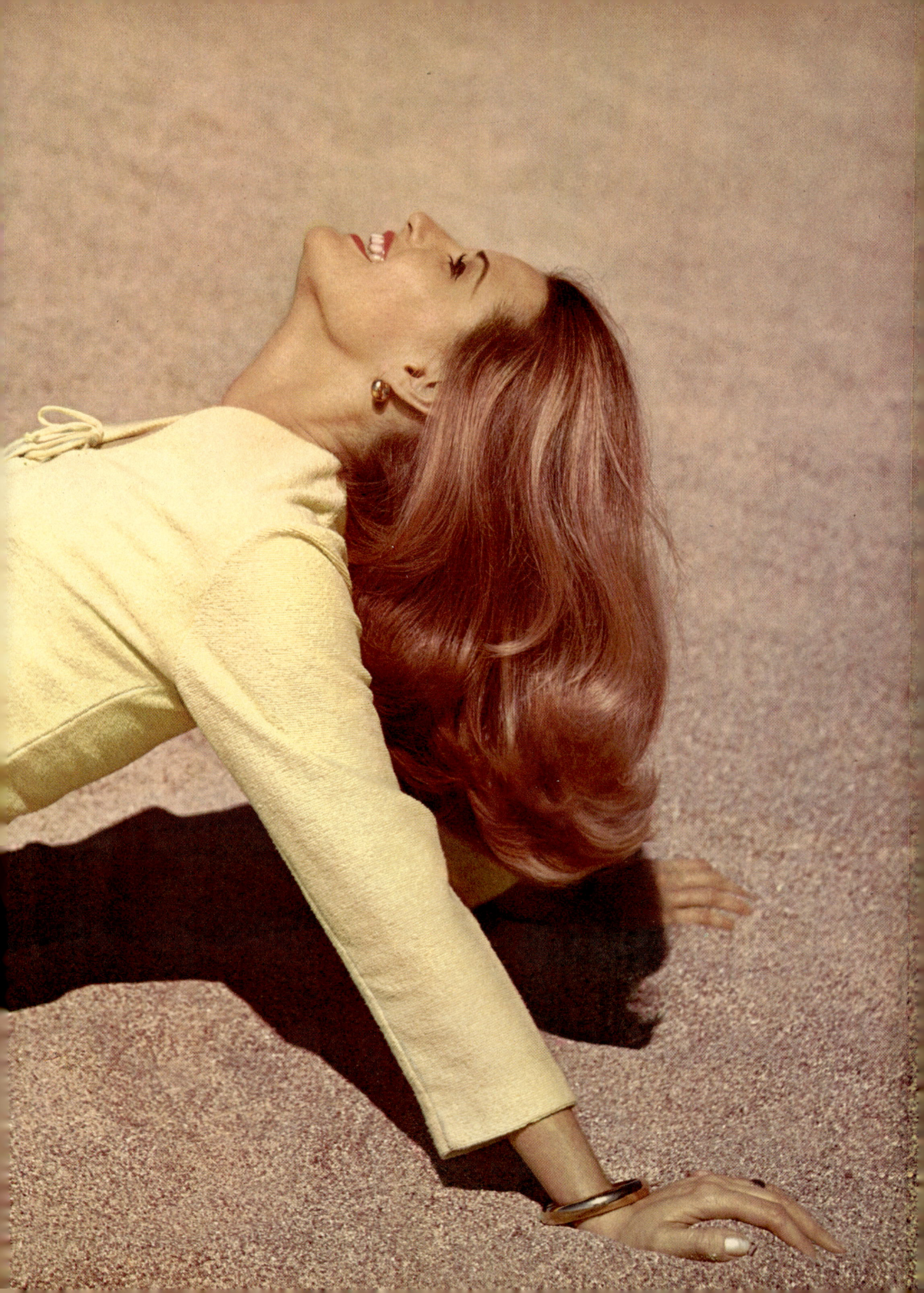

HOW MUCH SHOULD YOU WEIGH?

Today's "ideal" weights for health are close to what has long been considered "ideal" for beauty. It is now believed that you stay healthier if you are slim. But all too many women are considerably over the ideal.

How much should you eat? Even if you are close to the "ideal," weight control can be important to you. It is no longer considered natural or necessary to gain pounds as you grow older. It simply takes less food, as we get older, to run the machine, and anyone eating the same amount over a decade or two is bound to gain as the daily calorie need diminishes.

❧ A calorie is the unit of energy that nutritionists use in their food count. Think of a calorie as fuel and of the body as a house that needs heating; the larger the house, the more fuel it takes to run it. If you close off a few rooms or leave fewer doors and windows open, less fuel will be needed. If, however, you still take in the same amount of fuel, you have more than the house needs to warm it, and the extra fuel goes into storage.

❧ Your body's fuel-storage tanks are the deposits of fat beneath the skin and round the muscles. The only way you can dump this stored fuel is by cutting the amount of fuel you take in and using instead what you have in storage. When, on the other hand, you take in too little fuel, your body is like a heatless home; you are eventually forced to burn up the furniture—fat the body needs to support the vital organs and to provide a cushion for muscles and skin. So underweight, though less common, can be as unhealthful as overweight. The goal should be to take in just enough calories to keep the body running at its top capacity.

❧ We use fuel even when at rest. The body uses energy to keep its organs running—heart beating, lungs functioning, and so forth—and also to provide the power for such activities as work and play. We use on the average about five calories per hour even when asleep; about 50 calories per hour are used in normal housework.

❧ You may need more or fewer calories, depending on your daily activities and also depending on whether you wish to gain or to lose weight. Your doctor can give you an accurate estimate of what your calorie intake should be to maintain or to reach the weight that is "ideal" for you.

❧ If you wish to lose a pound a week (and this is considered a reasonable goal to set if you are only moderately overweight to start), you will have to cut 500 calories a day—3,500 calories a week—to lose it. And once you reach your desired weight—say 110 pounds—your daily allotment to maintain that weight will be smaller.

Increase your activity. You can also lose weight by increasing your activity; if you burn more calories a day, you need cut fewer from your diet in order to lose your pound a week. But you must walk briskly for an hour to use up even 200 calories, and most persons find they have to cut down on their calorie intake as well as increase their activities to do more than maintain their weight.

❧ On the other side of the scoreboard are creeping ounces that make pounds come upon you through minor changes in activity—a typist changing from a manual to an electric typewriter may gain one pound in 10 weeks if she doesn't compensate for the laborsaving by other activities or by cutting calories.

❧ The intelligent person will take a median course by cutting down on calorie-expensive items that ruin the weight budget (easy to wreck when you have only 1,000 to 1,200 calories to spend) and by also increasing activity, which puts calories in the bank.

TESTED WAYS TO LOSE WEIGHT

Do count calories. If you are on a close calorie budget, even small indulgences, seemingly harmless, can put you back on a weight gain.

❧ Stick to your diet for at least six weeks. It takes this long to reeducate your eating.

❧ Don't try to lose more than a pound to two pounds a week.

❧ See your doctor for a diet that you can rely on—one that is tailored to *your* needs.

❧ *Do* drink plenty of water. Many foods have high water content; as you cut your food intake, you may also be cutting your water intake. You may feel hungry when you're really dehydrated. Any liquid — low-calorie soft drinks, bouillon, tea, coffee—helps fill you.

❧ Do change your daily routine when you change your eating habits. If you usually eat breakfast with the family, wait and eat after they have left. If you usually eat breakfast alone, change and eat it with your family. Break up your routine so that meals fall at new times. But set up a new schedule and stick to it while dieting.

❧ Do get more exercise—activity helps you stay on your diet.

❧ Do eat a good breakfast; at least one fourth of your daily calorie allotment should be consumed at this meal.

HELPS IN GAINING WEIGHT

Be sure to check with your doctor to find out if there is any reason for your thinness other than undereating and overactivity. Sometimes a thyroid condition or other physical disorder may be at fault. Sometimes an excess of nervous energy may keep a woman slim. Sometimes a woman really enjoys being skinny. Or she may simply be of a body type whose metabolism runs to underweight.

❧ Gaining weight, if there is no medical problem, is a matter of discipline. Sometimes it can help if you eat with an "untwin." This would be a plumpy who is obviously eating too much. You eat exactly as much as she eats (or nearly as possible) and you will be sure to gain. Or do her a favor and order food for her, let her order for you, and you will be doing a Jack Sprat and his wife in reverse—plumpy eating the "lean" and skinny you, the "fat."

❧ Try to relax at mealtime and also to eat slowly and to get enough sleep at night. Don't burn yourself up with late hours and don't cheat yourself with hurried meals.

❧ Get regular exercise and learn to eat when you are hungry (after exercising) and to supplement your diet with between-meals eating.

❧ Eat foods that will build body tissue —milk, meat, eggs, bread, and butter.

❧ Avoid bulky foods; instead use foods that are high in calories, low in mass, such as cheese and ice cream.

❧ Eat even when you are not hungry; you have *to want to gain* to gain.

❧ Drink little water, tea, or coffee with your meals so you don't fill up on wasted bulk.

❧ Drink milk instead of water when you are thirsty.

❧ Consistency is more important than quick gains. Reeducate your eating habits.

WHAT SHOULD YOU EAT?

To maintain health we all—fat, thin, and normal—need basically the same foods. Here from the American Dietetic Association are the basics of a 1,500 calorie daily diet pattern.

   1 pint (2 cups) whole milk
   1 egg
   5 ounces of lean meat (liver once weekly), poultry, fish (broiled, boiled, or roasted) or cheese
   ½ cup enriched or whole-grain cereal, 1 small potato, 4 slices enriched or whole-wheat bread (or ½ cup of cooked spaghetti or noodles, cooked cereal, a muffin, biscuit, or 2-inch square of corn bread)

1 serving green or yellow vegetables
2 servings of other vegetables
1 serving citrus fruit or tomato (4-ounce glass grapefruit or orange juice, 8-ounce glass tomato juice)
2 servings other fruit, fresh or unsweetened
4 teaspoons butter or enriched margarine

To cut this to 1,200 calories, use skim milk or buttermilk instead of whole milk and cut out cereal, potato, or one slice of bread and one teaspoon of fat daily. Consult your physician before going on a drastic reducing diet.

1000-calorie diet. Many women need to go to a 1,000 calorie daily diet in order to lose weight. Here is a diet pattern for 1,000 calories a day:
  1 pint (2 cups) skim milk
  1 cup cottage cheese
  1 medium egg
  Selected meat, fish or poultry (liver once a week), 6-ounce portion
  1 serving green or yellow vegetable
  2 servings of other vegetables
Plus either:
  1 slice bread
  2 portions fruit
  3 portions other vegetables
Or:
  2 slices enriched whole-wheat or white bread
  2 portions fruit
  2 portions other vegetables
Or:
  1 portion cereal
  3 portions fruit
  2 portions vegetables

BASIC DIET PATTERN

BREAKFAST

1 serving high vitamin-C fruit
1 serving from bread-cereal group plus 1 egg or 2 servings from bread-cereal group (use part of skim milk with cereal)
1 pat butter or margarine
1 cup skim milk

LUNCH

2-unit serving from meat group
1 serving dark green or yellow vegetable
1 serving other 15-calorie vegetable
1 serving any 40-calorie fruit
1 cup skim milk

DINNER

3-unit serving from meat group
1 serving dark green or yellow vegetable
1 serving other 15-calorie vegetable
1 serving any 40-calorie fruit
Black coffee or tea with lemon

PREDICTED DAILY CALORIE NEEDS FOR WOMEN OF NORMAL WEIGHT

HEIGHT FEET	INCHES	AGE 15-19	AGE 20-29	AGE 30-39	AGE 40-49	AGE 50-59	AGE 60-69	AGE 70-79
4	9	2080	1890	1810	1760	1710	1480	1370
4	10	2110	1920	1840	1790	1740	1510	1400
4	11	2140	1950	1870	1820	1770	1530	1430
5	0	2190	1980	1900	1850	1800	1550	1450
5	1	2240	2020	1940	1890	1850	1590	1480
5	2	2290	2060	1980	1950	1900	1640	1510
5	3	2350	2100	2030	2000	1950	1690	1550
5	4	2400	2150	2080	2040	2000	1740	1590
5	5	2460	2200	2140	2080	2050	1780	1640
5	6	2520	2250	2190	2120	2100	1820	1690
5	7	2570	2300	2240	2160	2150	1860	1730
5	8	2620	2350	2290	2220	2200	1910	1770
5	9	2680	2400	2340	2260	2250	1950	1800
5	10	2740	2450	2400	2310	2300	1990	1830
5	11	2800	2500	2450	2360	2350	2040	1880
6	0	2860	2550	2500	2410	2400	2090	1930

Courtesy of Department of Health, City of New York.

DESIRABLE WEIGHTS FOR WOMEN AGE 25 AND OVER
weight in pounds according to frame (in indoor clothing)

HEIGHT in 2-inch heels FEET	INCHES	SMALL FRAME	MEDIUM FRAME	LARGE FRAME
4	10	92— 98	96—107	104—119
4	11	94—101	98—110	106—122
5	0	96—104	101—113	109—125
5	1	99—107	104—116	112—128
5	2	102—110	107—119	115—131
5	3	105—113	110—122	118—134
5	4	108—116	113—126	121—138
5	5	111—119	116—130	125—142
5	6	114—123	120—135	129—146
5	7	118—127	124—139	133—150
5	8	122—131	128—143	137—154
5	9	126—135	132—147	141—158
5	10	130—140	136—151	145—163
5	11	134—144	140—155	149—168
6	0	138—148	144—159	153—173

Desirable weights and average weights courtesy of Metropolitan Life Insurance Company

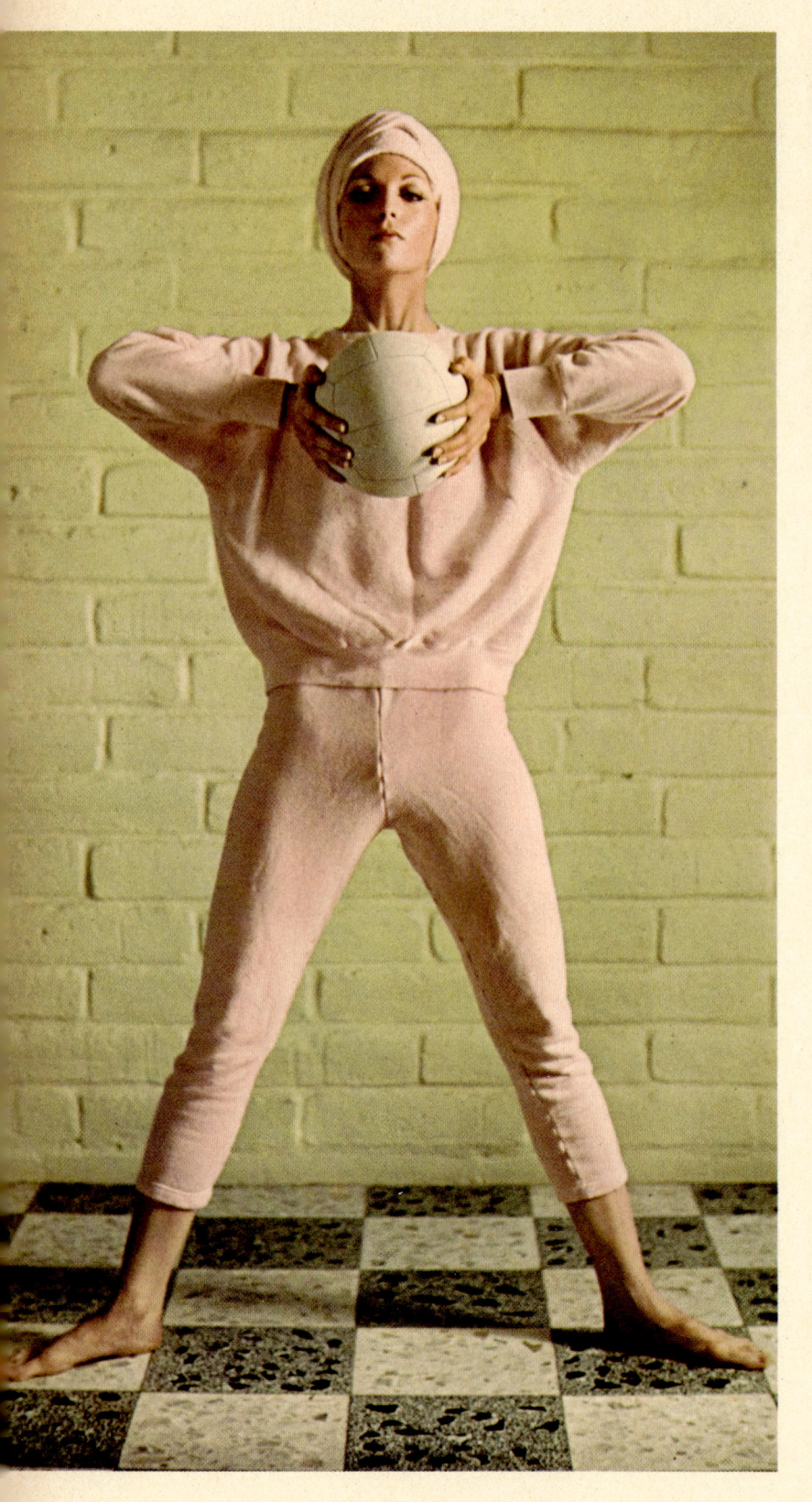

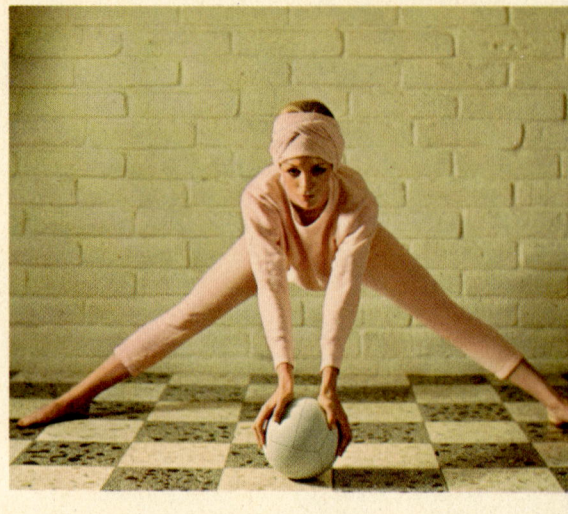

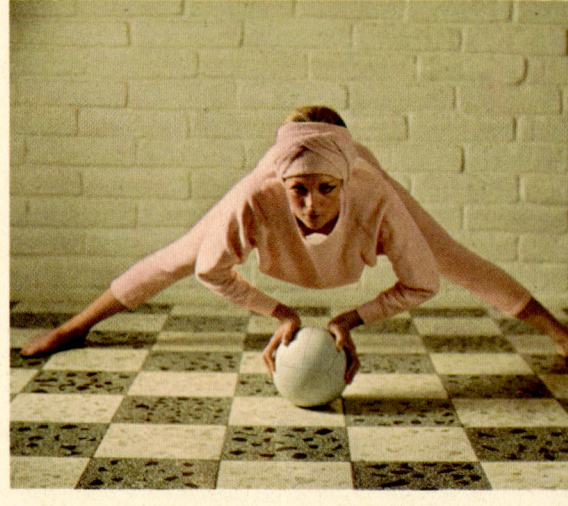

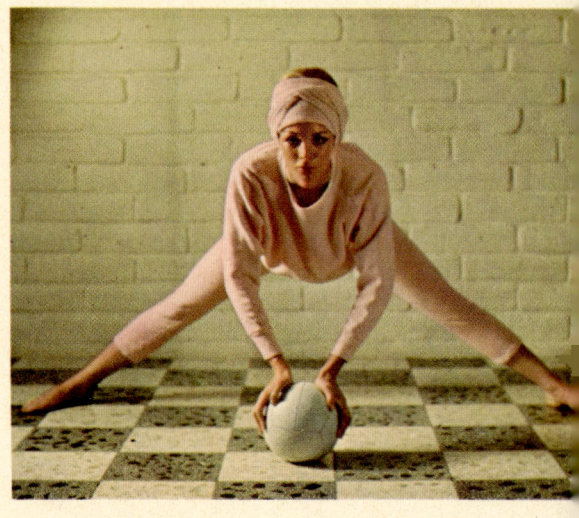

Exercise For Figure Beauty And Vitality

Figure control is easiest if you encourage activity in your daily life. The day can be started with a light cheerful wake-up—skipping around the garden or an early-day walk or jog. During the day household tasks can be broken up with 10-minute workouts—figure-shapers or simply jumping rope. Such exercise breaks (four or five a day) are as effective—and not so boring—as a steady 40-minute or hour-long endurance contest. In housework, too, active tasks should be alternated with sitting tasks so that you don't get tired of what you're doing. In fact, vary your work every 40 minutes—and the whole day's chores will go more easily.

❧ Here is a sample exercise break: Start with a gradual slow stretch, beginning with your toes and feet and legs and working up your back, vertebra by vertebra, till you have stretched your arms high above your head. Now, jog in place till you are breathing heavily—say about half a minute. Now switch to a few sit-ups. Then jog again for a half-minute, or till you are puffing. It is a good idea to do this warm-up stretching routine before beginning any exercise program. It also serves as a wake-up exercise.

❧ You will find that change-of-pace exercise—even vigorous exercise—can be as "restful" as sitting down. And the woman who gets into the habit of being active has won a large part of the figure-control battle. When you make a whole new habit of activating yourself—spending less time sitting, more time doing—figure fitness comes naturally.

❧ Vigorous exercise should be vigorous—it should put your heart to racing and make you breathe hard (with your own physician's approval, of course). If you extend yourself a little bit beyond what is easy for you to do, you soon find it is easy.

❧ And don't overlook the activity value of the simple things you have fun doing—swimming, bicycling, other sports that give you energy-plus and pounds-minus.

❧ Exercising to music during your regular workouts is another way to overcome boredom and to improve coordination while spot-reducing and figure-firming. The music should be cheerful and bouncy. Any of the popular records will keep you moving and pick up your spirits.

❧ Exercising in water also has a plus effect. The water is resistant, making greater effort necessary for any movement and thus giving the muscles added firming. Many of the simple exercises you ordinarily do—scissors kicks and so forth—can be done in water, either standing or while holding onto the pool edge. Crosswalking through the water, swinging the arms back and forth as you walk with legs crossing over, is effective. So is the belly flop. Throw arms and body forward while kicking feet up. Fun, too!

A ball makes figure-firming more fun. This ball routine from the Golden Door—the famous beauty spa in Escondido, California, firms the upper arms and abdomen and flattens the rear.

❧ Start by holding the ball before you at chest level, arms at shoulder height, spreading feet as wide as possible.

❧ Stretch arms to the front, reaching forward; lower the ball to the floor in front of you, keeping arms and back straight.

❧ Push forward against the ball by bending elbows.

❧ Still leaning on the ball, push up by straightening elbows.

❧ Push backward away from ball, elbows straight.

❧ Alternately push forward, up, and back four times as rhythmically as possible and return to starting position. Then repeat.

STICK EXERCISE FROM THE GOLDEN DOOR

Any smooth stick (that old broomstick, with the sweep removed) can be your accessory to this wonder-worker.

Waist-whittler. Stand, legs spread, holding stick at ends with both hands, and raise stick overhead, arms stretched high.

🌸 Bend to left.

🌸 Tightening buttocks and letting the stick slide through your hands but not letting go of it with either hand, bend farther, trying to touch the floor on the left side.

🌸 Bring stick overhead and repeat to right side.

🌸 Stand, raise stick overhead, and then bring it down behind the shoulders.

🌸 Twist to right; twist to left.

🌸 Stand, legs spread, holding stick overhead with both hands.

🌸 Bring stick down in front of you to hip height, bending forward from hips, with back straight. Raise stick over shoulders while leaning forward.

🌸 Bring it down in front of you again.

🌸 Repeat.

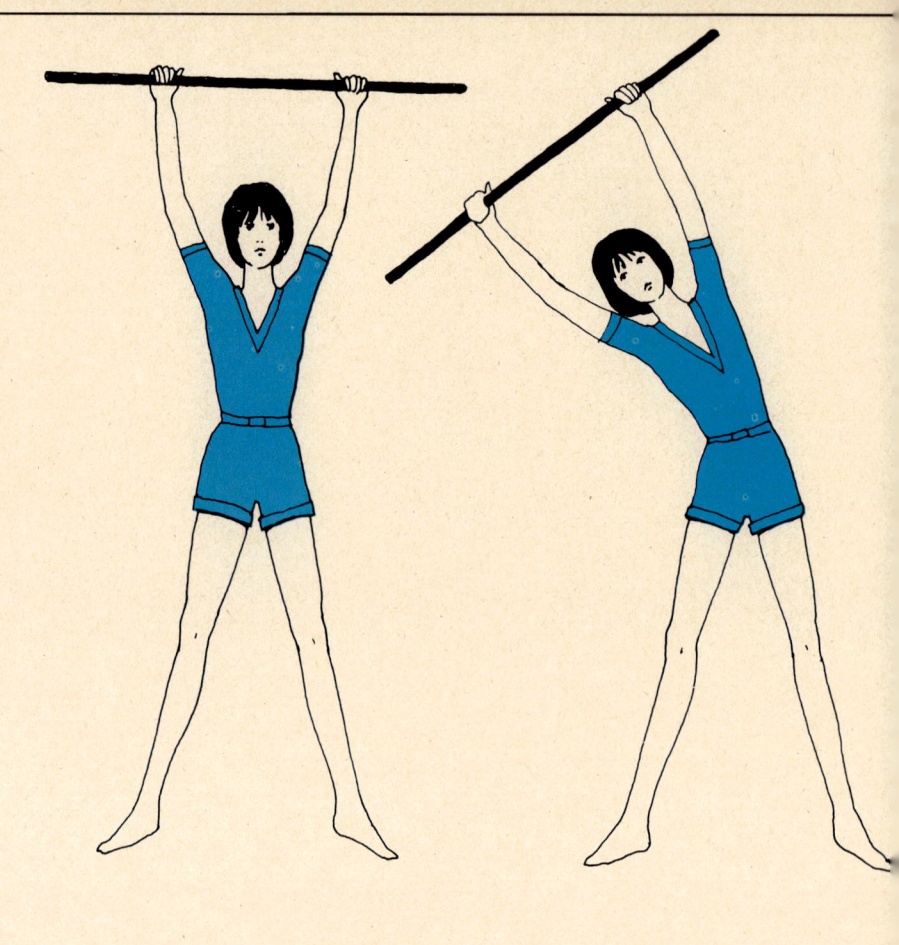

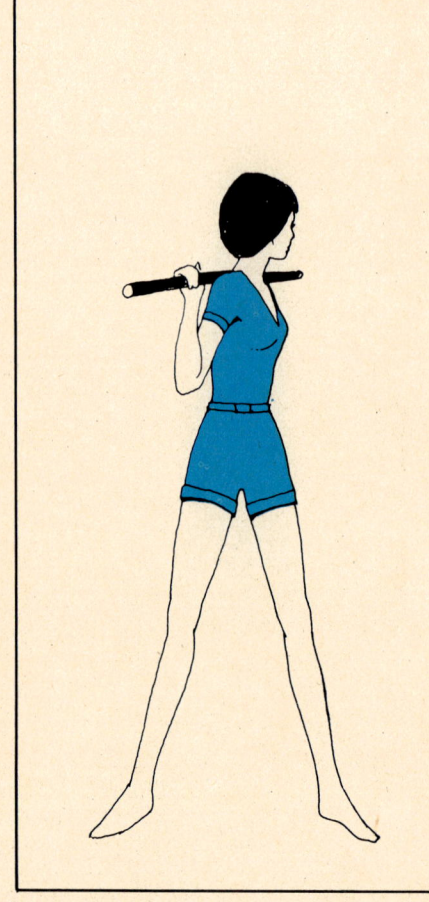

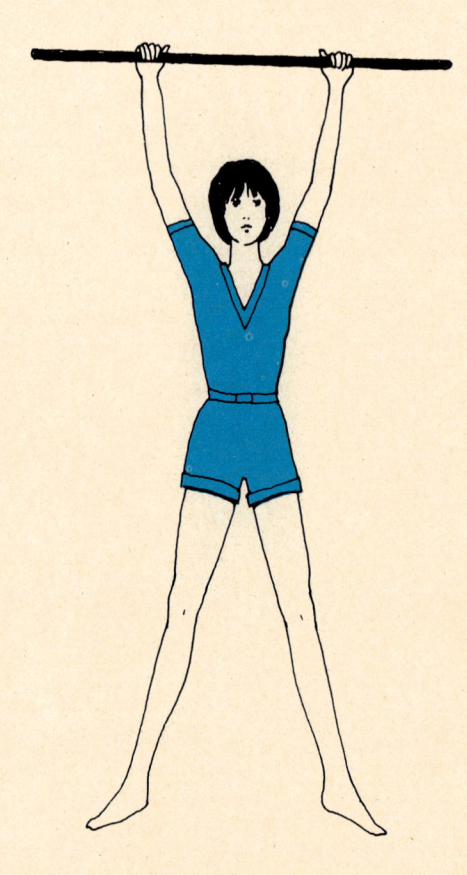

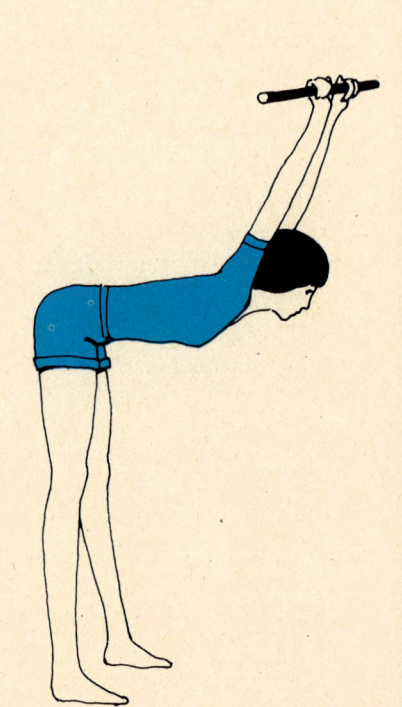

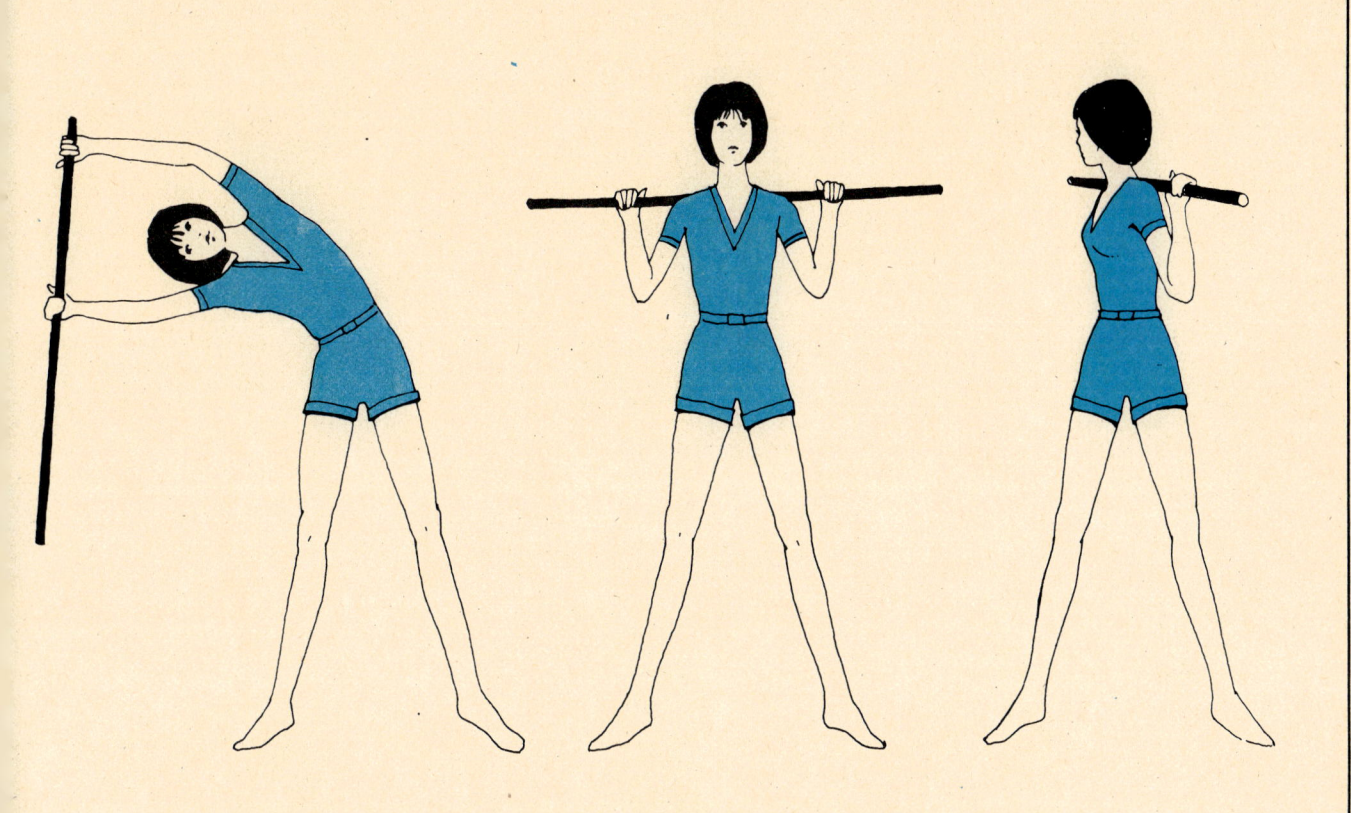

Thigh-stretcher. Sit on floor, with legs stretched out in front of you, and hold stick out in front of you. Place left foot on the stick.

- Bend knee and pull toward body.
- Lift stick, stretching leg forward.
- Slowly bring leg down by bending knee and lowering arms.
- Do 10 times and repeat with other leg.

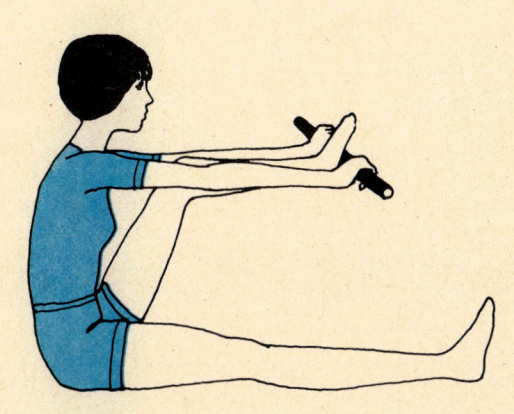

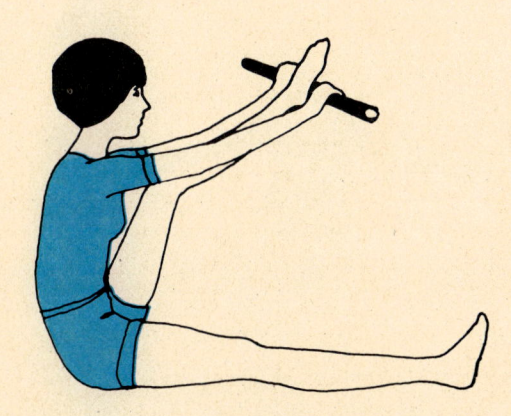

MISS CRAIG'S TENSION-FREEING EXERCISE BY MARJORIE CRAIG

Tension causes stiffness in the body. It leaves ugly lines on the face. So when you feel uptight and fatigued, an exercise that releases body tensions helps you feel more relaxed. Its good effects last for about two hours. Do this exercise in one continuous movement, keeping as loose and relaxed as possible. For homemaker or working girl, it should be repeated five times a day at two-hour intervals. You'll end the day refreshed and invigorated.

- Stand with feet 8 inches apart with the knees bent and the hips tucked under, arms raised overhead.
- Alternately stretch arms overhead, first one, then the other.
- Again stretch up the first arm.
- Then stretch up the other.
- Stretch both arms overhead.
- Swing arms outward . . . and down. At the same time let the upper part of your body relax and drop forward, knees bending.
- Bend knees more deeply and swing arms in front of the body, crossing each other.
- Swing arms back and out, gradually raising the body, arms out and up and as wide as you can.
- As you return to the original position with arms raised, again stretch arms up, first one and then the other.
- From arms-raised position, drop forward, bending knees and letting arms and head hang down, and bounce five times.

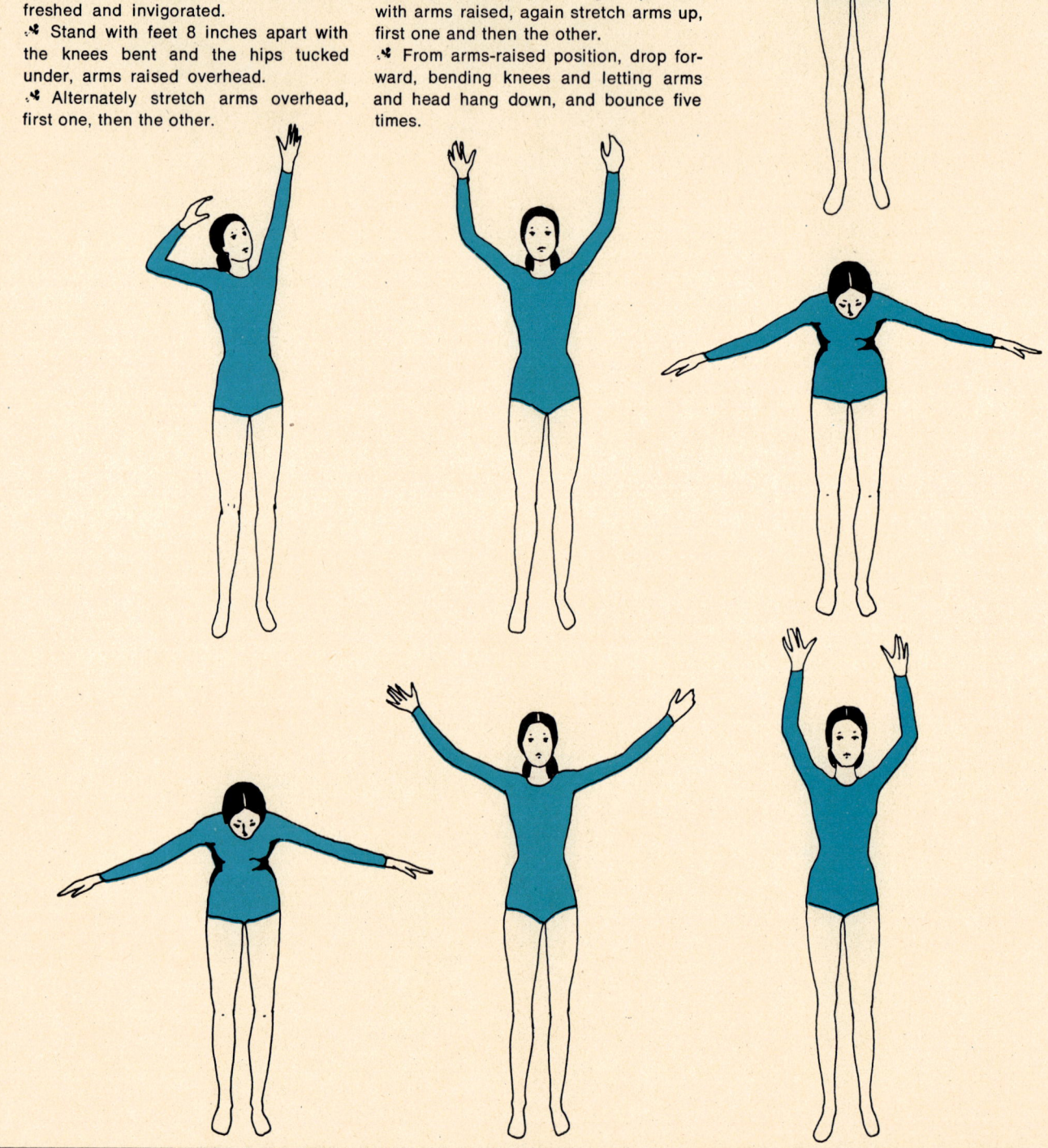

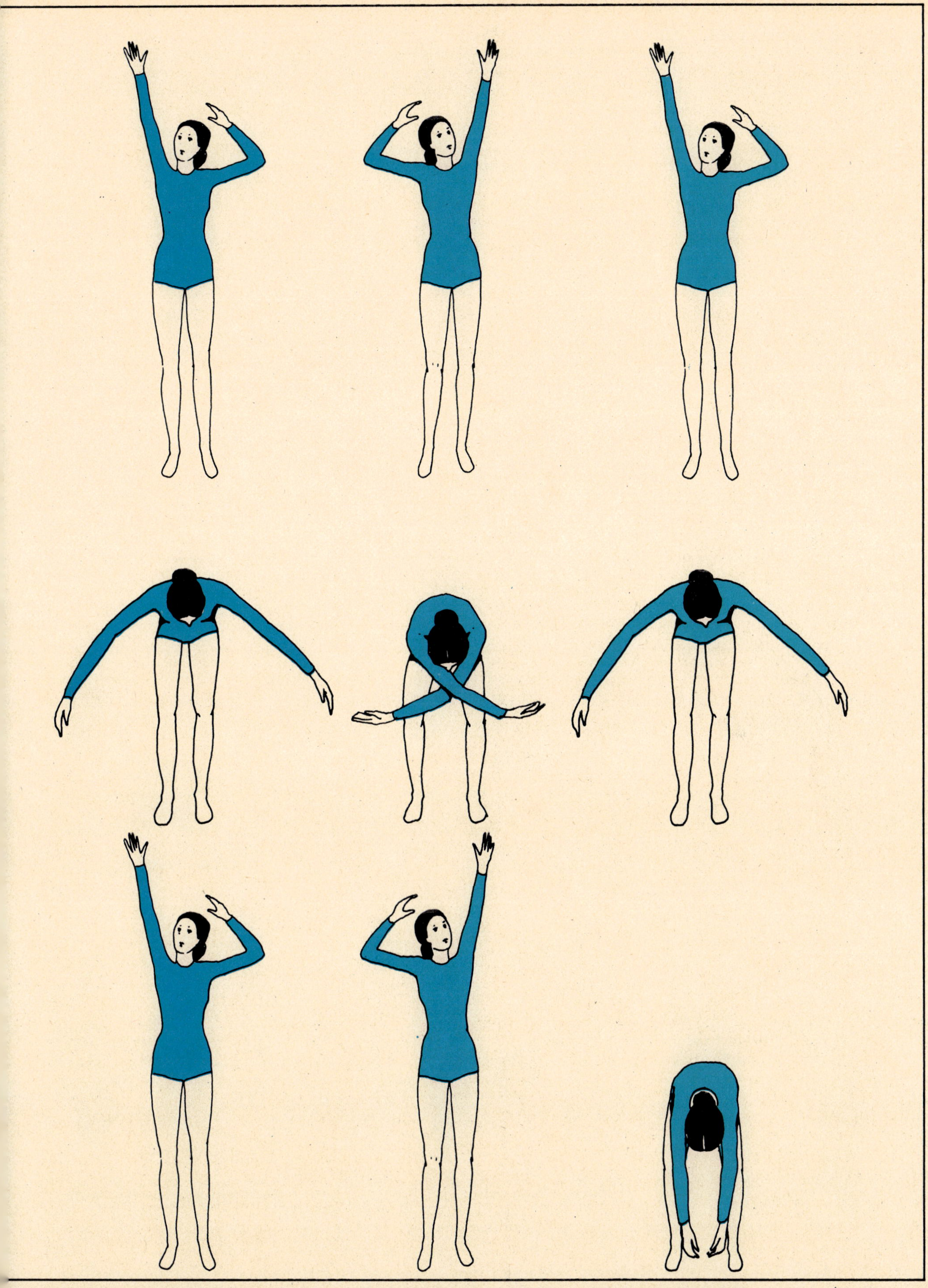

STRETCH EXERCISES
BY EVELYN LOEWENDAHL

Stretches are the simplest and most effective movements for improving circulation, for slimming and firming the body, and for giving you a general feeling of well-being. They make the back flexible, giving you beauty of posture and movement. They leave you refreshed, too, with no soreness.

* Do all these exercises daily. A brief period—10 to 30 minutes or so—of exercise every day is more helpful than sporadic exercise periods of long duration.
* A half hour after breakfast is an excellent exercise time. If possible, try to keep an appointment with yourself each day at the same time. This exercise period can then become routine.
* The floor is your best exercise mat. A thin pad or blanket can be used, if you like, for cleanliness and for comfort. After exercising, take a brief rest.

A full body stretch. Stand with legs spread apart, arms stretched out at sides.
* Swing the left arm, freely and wide, down to the right toe.
* Return to standing position.
* Swing the right arm to the left toe.
* Return to standing position.
Repeat 10 times.

To relieve tightness in the upper back, shoulders, and upper spine. Stand, feet together, with arms stretched out in front of you, hips forward.
* Keeping hips and legs in place, swing to the right from the waist, letting both arms swing loosely and easily.
* Swing to the left with the same loose and easy movement.
Repeat 10 times.

To relax a tired tense neck. Stand with arms at sides, one leg behind you.
* Pretending your head weighs 50 pounds, drop chin to chest.
* Let the head hang as loosely as possible for a count of five.
* Straighten.
Repeat five times.

To firm sides of abdomen. Lie on back with legs together and straight, arms stretched out, shoulder height, at sides.
* Raise left leg and at the same time stretch right arm toward it.
* Return to starting position.
* Raise right leg, stretching left arm toward it.
Repeat 10 times.

To firm abdomen muscles. Lie on back with knees bent, feet flat on the floor, arms at sides, palms down.
* Keeping arms on the floor, raise hips, straightening the lower back to flatten the abdomen as much as possible.
* Keeping the abdomen as flat as possible, rotate raised hips in a perfect circle—up, around to right side, down, up to the left side—for five complete circles.
* Relax.
Repeat. With practice, you will make more nearly perfect circles.

To firm upper abdomen. Sit on floor with legs crossed. Clasp hands at back of head, elbows back and high and out at sides.

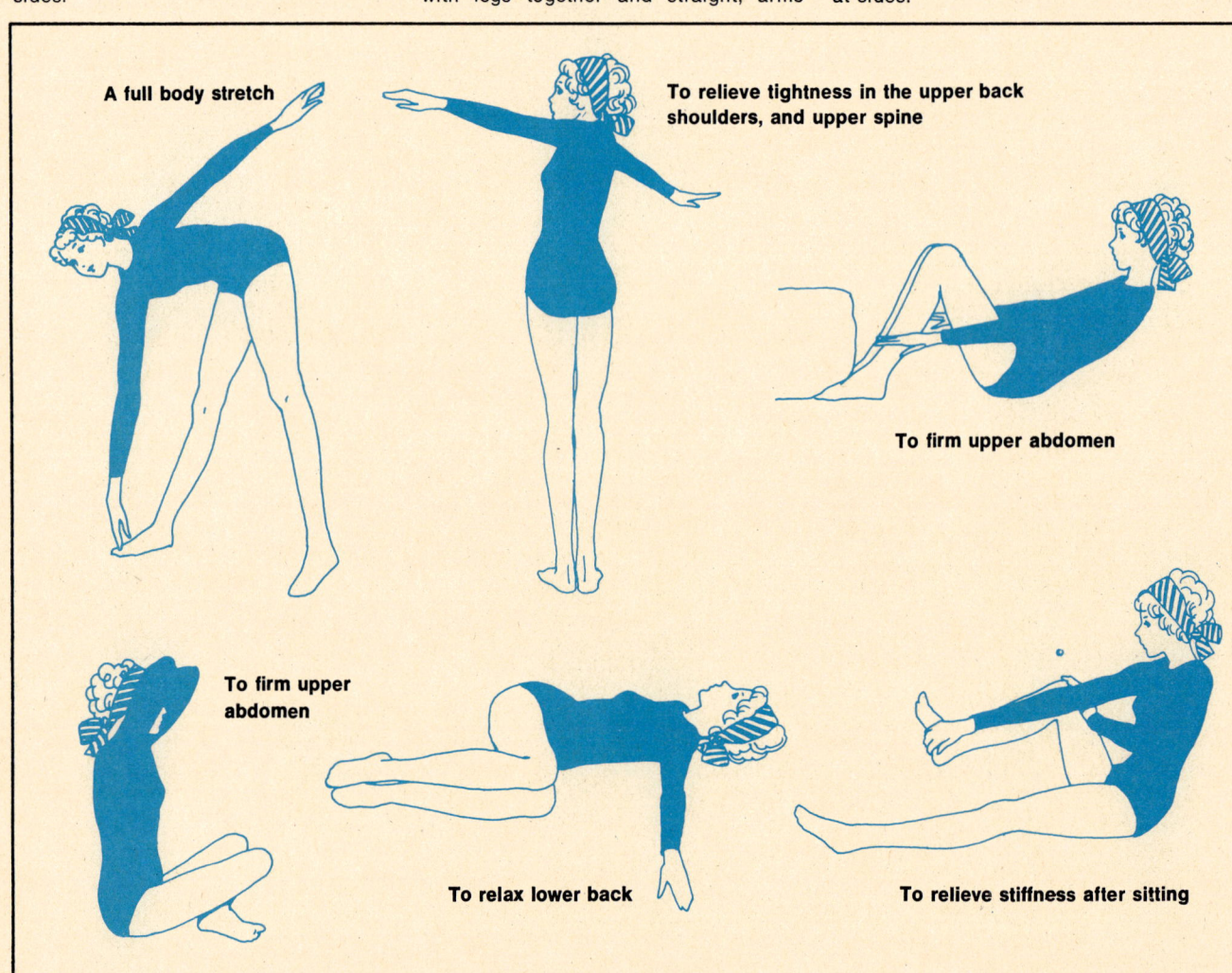

A full body stretch

To relieve tightness in the upper back shoulders, and upper spine

To firm upper abdomen

To firm upper abdomen

To relax lower back

To relieve stiffness after sitting

✤ Pull in the abdomen, and at the same time bring elbows forward till they touch.
✤ Release, elbows out.
Repeat 10 times.

To test for a tight lower back. Stand with back to a wall, heels about two inches away. Back of head, the shoulders, and the back of hips should touch the wall.
✤ Try to roll your lower back toward the wall, so that the entire spine is as flat as possible against it.
✤ With one hand, feel to see if there is any more than a slight hollow at the lower part of the spine. A tight lower back cannot touch the wall; a mobile back can.

To relax lower back. Lie on back, with legs straight. Stretch arms out to the sides at shoulder height.
✤ Keeping legs together, bend and lift knees and then gently drop them to the right, trying to touch the floor.
✤ Bring knees back up to middle and then drop them to the left.
Repeat 10 times on each side.

To relieve stiffness after sitting. Sit on the floor with left leg stretched out; hold right foot with right hand.
✤ Lift the right leg with knee bent.
✤ With left palm, gently push right knee down as far as possible, holding for a count of five. Release.
✤ Repeat with left leg, holding left foot with left hand.
Do only once with each leg. With daily stretches you will be able to straighten the knee. Practice till you can comfortably straighten the entire leg.

Gentle stretch for low back. Kneel, sitting on your heels.
✤ Stretch arms forward on the floor, fingers outstretched.
✤ Reach forward as far as possible till your forehead touches the floor.
✤ Hold for a count of five, keeping knees close to chest throughout the stretch.
✤ Relax.
Repeat five times.

Moderate stretch for low back. Sit on floor, legs spread apart, knees straight.
✤ Clasp right ankle with the right hand and try to touch the forehead to the right knee.
✤ Come up slowly to a sitting position and relax.
✤ Repeat, holding left ankle with left hand.
Repeat five times on each side. As you practice, it will become easier for you to lower forehead farther.

To stretch low back and sides of hips. Kneel, with arms stretched overhead.
✤ Bend from hips to the right side as far as possible.
✤ Hold for a count of five, then come up straight.
✤ Bend to the left side, holding for a count of five.
✤ Come up straight.
Repeat 10 times on each side.

Stretch for low back. Stand with right leg stretched out to rest on a chair seat in front of you.
✤ Drop torso forward from waist and try to touch forehead to knee.
✤ Change legs and repeat.
Repeat three times for each leg.

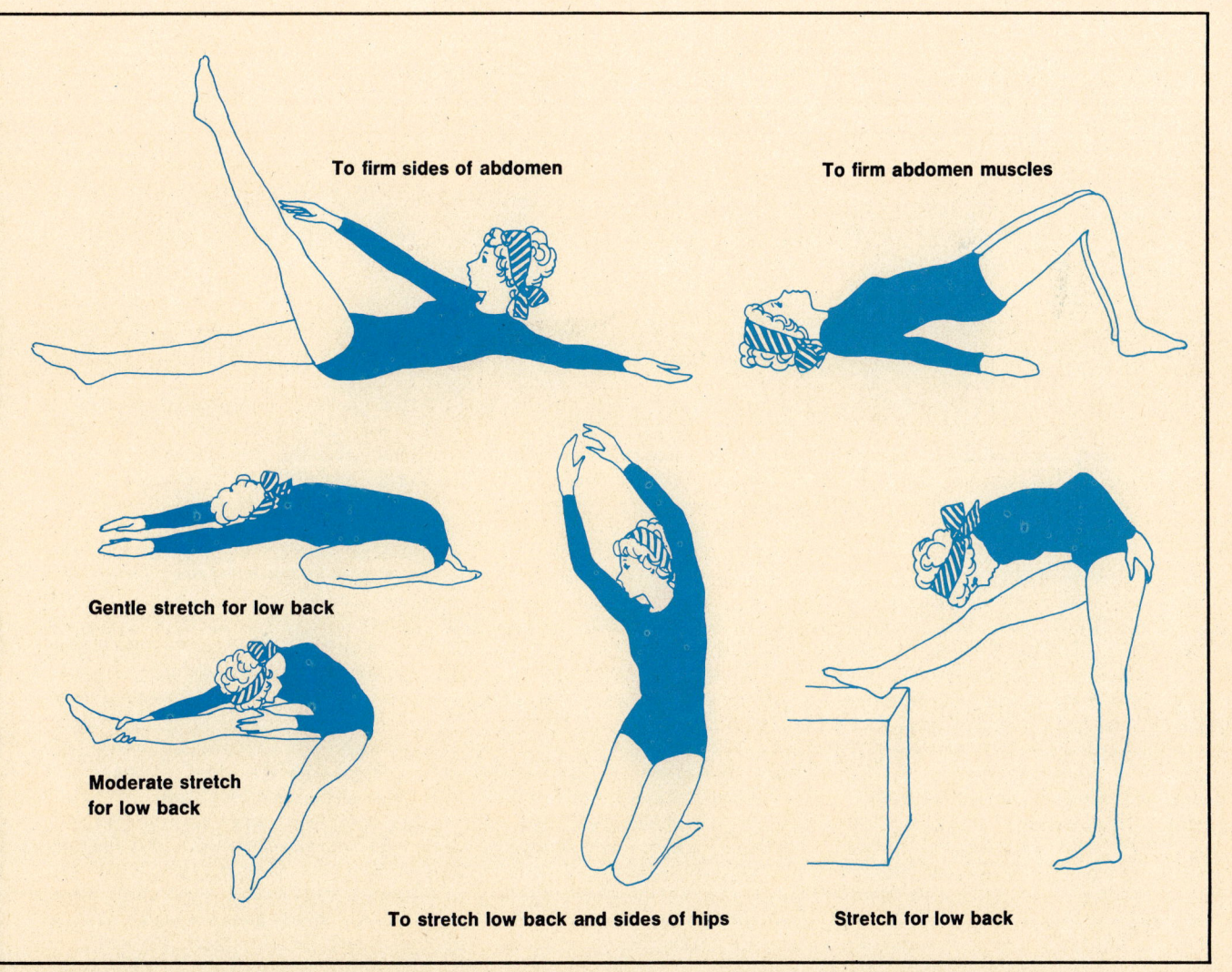

To firm sides of abdomen

To firm abdomen muscles

Gentle stretch for low back

Moderate stretch for low back

To stretch low back and sides of hips

Stretch for low back

SLIM-WHILE-YOU-SIT YOGA
BY RACHEL E. CARR

Breathe deeply and rhythmically. You will be able to relax more easily once you learn to breathe deeply and rhythmically, using your diaphragm. Deep breathing is an important physical function. It stimulates the circulatory system, exercises lungs and midriff.

☙ Before you begin, sit comfortably erect, with knees slightly apart and hands resting on your lap. Loosen clothing around the waist. Close your eyes.

☙ Now exhale, pulling your abdomen to empty your lungs. Then inhale slowly and deeply. Expand your abdomen and pull in air through your nostrils. Feel your lungs expanding, your chest inflated with air, and your shoulders rising. Then slowly let the air out through your nostrils with mouth closed. Repeat five times in a long unbroken wave.

This is the correct way to breathe—diaphragmatically. Repeat several times a day till you are able to breathe deeply and rhythmically without conscious effort. The abdomen should move in and out as far as possible to provide strong breath control, thus toning the abdominal muscles. Breathe through nostrils with mouth closed.

These exercises have a twofold benefit. They stimulate circulation through deep breathing and tone muscles in upper arms, chest, and shoulders by a play of resistance. For added benefit, sit cross-legged to limber the knees as you do these exercises. You should feel the pull in your arms, chest, shoulders, and upper back. Repeat each exercise three times while holding your breath for approximately 20 seconds.

Horizontal stretch. Clasp hands close to chest. With eyes closed, inhale deeply (expanding abdomen) and stretch your arms forward. With resistance, slowly pull arms toward you, touching the chest. Repeat three times while holding your breath, mouth closed.

Vertical stretch. Place your hands behind your head, with palms clasped. Close your eyes. Inhale deeply (expanding your abdomen) and stretch the arms upward. With resistance, slowly pull your arms down behind the head. Repeat three times while holding your breath, mouth closed. Then relax.

Beauty treatment. Practice this invigorating facial exercise before a mirror to see the effect of muscles in action. Called in yoga the lion posture, the facial movements imitate the fierceness of a lion springing; this prevents the sagging of facial and neck muscles. Emphasis is on the forceful expulsion of breath through the mouth; then the breath is held for a few seconds as the muscles are tautly pulled.

☙ Sit in a chair with hands resting on your knees or sit cross-legged. Inhale deeply and then forcefully exhale through your mouth. While exhaling with mouth wide open and eyes wide and staring, thrust out your tongue and stretch your arms down with fingers stiff and spread tautly apart. Hold the breath for a few seconds and then close your mouth and inhale deeply through the nostrils (expanding the abdomen). Exhale again slowly through nostrils and relax. Repeat three times.

Tone neck and chin line. These movements, done slowly and rhythmically, limber tight muscles of the neck and also tone throat and chin line.

☙ First, close eyes and then roll your head in a wide circle to the left and then to the right.

☙ Then place clasped hands on your forehead, elbows out. Press backward, using resistance; then relax. Repeat three times.

Firming the bustline. Sit straight with arms across the chest. Place right fist inside the palm of the other hand. Press the hands together, using forcible strength of arms and shoulders. You should feel the pull in arms, chest, and shoulders.

Tone shoulders and back. These exercises help if you tend to slouch.

☙ Raise your right arm and bend it back over your right shoulder with the palm flat, just below the neck. Cross the left hand behind the back, with the back of the hand resting on the spine, fingers upward. Now try to make the fingertips meet. With practice, as muscles are stretched and limbered, you will be able to lock your fingers.

☙ Keep your arms in this position, head straight, and inhale deeply (expanding the abdomen), contracting your back muscles to feel the pull. Keep stretching to bring both hands close together, but don't strain. Exhale, arms down, and relax. Repeat four times, alternating right and left arm over the shoulder, with the other hand behind the back.

Flabby underarms. Flabby underarms will quietly firm if you do this exercise faithfully. Sit straight with feet flat on the floor. Grasp the bottom edge of the chair with the fingertips of both hands. Then try to lift the chair, exerting as much strength as possible, while holding your breath. You should feel the pull in shoulders and underarms. Repeat three times.

Slim and shape. Sit erect with feet flat on the floor. Slowly raise right leg till knee is straight. Contract kneecap by pulling muscles upward, keeping knee straight. Hold for a few seconds and then bend the leg down and as far back as you can, without breaking the rhythm of motion. Do the same movements with the left leg. Repeat six times, alternating right and left leg, contracting and holding the muscles with the leg raised.

Tone legs, abdomen, and buttocks. Play of resistance is the key to this exercise. Sit with legs rigidly outstretched and crossed at the ankles.

☙ Hold onto the seat of your chair and try to pull feet apart, using resistance. Then relax. Repeat three times.

Reduce buttocks. The play of resistance in this exercise has many benefits. It reduces buttocks, firms arms, and strengthens weak back muscles.

☙ Lean forward to grasp your legs as far down as you can. Then, with the breath held and still grasping the legs, pull straight up, using only your back muscles. You should feel the pull in your buttocks, arms, and back. Repeat three times.

Reduce inner thighs. Hard-to-firm inner-thigh muscles will respond to this exercise. Lean slightly forward in a chair with feet a few inches apart. Cross arms and place hands inside opposite knee. Then try to press your knees together, using resistance. Repeat three times. This exercise also firms hollow inner thighs.

Slim ankles and strengthen arches. These foot movements can become a habit whenever you sit for a few minutes—especially while televiewing.

☙ Raise right foot about 10 inches off the floor. Rotate it slowly with the ankle relaxed—five times to the right and then five times to the left. Lower the leg. Repeat with the left foot.

☙ Raise right foot about 10 inches off the floor. Curl toes under the foot. Hold for a few seconds and then relax the foot and lower it to the floor. Repeat with left foot. Repeat 10 times, alternating first right, then left foot.

☙ Hold onto the sides of the chair. Raise both heels, with toes resting on the floor. Press down on your toes. The higher you raise the heels, with the toes on floor, the more pull you feel in the insteps and ankles. Hold the stretch and your breath for a few seconds. Then relax feet. Repeat slowly, five times.

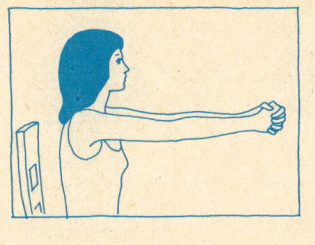

Horizontal stretch **Vertical stretch** **Beauty treatment for face** **Firming the bustline** **Tone neck and chin line** **Tone shoulders and back**

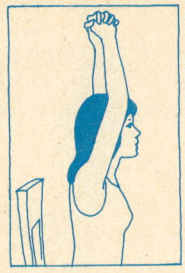

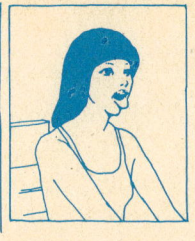

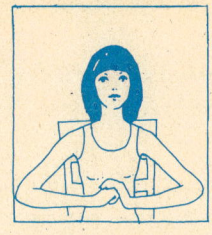

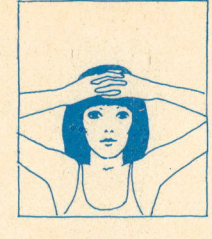

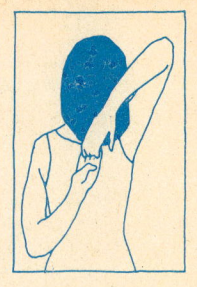

Tone legs, abdomen, and buttocks

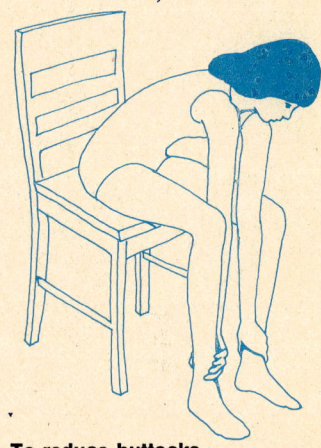

To reduce buttocks

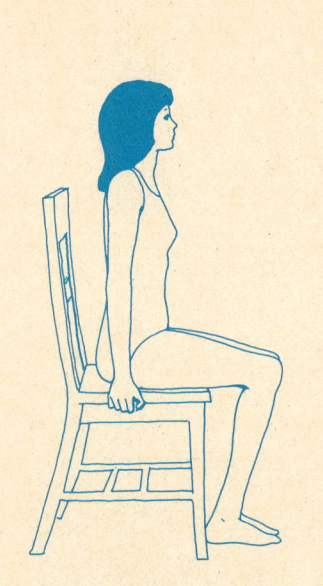

Get rid of flabby underarms 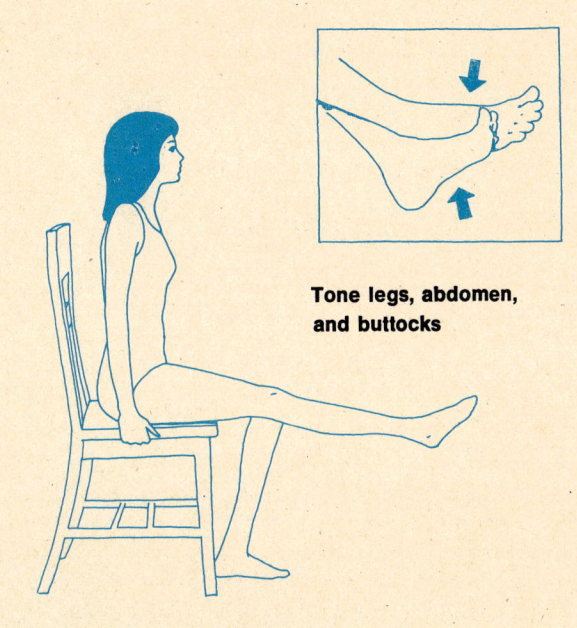 **Slim and shape your knees**

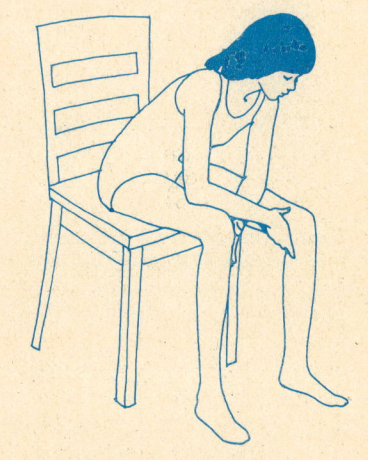

To reduce inner thighs

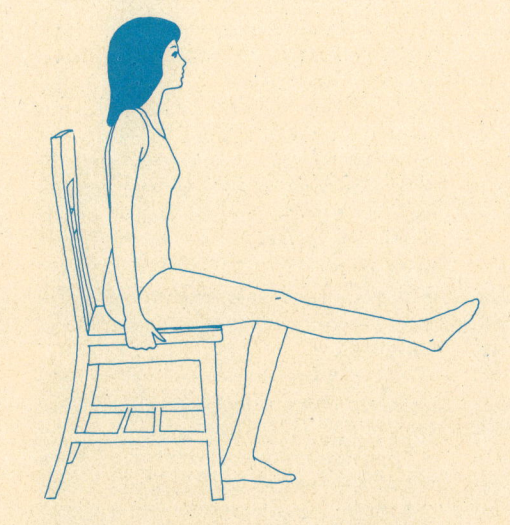

Slim and strengthen arches of the feet

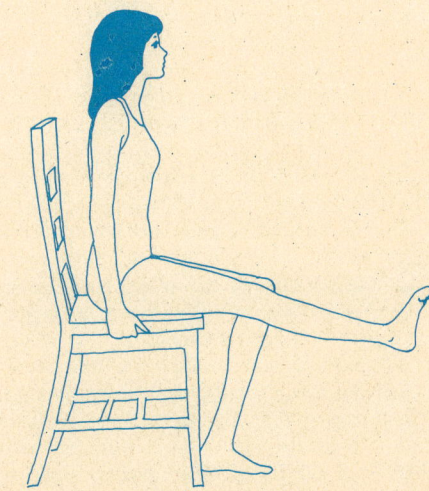

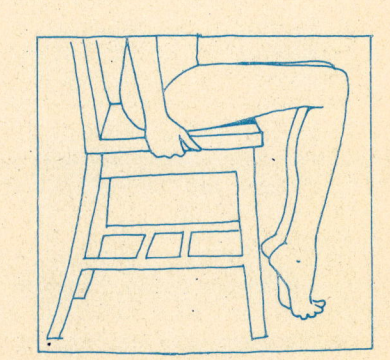

145

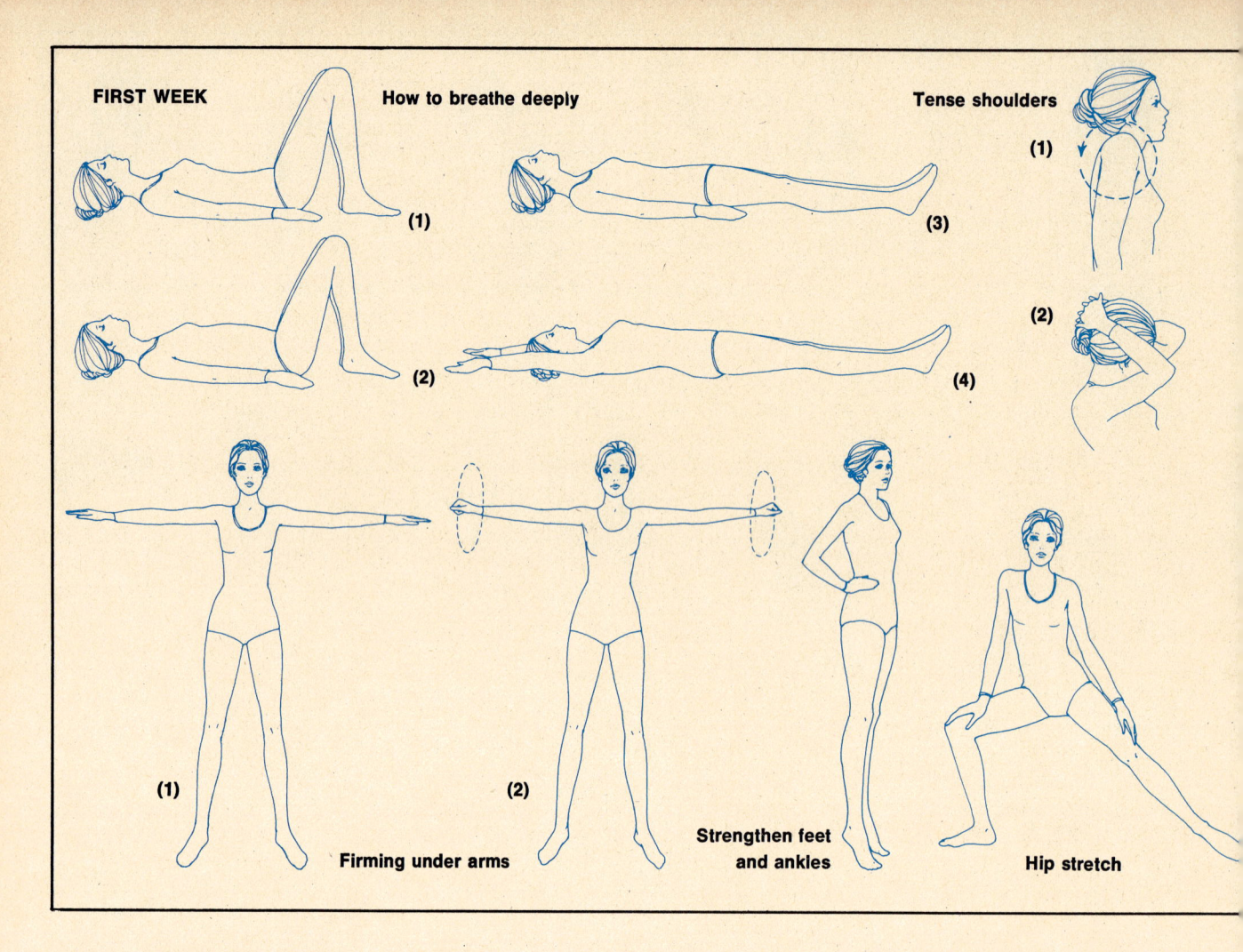

4-WEEK EXERCISE PLAN FOR INNER STRENGTH, OUTER BEAUTY
BY RACHEL E. CARR

The ideal way to practice yoga is in a quiet environment to develop the harmony of body and mind in action. The breathing, particularly, should be done calmly and rhythmically, with your mind completely in control. It is best to practice yoga in the early morning, before you are caught up in the whirl of the day's activities. Exercise on a thick firm surface in a well-ventilated area. Your clothing should be light and loose to give you maximum freedom. Following a heavy meal, wait at least two hours before practicing. You will find that exercising just 10 minutes a day will boost your energy and relieve tired aching muscles—and will relax you in mind, body, and feelings.

FIRST WEEK

How to breathe deeply. All breathing in yoga is done diaphragmatically so air can be drawn deep into the lungs. This is the key: Inhale and expand abdomen; exhale and pull in abdomen.

✲ Lie on your back, with legs bent and feet drawn close to your buttocks, palms down by sides. Close your eyes and, as much as possible, free your mind of all thought. Concentrate only on the flow of breath, breathing in and out through your nostrils. Exhale and pull in abdomen (1).

✲ Inhale and expand your abdomen (2), keeping chest still. Continue to inhale and exhale rhythmically 20 times. Then relax.

✲ When you can breathe diaphragmatically without conscious effort, follow this rhythmic pattern: Inhale for the count of five seconds, exhale for the count of 10 seconds, and hold your breath for 15 seconds. Repeat five times.

✲ For complete breathing, practice first in the lying position (3) legs outstretched and together; hands at sides.

✲ Exhale to empty your lungs as you pull in your abdomen. Slowly inhale, expanding your abdomen a little; then pull the air up into your rib cage and, finally, trap the air in your chest. When your lungs are fully inflated, gradually release the air by slowly relaxing your chest and rib cage as you pull in your abdomen. Repeat five times.

✲ Next, as you breathe in, raise your arms (4) over your head till the backs of your hands touch the floor. Hold your breath for 10 seconds and stretch like a cat from head to toe. Then slowly release the air as you drop your arms forward and down to your sides. Repeat five times.

Firming underarms. Synchronize breathing with these exercises so your lungs, too, benefit from the coordinated movements.

✲ Stand with your feet apart and arms outstretched to the sides.

✲ Inhale deeply and stretch arms as far out as you can (1) without tensing your neck. You should feel the pull under your arms and in the shoulders and back.

✲ Hold your breath and the pose 10 seconds; then exhale and relax. Repeat five times.

✲ Stand with feet apart, arms outstretched, fists clenched (2). Inhale deeply.

✲ Hold breath and slowly rotate arms in five continuous wide circles, pulling as hard as you can on your arm muscles. Then exhale and relax. Each rotating

SECOND WEEK   Flight   Dance of the legs

Limbering knees

First steps to the headstand

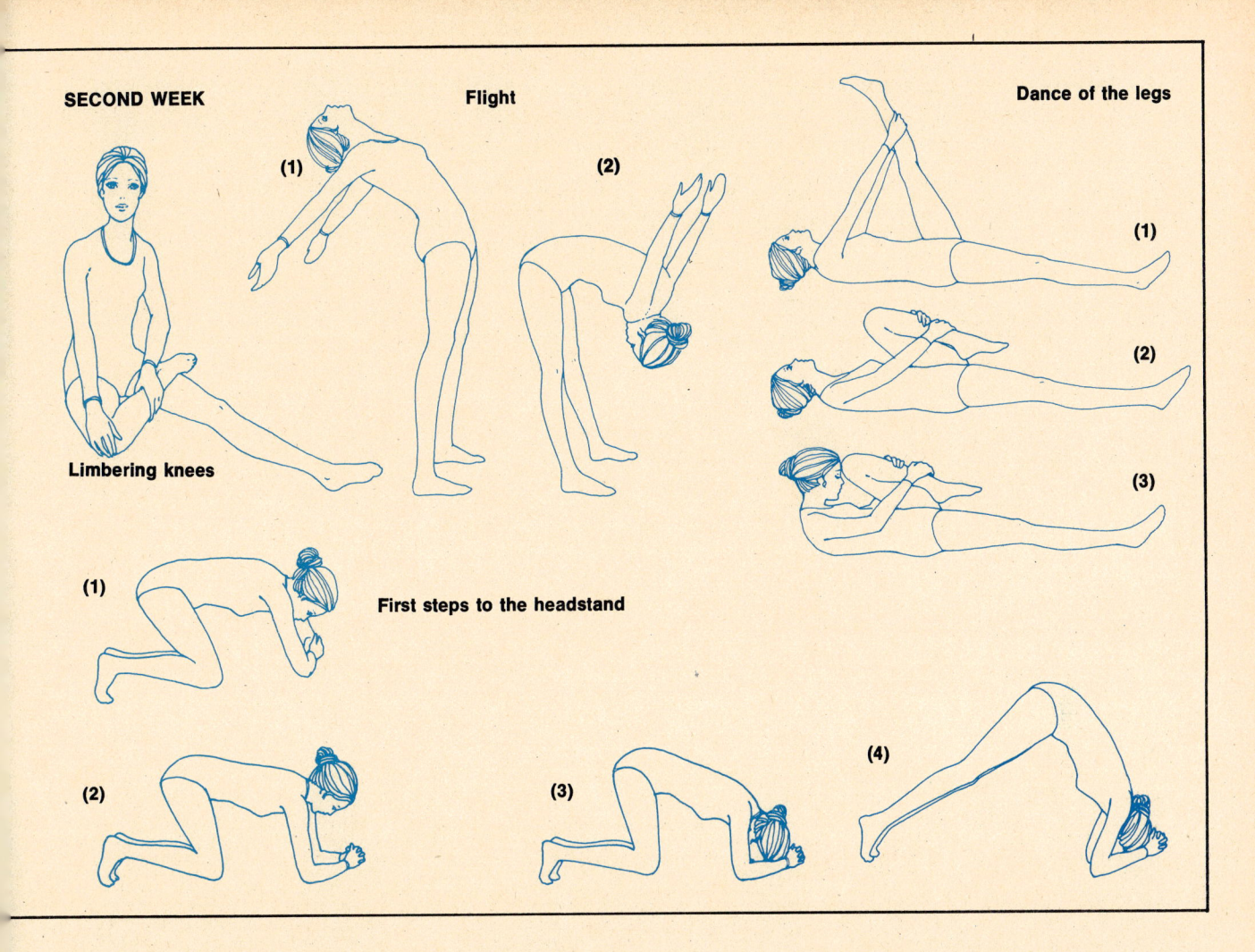

movement should take approximately one second. Repeat five times.

For tense shoulders. Stand with arms completely relaxed. Keep the spine straight.

✿ Raise shoulders high as you can, then far back, contracting the muscles; then drop the shoulders, down and forward. Each rotation of the shoulders **(1)** should take about five seconds. Repeat 10 times.

✿ Kneel or sit. Clasp hands together and press firmly on the back of the head, putting head forward as far down as you can **(2)**. There should be a play of resistance. Hold for 10 seconds, then relax. Repeat five times.

To strengthen feet and ankles. Stand with feet together, hands on hips.

✿ Rise on toes and balance for five seconds. Then lower heels. Repeat 10 times.

✿ Stand with feet about six inches apart, hands on hips. Rise on toes; rotate your feet to the outer sides, back on heels, to the inner sides, and return to tiptoe position. Repeat 10 times, feeling the stretch and pull in your arches and ankles and then relax.

Hip stretch. Stand with feet far apart, hands on thighs, and spine straight.

✿ Turn right foot out; bend the knee with the right hand resting on it.

✿ Then stretch the left leg away from you till the knee is perfectly straight, left hand on the thigh.

✿ Hold for five seconds, pressing right hand on right knee. Repeat three times; then do the same movement, bending your left knee.

SECOND WEEK

Limbering knees. This prepares you for traditional yoga sitting postures. At first your knees may stubbornly rest in the air, but with practice the joints in ankles, knees, and hips will be well-toned.

✿ Sit on the floor with legs apart, spine straight, and arms at sides.

✿ Bend the right leg, with the foot resting on the left thigh. Grasp the bent right knee and ankle with both hands.

✿ Gently press the right knee down to the floor—or as far as it will go without straining. Hold the pose for a few seconds while gently pressing the knee down.

✿ Then relax and stretch out the leg. Bounce it lightly to increase circulation. Repeat three times. Then repeat with the left leg resting on the right thigh.

Flight. There is a feeling of flight in this exercise as your arms are thrust backward and forward in rhythmic motion, with synchronized diaphragmatic breathing.

✿ Stand with feet apart and arms outstretched at sides. Close eyes. Inhale deeply and bend as far back as you can **(1)**, with your arms thrust back.

✿ Exhale and bend forward and down **(2)**, keeping arms back and up. Repeat five times; then return to the standing position.

First steps to the headstand. Even if you have no intention of ever standing on your head, these preliminary steps to the headstand will limber the spine, strengthen neck muscles, and tone legs. Do this exercise on a soft thick surface.

✿ Kneel with legs together **(1)**. To measure the right distance for your

147

THIRD WEEK

Perfect posture

The camel pose

The bridge

The shoulder stand

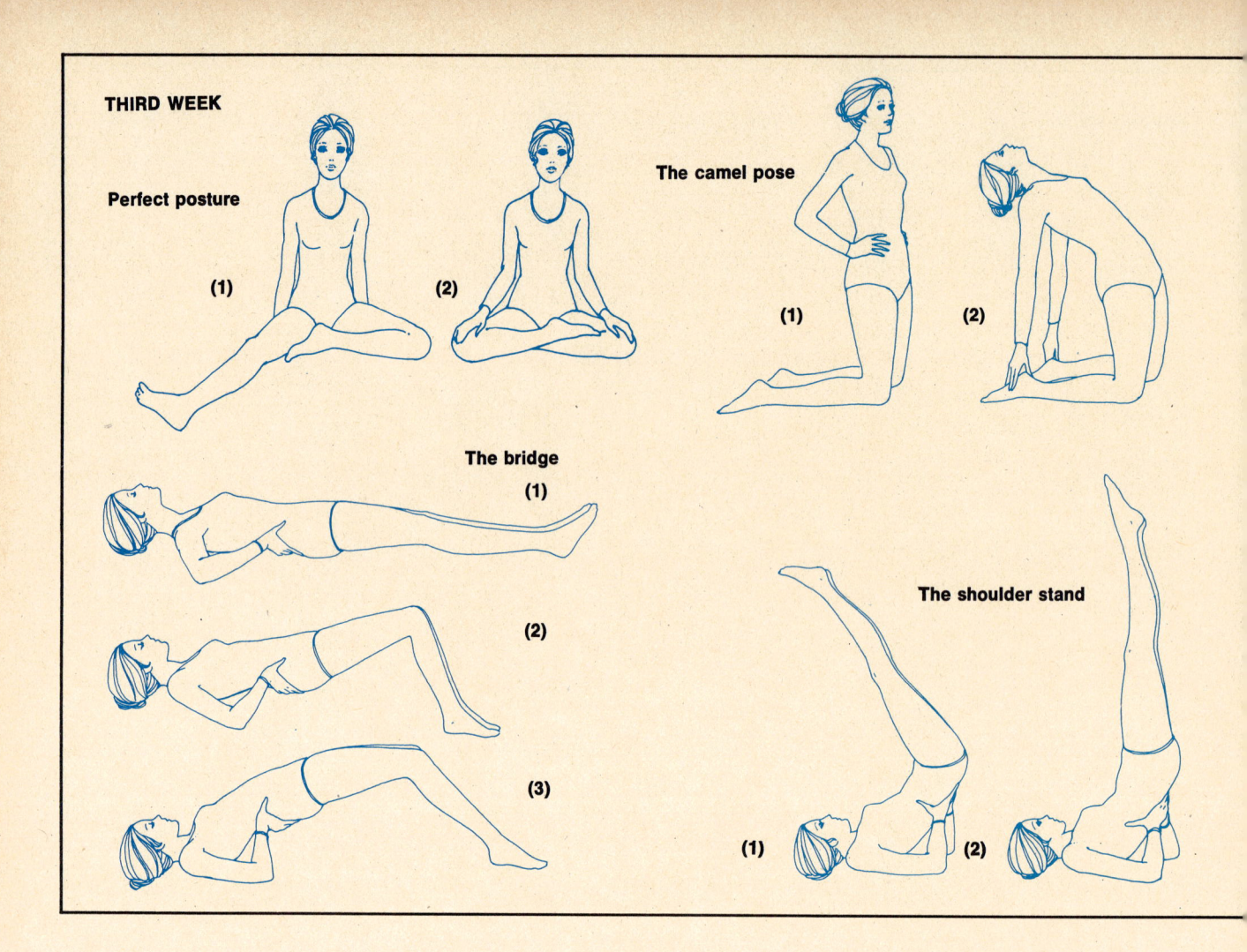

arms, bend them so the fingertips touch the elbows.

☙ Without moving elbows, stretch out arms and interlock fingers **(2)**. You now have the correct distance. Bend head down, encircling it with clasped hands **(3)**.

☙ Straighten legs by unbending the knees and resting on your toes **(4)**. Take a few steps, "walking" in toward your head, then a few steps back. Repeat slowly five times.

☙ Remain in this position and rock back and forth on your toes by raising and lowering your feet. Repeat 10 times. Then bend knees and slowly come out of the headstand position.

Dance of the legs. Lie flat on your back, arms overhead and eyes closed.

☙ Inhale deeply while raising left leg **(1)** as straight as possible. At the same time bring arms up to grasp the left ankle (or as far as you can reach without straining). Right leg remains on the floor.

☙ Exhale. Still grasping the left leg, bend and clasp it close to your chest **(2)**. Hold breath.

☙ Raise head to meet the knee **(3)**. Hold the pose and your breath for a few seconds.

☙ Then inhale slowly while lowering head, with arms overhead and leg returning forward to the floor. Exhale and relax.

☙ Repeat with both legs.

THIRD WEEK

Perfect posture. This traditional sitting posture puts the body in good physical balance for breathing and meditation. At first you may find it easier to sit on a flat cushion to raise your legs a little off the floor.

☙ Sit with legs outstretched, spine straight, hands at sides. Bend left leg so the sole of the foot rests against the inner right thigh **(1)**.

☙ Place the right leg over the left so the foot rests against the inner left thigh, and the ankles meet—right over left **(2)**.

☙ Rest hands on knees. Close eyes and hold this pose for a few seconds while breathing rhythmically.

☙ Then relax legs and reverse the position, crossing the left leg over the right.

☙ Repeat four times, alternating legs.

☙ When you become more relaxed in this posture, do the complete breathing a few times and concentrate on the rhythmic flow of your breath.

Camel pose. Take this exercise in easy stages to limber your spine. First bend only as far back as you can. Repeat a few times. Then bend back, reaching for your ankles, and synchronize breathing with the movements.

☙ Kneel with legs apart and hands on hips. Close eyes **(1)**. Inhale deeply and bend as far back as you can.

☙ Exhale and reach for your ankles **(2)**. Breath freely and hold the pose for a few seconds.

☙ Then inhale and come up slowly to the kneeling position.

☙ Exhale, relax. Repeat three times.

The bridge. Lie flat on your back, hands on waist, thumbs up, elbows bent and resting on the floor **(1)**.

☙ Inhale deeply, bending knees, and, with the help of your arms, arch your spine **(2)** as high as possible; keep head on the floor without straining neck.

☙ Slide your feet forward to create a wide bridge between your head and

FOURTH WEEK

Sun salutation

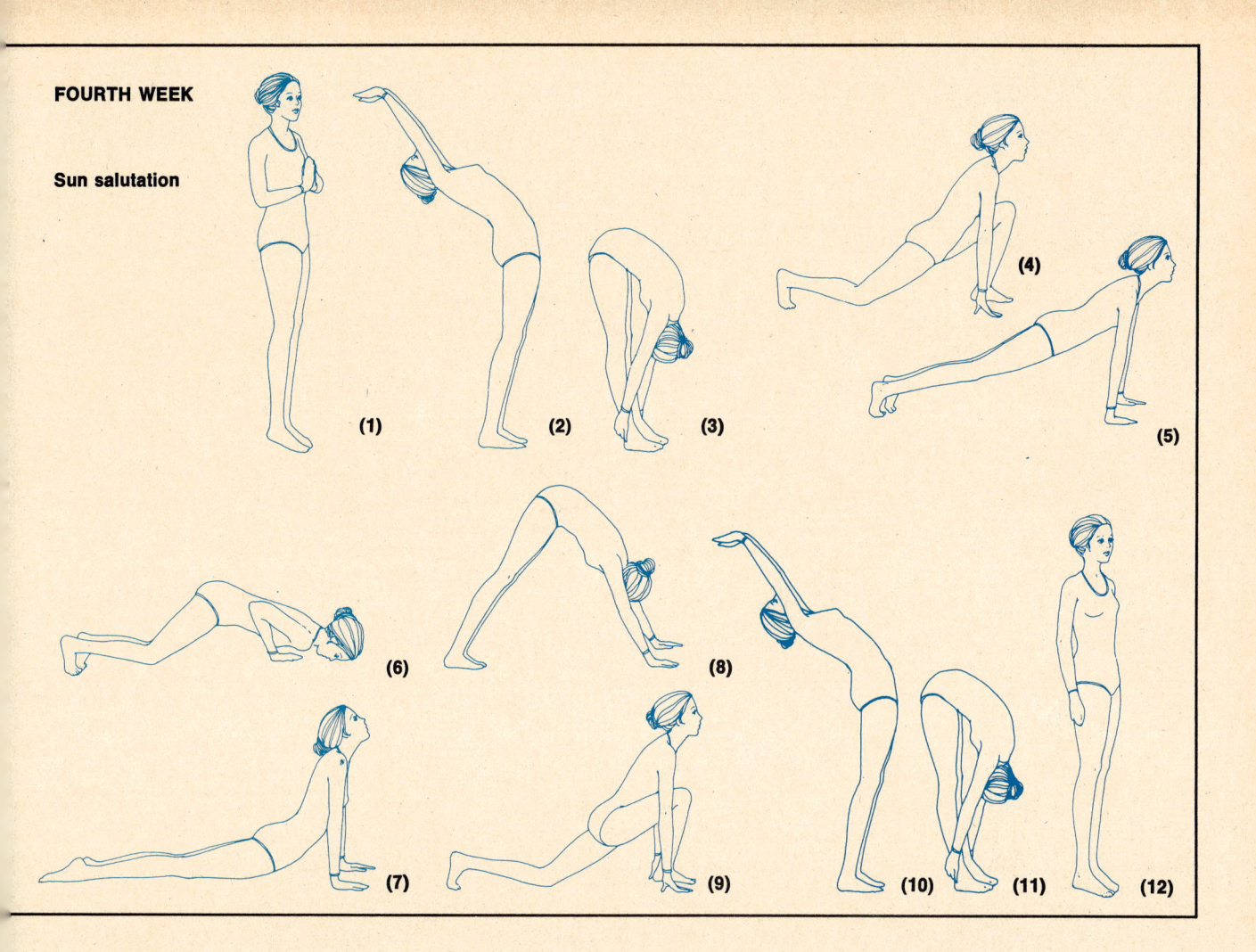

feet **(3)**. Breathe rhythmically while holding the pose for a few seconds.

❧ Inhale and lower the spine and legs. Exhale and relax. Repeat three times, slowly increasing the hold.

Shoulder stand. Lie flat on back, with legs together, arms at sides, and palms down. Close eyes.

❧ Inhale deeply and raise legs over head **(1)** by pushing hips up with your hands, elbows bent on the floor.

❧ Breathe freely and continue to raise legs till they are in a vertical position **(2)**, with spine straight and legs together. The weight should be on your shoulders and arms, with chin pressing against the jugular notch.

❧ Hold the pose for approximately 30 seconds, breathing rhythmically.

❧ Inhale deeply, and slowly lower your legs in gradual stages. Let your hands slip farther down along the hips till your back is on the floor, with palms down. Keep head on the floor by arching the neck backward as you lower legs. Exhale.

❧ With palms pressed down, continue to lower your legs to the floor, keeping knees straight. Repeat three times.

FOURTH WEEK

Sun salutation. Traditionally this exercise is practiced in the early morning. First practice the different postures individually; then incorporate them into one continuous rhythmic motion with synchronized breathing.

❧ Stand erect with legs together, hands close to chest, palms touching **(1)**.

❧ Inhale deeply while raising arms overhead. Bend back to arch spine **(2)**.

❧ Exhale while bending forward till hands are in line with feet **(3)**. (Don't strain. Bend only as far as you can.) Contract the abdomen and bring head close to knees. Knees are straight.

❧ Inhale and move right leg in a backward step with the knee touching the floor and toes turned in **(4)**. Fingers are held tautly on the floor to support your body. Keep left foot firmly on the floor, with left knee between both hands. Bend head back, arching spine as you look up.

❧ Inhale and hold breath. Without shifting the right leg, raise the knee off the floor; then move left leg in a backward step to meet right foot **(5)**. Toes are turned in, and body is elevated, with arms straight and hands firmly on the floor. Look straight ahead.

❧ Exhale. Bend knees to touch the floor without shifting palms. Then move your body slightly backward so your forehead and chest come in contact with the floor **(6)**. Buttocks, shins, and nose are off the floor.

❧ Inhale; bend backward with arms straight and palms firmly on the floor **(7)**. Contract the back muscles.

❧ Exhale. Without moving your feet and hands, arch the back in a cat's stretch **(8)**, head down between arms.

❧ Inhale and bring the right foot forward, alongside your palms **(9)**. Left foot and knee touch the floor. Look up, bending your spine slightly.

❧ Exhale and bring your left leg forward without moving the right. Keep the knees straight and bring your head down to your knees **(10)**. Contract abdomen.

❧ Inhale deeply while raising arms overhead. Bend back to arch spine **(11)**.

❧ Exhale and lower your arms to the sides **(12)**.

❧ Repeat the movements, moving your left leg back. Do each series of exercises twice.

149

**4-WEEK FIGURE-FIRMING PLAN
BY BONNIE PRUDDEN**

Diet is certainly half the task in figure control, but to make your program a success and to speed it up—to take up the slack, to smooth out the hollows, to firm and to curve, to banish fatigue forever, and to add that all-important glow of vitality—you add exercise.

If you think you are too heavy, too rusty, too old, or too dignified, you aren't. Start easy for the first three weeks and work alone for the fourth. The key to a successful exercise program is every day a little more, even if it is only one step. Get a notebook and a tape measure and chart your progress and your inches. Remember that inches will come off faster than pounds. That is because you are replacing slabby flab with smooth, curving, vital muscle—and muscle, though it looks less, weighs a bit more. Diet is indeed half the battle, but it is exercise that will get you there.

**FIRST WEEK
BASIC EXERCISES**

There are five basic exercises, and they are not just for now. These exercises are for you forever and always. They will keep you limber and strong, help with proportion, and, most important, serve to release tension, especially in your shoulders and back. Tie them into habits that turn up often in your day. For example, keep a notebook in the bathroom and each time you go there, do this simple series. It will take you less than three minutes each time, but if you multiply those three minutes by five times, you have 15 minutes a day or *almost two hours of exercise a week.* The effect of exercise, like that of calories, accumulates. Three times five is just as good as 15 at a time.

Waist twist. Stand with feet well apart and arms at shoulder level. Twist the upper body left and right as far as possible **(1)**, letting the arms droop slightly as you twist but always ending at shoulder level. Do 25 (a complete left-right twist to a count). This exercise will slim the waist and upper torso and will release tension in the shoulders and upper back. Keep the same standing position **(2)** and, with *knees straight,* bend forward from the hips. Pretend a small dwarf is standing in front of you and, keeping elbows bent, box both of his ears, first one side and then the other, 25 times. Pull elbows high to increase the twist action. This will work fat or fibrositic areas (a thickening of tissue due to stress) and prevent unsightly lumps as well as stiffness and sometimes pain.

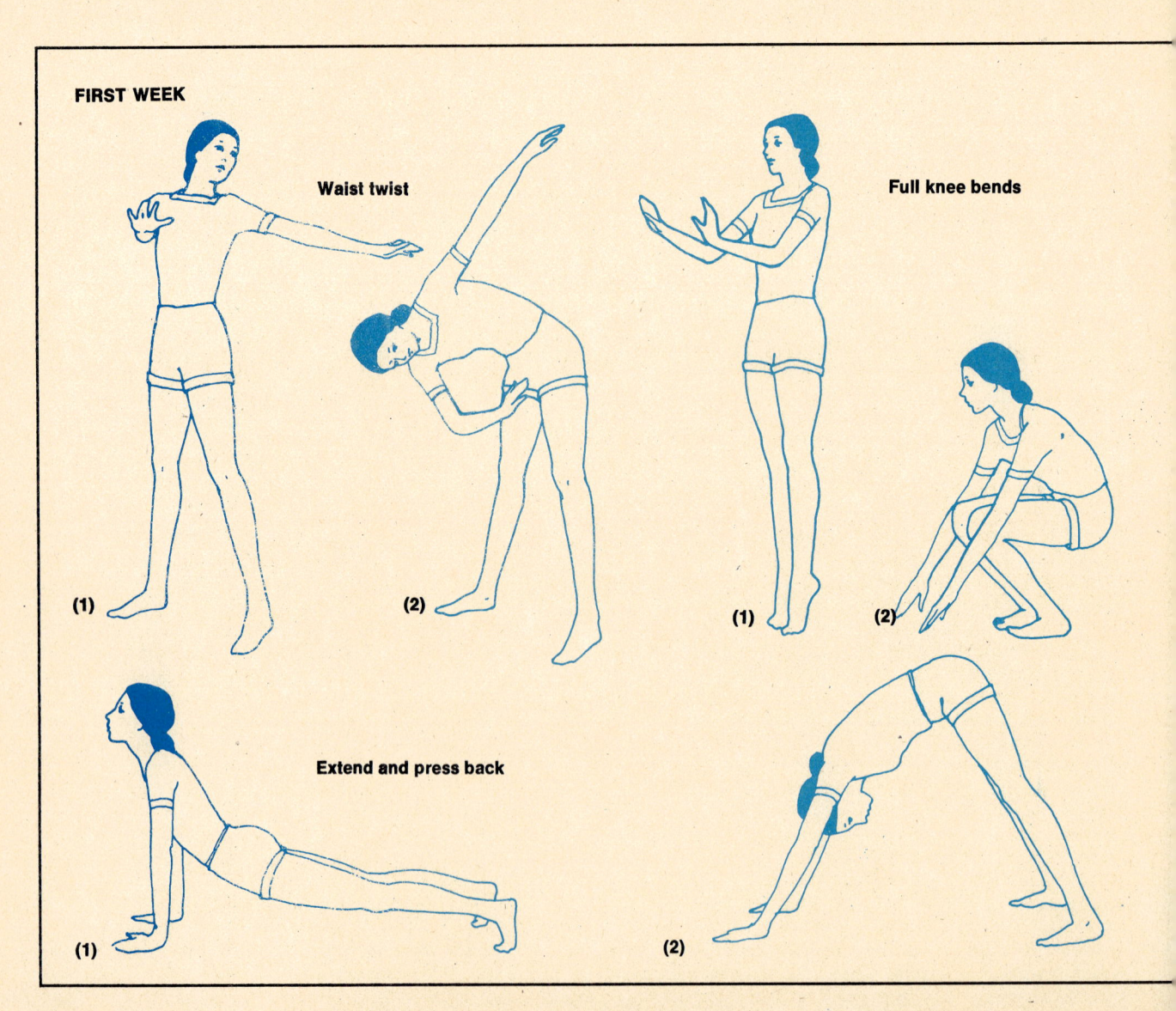

Full knee bends. Stand with feet together and arms stretched forward. Rise *slowly* high on your toes **(1)**. Go down slowly into a deep knee bend **(2)** till you touch the floor with your fingertips. Rise to tiptoe standing position and then lower heels to starting position. Do all moves *slowly,* starting with five and working up to 10 by adding two a week. Note: If thighs are heavy, spend one minute on each thigh, kneading the tight and sometimes tender flesh to loosen the fibrositic tissue. Do not be gentle and don't worry about bruising.

Bent-knee sit-ups. Lie on your back, hands clasped behind head, *knees bent,* and feet held down with a weight **(1)** or thrust under a chair. Keeping your chin on your chest and your back rounded, roll up to a sitting position **(2).** At the top of the sit-up, straighten your back, lift your head, and press the elbows back. Hold for a second or two; then drop your head, round your back, and roll *slowly* down to the starting position. Start with five and add two a week till you are doing 10. If you find you can't do even one sit-up, reverse the process. Start at the top of the sit-up and roll *slowly* down. Get up any way you can and repeat. Do five down-rolls three times a day till you can do one sit-up. Add the sit-ups as fast as strength improves. Note: This is your most important single exercise. It works *for* a figure and *against* fatigue and backache.

Extend and press back. Start on hands and feet with the body fully extended **(1).** Feet should be spread apart; head should be up; and there should be a slight downward arch in the back. *Keeping the feet facing forward* (not turned out), press the seat backward **(2),** keeping the legs straight to arch the body upward, till the heels touch, or almost touch, the floor. At the same time press your head down and back between your arms. This exercise will release tension in the shoulders and the legs, strengthen the arms, chest, and shoulders, and will also stretch the heel cords to improve your walk. Start with four complete exercises and add two a week till you are doing 10.

Back and hamstring flexibility. Stand with feet well apart, knees straight, and hands clasped behind your back. *Keeping your head up,* bend forward from the hips. From the bent position **(1),** bounce the upper body downward in eight short easy bounces. Let gravity do the work. Then drop the entire body downward **(2)** and let it hang loose. From this position, again letting gravity do the work, bounce downward for eight easy bounces. These 16 bounces comprise a set. Do two such sets and add one a week till you are doing four sets a day. **NOTE:** An inflexible back contributes to backache and an aging look (at any age). If you can't stand with legs straight and feet together and lean over to touch the floor with your fingertips, you are a candidate for both. In that case, do this exercise often throughout the day to offset the tension you are living with. (No, reaching the floor has nothing to do with the length of your arms.)

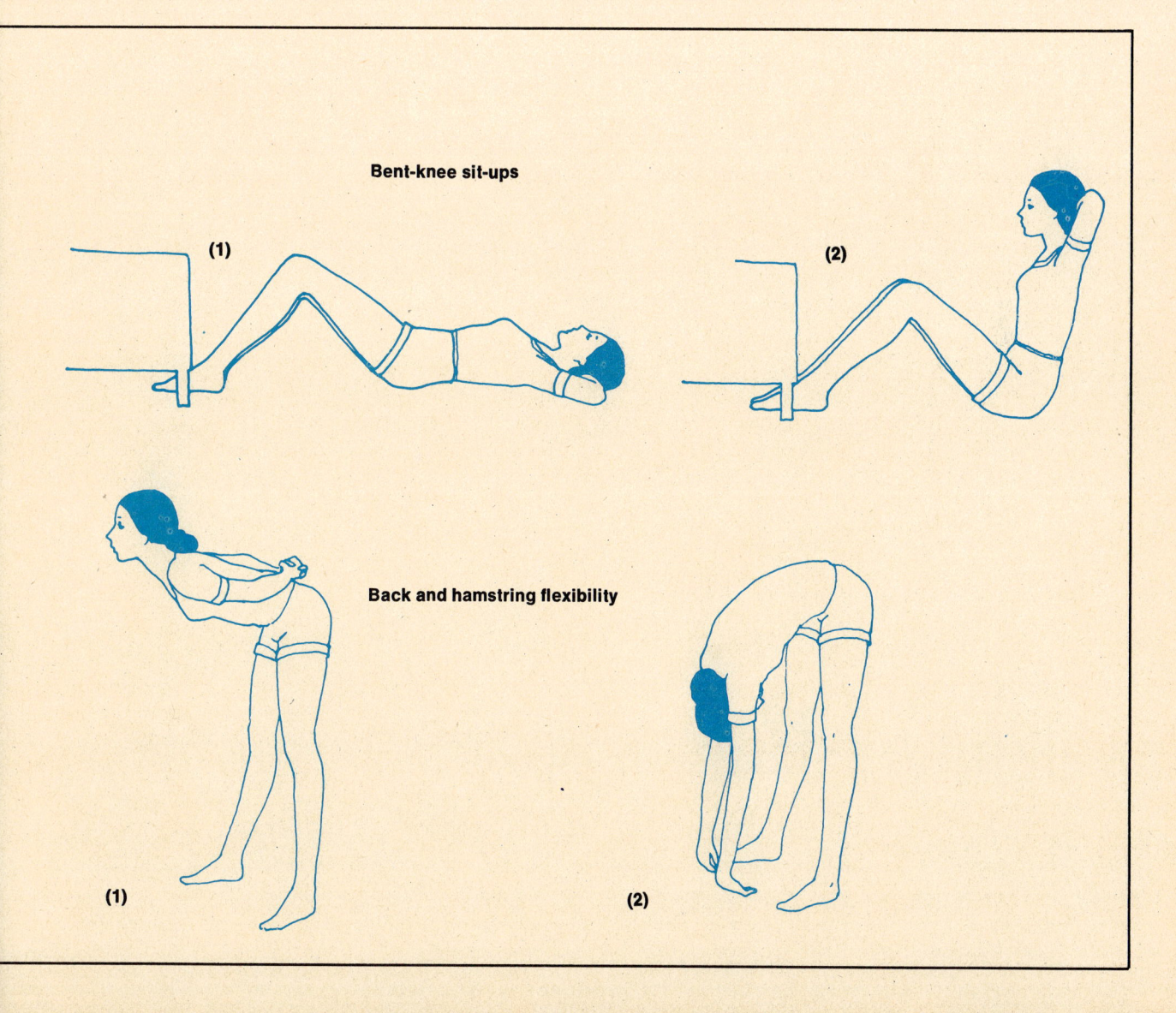

Bent-knee sit-ups

(1) (2)

Back and hamstring flexibility

(1) (2)

151

SECOND WEEK ADD-ONS FOR FIGURE PROBLEMS

Everyone has at least *one* figure problem. Pick out the one that annoys you the most and work hard on that *one*. When you have it under control, pick out the next. Give all of the areas at least a little attention simply to keep what you like as you like it.

The flagpole for protruding abdominals and "spare tires." Lie on back, left leg raised (1) and right leg at full stretch just off the floor. Stretch arms overhead and, keeping the raised leg vertical, swing up to grasp the ankle (2). Keeping the leg vertical, roll slowly back to rest on the floor (1). Repeat four times and then change legs and do four more. These comprise a set. Add a set a week till you can do four. Note: If you cannot swing up all in one movement at first, simply grasp your leg at the thigh and walk your hands up to the ankle, hand over hand.

The crossover for thick or thin thighs. If your thighs are heavy or the tissue stiff and thick, spend a minute in kneading-and-pinching massage on each leg *before* the exercise. Sit with legs spread and lean back on straight arms. Carry the left leg across over the right (1) and touch the big toe to the floor. Then, keeping the leg in the crossed position, rotate the foot so that the toes point to the ceiling. Carry the left leg back over to the spread-leg position and touch the floor with the little toe (2). Repeat the crossing four times with each leg to make a set. Start with two sets and work up to four. If you *really* have problem thighs, do as many as you can each day. This is *the* exercise for thighs.

Knee-to-nose kick for problem hips. Get down on all fours (using the bathroom rug if you have tender knees). Bring the left knee as close to your nose as possible (1). This strengthens the abdominals and stretches the back. Next, extend the left leg back and up (2) and at the same time bring your head up. This slims the seat and stretches the abdominals. Do eight with each leg to make a set. Add a set a week for problem hips.

The hydrant for the "saddlebags" at the sides of the hips. Start on hands and knees. Keeping the left knee bent, raise it to the side till level with the hips (1). Extend the leg straight out to the side (2), trying to maintain the hip level. (This miserable exercise has only one thing going for it—it works.) Then bend the knee back (1) and replace on the floor as in the starting position. Do two to a side for a set. Do two sets and work up to four.

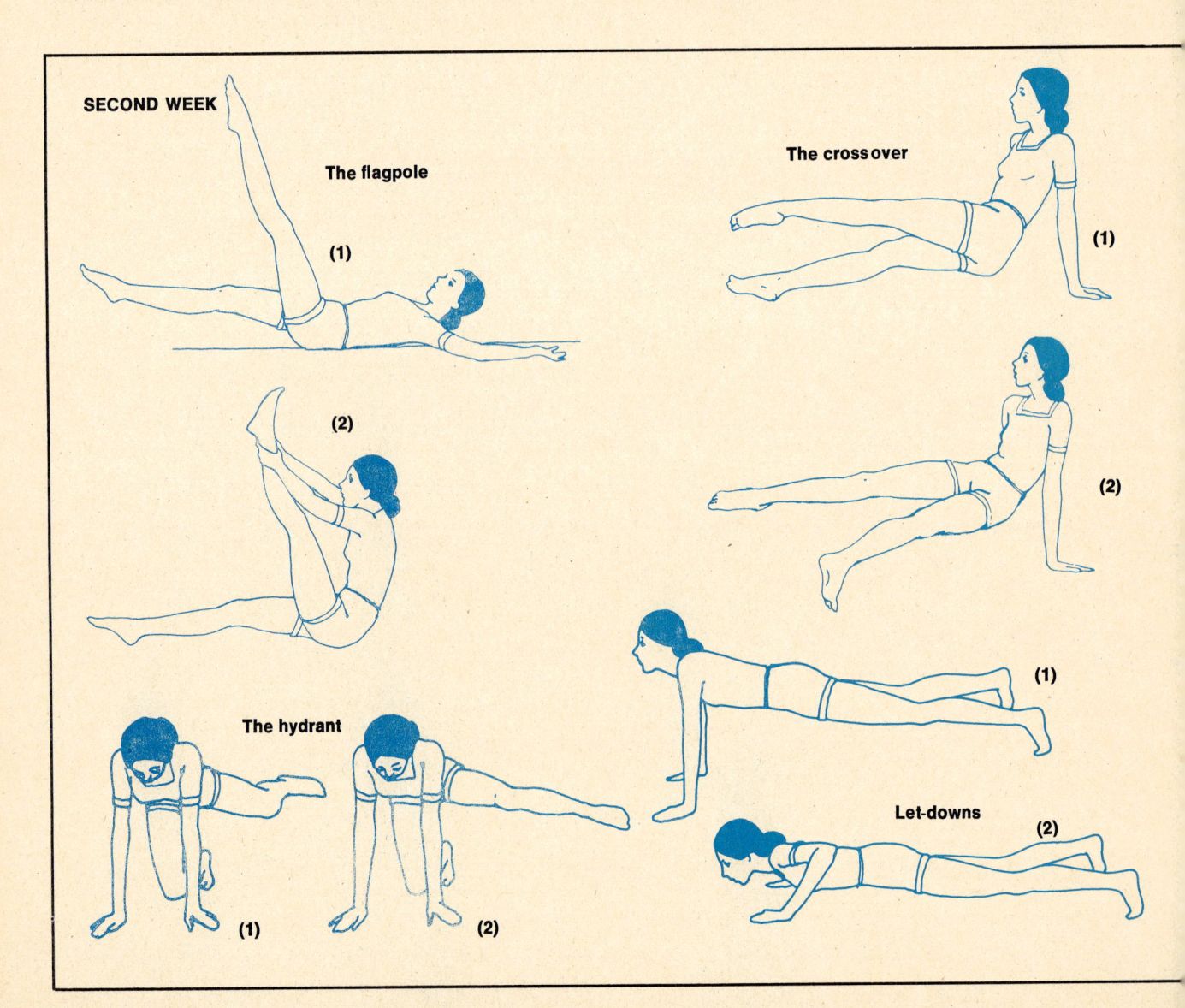

Let-downs for problem arms and bustline. Weak and flabby arms soon begin to show as weak and flabby even when they are slender. Upper arms and shoulders are also favorite targets of tension with accompanying stiffness and pain. Start on hands and feet **(1)** with body held straight and legs well spread. Lower your body slowly **(2),** taking five full counts to reach a position one inch above the floor. Then collapse and rest. Get up any way you can and repeat. Start with three and add one a week till you are doing 10.

Shoulder twist to shape heavy or flabby upper arms. Rest most of the weight on the right foot, twist the right arm under as far as possible **(1)** and watch your thumb as it comes around. You should feel the pull in the back of the arm and shoulder. Then open and twist the arm out and back as far as possible **(2),** keeping your eyes on the thumb. Each time you open, take a breath in. Start with four to each side and then eight together. Do three sets.

**THIRD WEEK
ADD-ONS FOR POSTURE PROBLEMS**

Posture, good or bad, is the result of many things, and those things usually begin in childhood. As people think, worry, fear, hate, love, and even dream, so do they sit, stand, walk, and run. One can, working with the right exercises, pull a body up, change a stance, a walk, a way of moving. And suddenly the person inside feels different and stronger.

Shrugs for tension in shoulder and neck. The shrug series should be tied into sedentary and stress-contributing habits such as watching TV, typewriting, driving, ironing, telephoning, practicing a musical instrument, and even playing bridge. Tension from concentration alone attacks the neck and shoulders all day long. We tighten those areas without even knowing it. Then a muscle goes into spasm. This causes pain and more spasm—and soon a headache is raging. To avoid this entirely everyday occurrence, prevent the first muscle spasm with shrugs. Use them often so that a spasm does not sneak up on you. You may appear to have St. Vitus's dance, but at least you won't have a pain in the neck. **Shrug up (1),** pulling shoulders up to almost touch ears. **Shrug down (2),** pressing shoulders down to make a long neck. **Shrug forward (3),** rounding shoulders forward to stretch the back. **Shrug back (4),** pressing arms back to stretch chest.

Snap and stretch for round back or shoulders. Stand with feet well apart and raise bent elbows to shoulder level with fingertips touching. Snap the elbows back **(1),** keeping the hands at shoulder level. Then bring the hands forward again—only this time do not stop at fingertip touch but allow the hands to overlap (the farther the over-

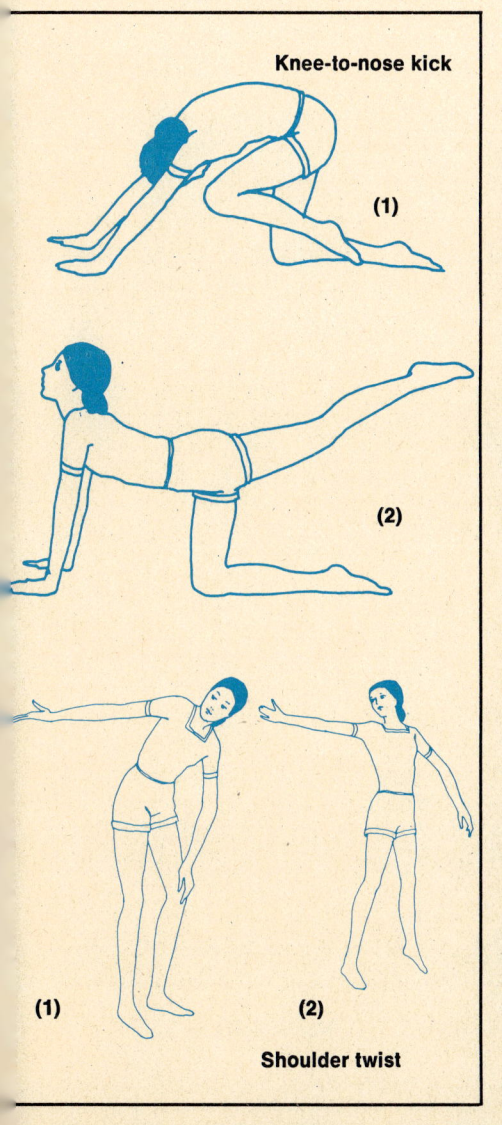

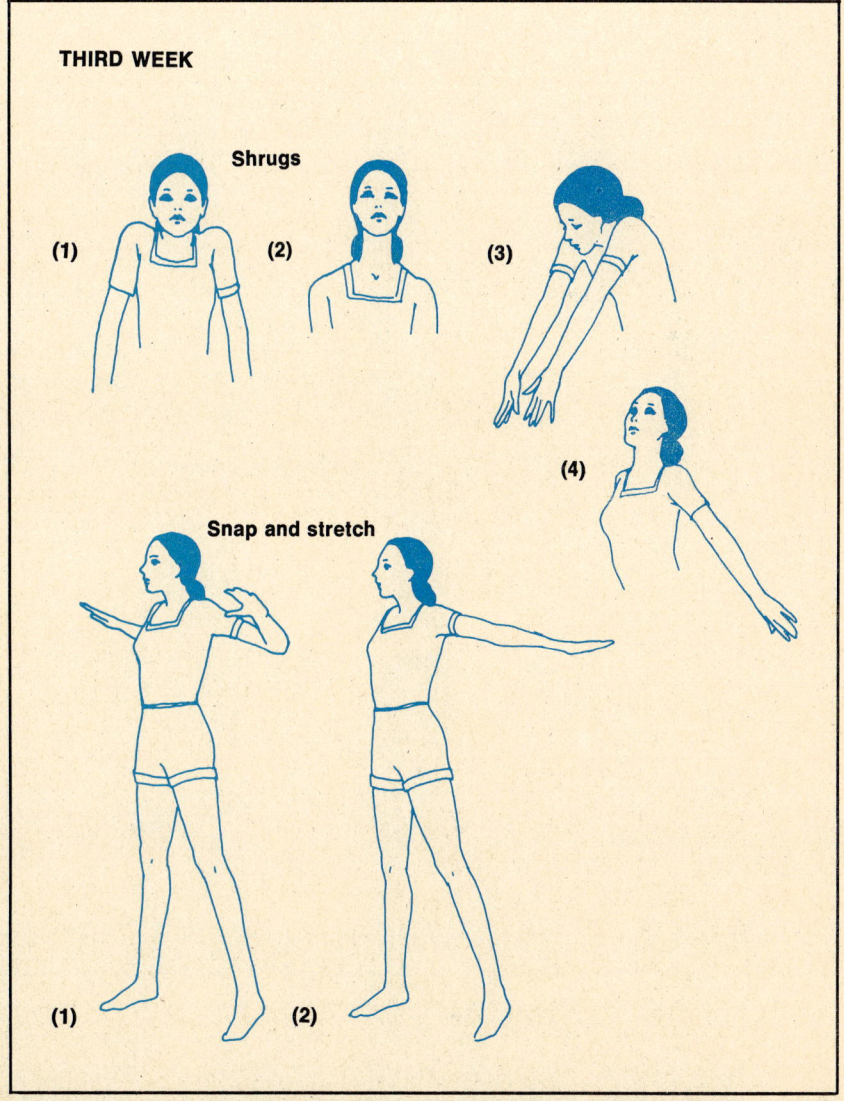

Knee-to-nose kick

(1)

(2)

(1) (2)

Shoulder twist

THIRD WEEK

Shrugs

(1) (2) (3)

(4)

Snap and stretch

(1) (2)

lap, the better). This stretches the back. Swing the arms wide **(2)** to full back stretch. Be careful not to drop below the shoulder. Do eight to a set and start with four sets.

Spine-down stretch for sway-backs and abdominals. Lie on your back with knees bent **(1)**. Check to see that your spine is flat on the floor. Raise both legs straight up **(2)** and point your toes. Return to the first, or resting, position and do several extensions. Next, extend the legs a little lower **(3)**, *but be sure your spine is still flat on the floor.* If there is an arch under your back, you have lowered the legs too far. Go back to second position **(2)** and try a much smaller distance down for your next extension. When you have gone down as far as you can with the back still flat, do five extensions. Work to lower the extensions week by week 'till your legs will extend parallel to the floor without touching it.

Side knee-to-chest for tense, tight, and bothersome low backs. Lie on your left side. Draw the right leg up as close to your chest as possible **(1)**. Then stretch it back down **(2)** as far as you can but *above* the resting leg. Then bring it to rest *on* the resting leg and *relax.* Do four with the right leg and then roll over and do four with the left to make up a set. *If you have a bothersome back,* do this set several times a day and begin and end your day doing this exercise in bed.

Thigh twist for hip and leg tension, balance, and gait. Stand on your right foot and twist the left foot **(1)**, leg, *and hip* inward. Twist the foot, leg, and hip outward **(2)**. Start with a slow beat, doing eight with each leg. As you improve, step up the time. Today's swinging music is just right for this exercise (and for the others as well), and you should do this twist often throughout the day.

FOURTH WEEK ADD-ONS FOR VITALITY

People get tired mostly because what they are doing bores them. Don't *walk* through the house; follow these suggestions. Keep music going and fit one of these to the music as you hear it.

Walks for feet, legs, hips and thighs.
Turned-in walk **(1)** is especially good for lower legs and flat feet. Turn your toes in as far as possible as you walk across the room or around the room. Take 16 steps in this position.
Turned-out walk—**(2)** This is good for inner-thigh flab, abdominals, and seat. Walk with feet well apart, knees turned out, and *seat tucked under* for 16 steps.
On-your-toes walk—**(3)** A foot-and-leg strengthener; good for balance. Get up high on your toes with a straight body and a proud head. Tightening the muscles of your thighs, seat, and abdomen will help you stay there. Take a small bounce with each step for 16.

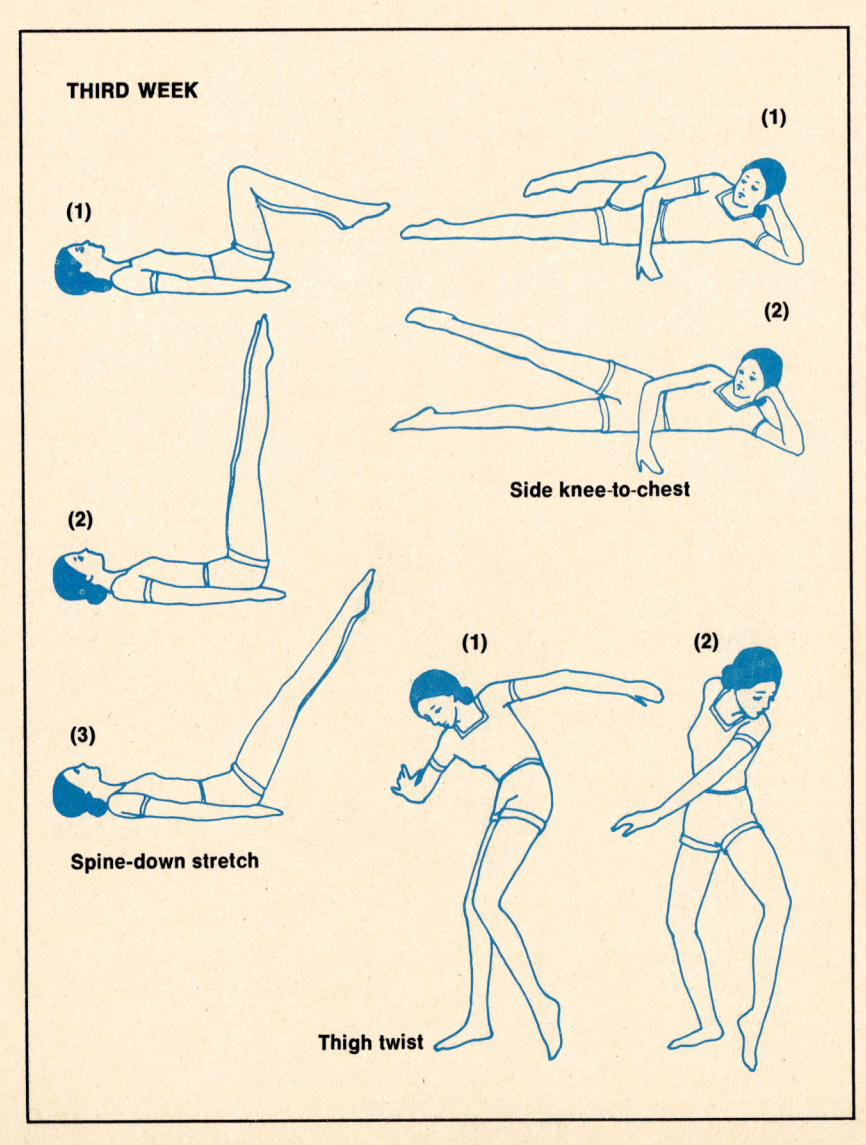

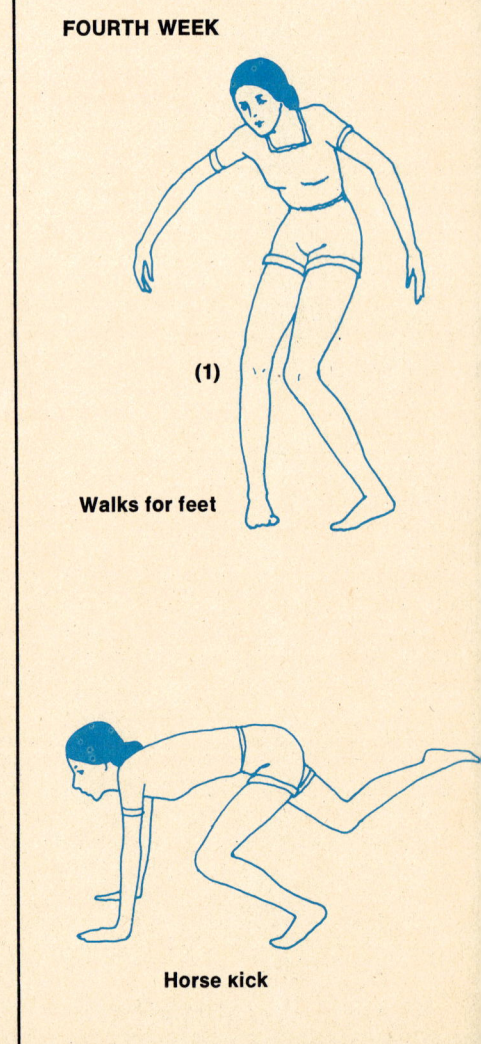

THIRD WEEK

Spine-down stretch

Side knee-to-chest

Thigh twist

FOURTH WEEK

Walks for feet

Horse kick

***Dropover walk*—(4)** Strengthens legs and back. Drop over well-bent knees and walk with small steps, feet facing straight forward—*not turned out*. Try to get down far enough to drag your fingertips. Walk 16 steps. When you have completed the walk series, start all over again. Try to keep this up through a full record-band, or about three-and-one-half minutes.

Running to strengthen leg muscles, heart, and lungs. Running is probably the best single exercise for leg muscles as well as heart and lungs (which means circulation and endurance), but do it right. If you just run in place for hundreds of beats, you will get bored and you will get leg cramps—then you will quit. Instead, put on a good swinging record *and change your step every 16 beats.*

***Straight run*—**You run 16 steps in place. Keep your knees fairly close together and feet pointing forward. On each step bring your heel down to touch the floor. *Do not run on tiptoe.*

***Scissors*—**Place one foot in front of the other and jump, changing both foot positions at the same time to cause a scissors action with your legs. Do 16 jumps. Relax.

***Side to side*—**With feet fairly close together, jump both feet from side to side. Forget about your arms, but as you become used to the jump, raise the shoulder on the side away from the jumping direction. This will work the entire torso as well as the arms and shoulders. Do 16 jumps. To these, you can also add one-foot hops (four to a foot), apart-together jumps, and forward-and-back jumps. If you keep changing from one to another, you will get the workout without the stiffness.

Horse kick for shoulders, arms, back, seat, and legs. Start out in the four-foot position, trying to keep the arms fairly straight. At first just try to run in place with little steps and to a beat. Four little steps would be a start—and, yes, it's normal to see stars, be breathless, and have a ringing in your ears. Those things mean its been too long since you've been in this position. Little by little, take slower steps and get those legs kicking high in the air. Believe it or not, you *do* need this. Work up to 16 steps at a time.

Tri-bike. Lie back on your elbows and use legs in a bicycle motion **(1)** for 16 circles. Then roll back onto your shoulders and, *supporting yourself at the waist,* do 16 more. When you are strong enough, push your legs farther over your head **(2)** to take away the necessity for waist support, stretch your arms flat, and bike in this position. Now—this is the really tough one—balance yourself on your seat **(3)** and, using no hand support, start the biking with four circles and gradually work up to 16 circles. Relax.

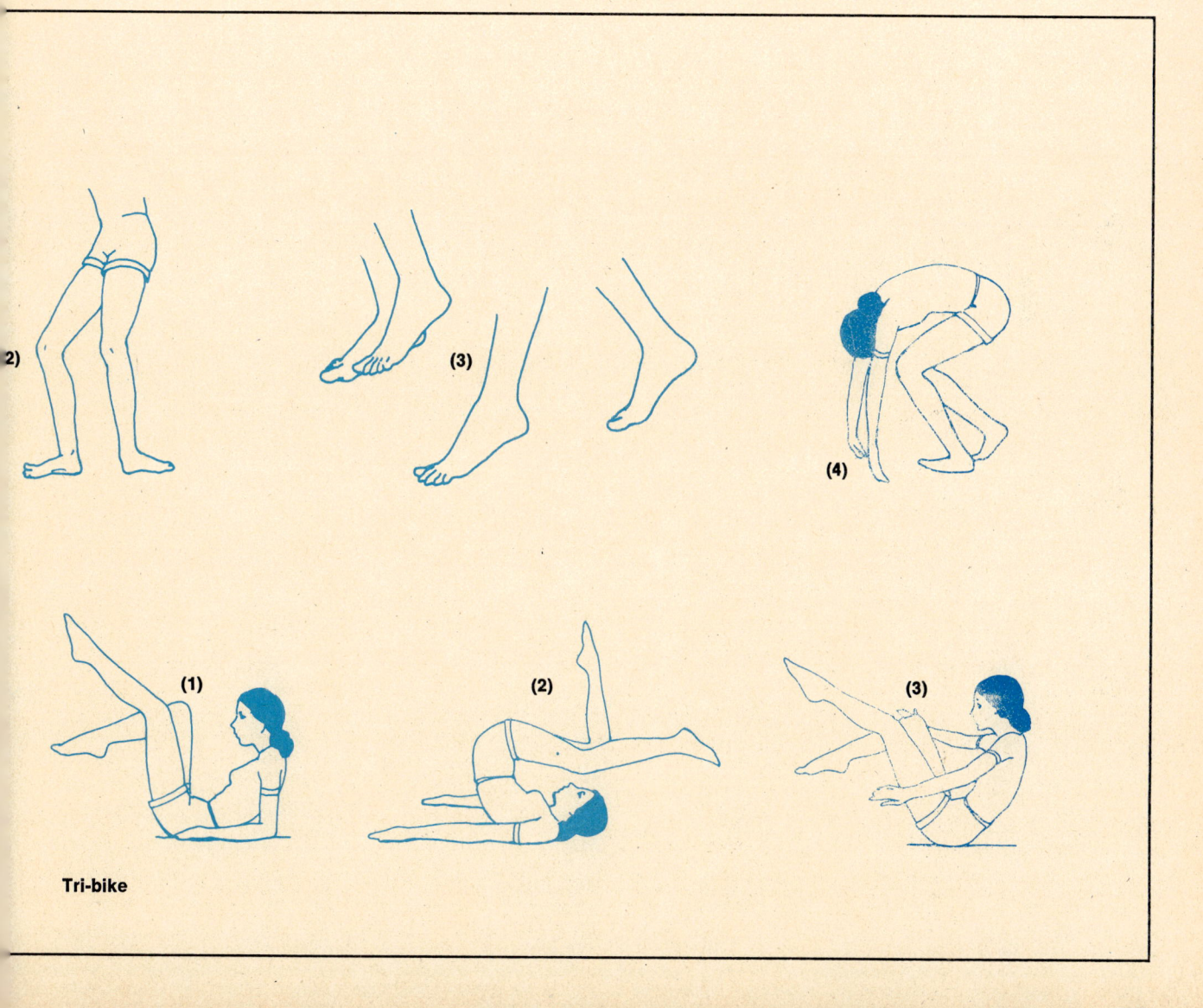

Tri-bike

INDEX

A

Abrasives, 122
Accessories, 115, 131
    bath, 118
Acne, 70, 73, 82, 89
    scars, 70, 73
Activity, outdoor, 80
Afro, curly, 29
Age, 112, 113
Aging skin, 90, 95
American Dietetic Association, 134
Ankles, 106, 130, 144, 145
Antiperspirants, 122
Arden, Elizabeth, 104
Arms, 115, 127, 152, 153
Astringents, 83
Automobile, 55, 83, 115

B

Back, 124, 142, 143, 144, 145, 151, 152, 153, 154
Ball exercise, 137
Bath, 112, 118-120
    aftersunning, 119
    afterswim shower, 119
    backache reliever, 119
    bedtime, 118
    cool-off, 119
    daytime relaxer, 118
    grooming, 120
    invigorating, 119
    preparations, 118
    quick freshup, 119
    shower, 51, 112, 119
    skin soother, 119
    temperature, 118
    wakeup, 118
    warmup, 119
Bath oil, 123
Beauty aids, instant, 129
Beauty flaws, 71-73
Beauty for the working wife, 112
Beauty guide, skin, 80
Beauty, outdoor, 56-57
Birthmarks, 99
Black, makeup, 53
Blackheads, 82
Bleach, facial hair, 70
Blemish covers, 46
Blush, natural, 50
Blusher, 46, 50, 54, 57
Boaters, 55
Body hair, 124-125
Body movement, 114-115
Body permanent, 6
Bosom, 106, 115
Braids, 22
Breasts, 73, 106, 115
Brushing hair, 17
Bustline, 144, 152-153
Buttocks, 144, 145

C

Calluses, 30, 127, 129
Calorie needs, 135
Camper, 55
Carr, Rachel E., 144, 146
Chapping, 91, 130
Cheekbones, 27, 66
Cheeks, 27, 47, 74, 75, 82, 84
Chignon, 22
Chin, 27, 65, 66, 72, 74, 75, 85, 144, 145
Circles, under-eye, 76-77
City, 55
Closeups, 111
Clothes, 51, 104-109, 131
Cocoa butter, 124
Colognes, 122, 123

Colors, makeup, 47, 58
Colors, slimming, 107
Combing hair, 17
Comb-out, 18
Compact powder, 54
Complexion, 67, 80-103
    normalize, 97
Conditioners, hair, 32-33
Conditioning, skin, 80-83, 93, 98-99
Contact lenses, 70
Contour cream, 42
Contouring cosmetics, 42, 46, 50, 113
Corns, 129, 130
Cosmetic surgery, 71-73
Cosmetics for your complexion, 46
Cotton, 30
Cover-up makeup, 43
Cowlick, 7
Craig, Marjorie, 117, 140
Cream, structured, technique, 103
Creme rinse, 32
Crow's feet, 78-79, 82
Curl, strength of, 30
Curls, clip, 30, 31
Curls, pin, 30-31
Curls, pin-on, 22
Cuticle, 126, 130

D

Dandruff, 31, 33
Daytime makeup, 54
Dental floss, 123
Dentifrice, 123
Dentistry, cosmetic, 70
Deodorants, 122
Depilatories, 122
Dermabrasion, 70
Diet, 80, 134-135
Dining out, 55
Double chin, 65, 113
Dress sizes, 108

E

Ears, 27, 72, 99
    hairdo to cover, 27
    pierced, 99
    surgery, 72
Egg shampoo, 32
Elbows, 127
Electric shaver, 125
Electrolysis, 70
Elizabeth Arden, 104
Evening makeup, 49-50
Exercises, 74-79, 137-155
    abdomen, 142, 143, 144, 145, 152, 154
    ankles, 144, 145
    arches, 144, 145
    arms, 146, 152-153
    back, 142, 143, 144, 145, 151, 152, 153, 154
    ball, 137
    bent-knee sit-ups, 151
    body stretch, 142
    breathing, 144, 146
    bridge, 148
    bustline, 144, 152-153
    buttocks, 144, 145
    camel pose, 148
    chinline, 144, 145
    combined eye, 79
    crow's feet, 78-79
    eye, 77-79
    face-saving, 74-75
    facial, 144, 145
    feet, 144, 145, 146, 147-148, 154
    feet and ankles, 146, 147-148
    feet and arches, 144, 145
    figure problems, 152
    flagpole, 152
    flight, 147
    hamstring flexibility, 151
    headstand, first steps to, 147-148
    heart, to strengthen, 155
    hip and leg tension, 154

    hip stretch, 146
    hips, 138, 152
    knee bends, 150
    knees, 144, 145, 147
    legs, 147, 154, 155
    legs, dance of, 147
    legs, horse kick for, 155
    lungs, to strengthen, 155
    neck and chinline, 144, 145
    neck, tension in, 153
    perfect posture, 148
    posture, 116-117, 153-154
    running, 155
    seat, horse kick for, 155
    shoulder stand, 148-149
    shoulders, 142, 144, 145, 146, 153
    shrugs, 153
    sit-ups, bent-knee, 151
    stick, 138-139
    stretch, 142-143, 144-145
    stretch, horizontal, 144-145
    stretch, vertical, 144, 145
    stretcher, thigh, 139
    stroking, 100-103
    sun salutation, 149
    sway back, 154
    tension-freeing, 140-141, 153
    thigh-stretcher, 139
    thighs, 144, 145, 152
    tri-bike, 155
    underarms, 145, 146
    under-eye circles, 76-77
    vitality, for, 154-155
    waist twist, 150
    waist-whittler, 138
    walks, 154
Eyebrows, 50, 57, 68-69, 113
    color, 47
    pencil, 54
    makeup, 42, 43, 59-60
    shaping, 59, 60
    well-groomed, 66, 67
Eye drops, 123
Eyeglasses, 27, 68-69
    hairdo for, 27
    hair styles with, 68-69
    makeup with, 68-69
Eyelashes, 50, 54, 68-69
    false, 46, 57, 62-63
    lengthener, 57
Eyelids, surgery, 72
Eye liner, 42, 47, 60, 61
Eye pads, 123
Eyes, 67, 82, 85, 113, 123
    care, 123
    circles, 60, 61, 76-77
    close together, 60, 61
    crow's feet, 78-79
    exercises for, 75, 77-79
    eyelids, 72
    glasses, 27, 68-69, 70, 113
    highlight, 50
    makeup, 42, 50, 57
    muscles, to relax, 80-81
    pouches, 60, 61
    round, 60, 61
    shape, improving, 60
    small, 60
    surgery, eyelids, 72
    under-eye circles, 76-77
    under-eye shadows, 50
Eye shadow, 42, 47, 54, 57, 60

F

Face, 58-63, 112
    balance, 58-63
    beauty treatment, 145
    diamond-shape, 24, 25
    fat, 26-27
    heart-shape, 24
    large, 26
    long, 24, 26
    pale, 51
    plain, 26
    round, 24

thin, 64
wide, 24, 64
Face-changers, 66-67
Face fresheners, 50-51
Face-freshening makeup, 51
Face lift, 73
"Face lift" makeup, 50
Face peeling, 70
Face planing, 70
Face-saving facial exercises, 74-75
Face shape, 24-25, 64-65, 66, 69
    eyeglasses and, 69
    hairdos for, 24-25
    how to analyze, 24
    makeup for, 64-65
Facial, 87, 88, 91, 92-93
    fast, 87
    home, 88
    salon, 91, 92-93
    water, 90
Facial exercises, 74-75, 144, 145
Facial flaws, 71-73, 113
Facial hair, 70, 113
Fall, 22
False lashes, 46, 62-63, 68-69, 113
Fatigue-reliever bath, 118, 119
Feet, 51, 112, 130, 144, 145, 146, 147-148
Figure, 109, 113, 131, 132-155
    type, 109
Fingernails, 126-27
    instant, 129
Flabby tissue, 82
Flaws, beauty, 71-73
Flip, 29
Flying, 55
Foot bath, 130
Foot beauty, 129-130
Foot burn, 130
Foot care, 130
Foot cream, 129
Foot massage, 130
Foot problems, 130
Foot relaxers, 130
Foot rest, 130
Forehead, 26-27, 66, 72, 73, 82, 85
Forty-plus, looking pretty at, 112-113
Foundation, makeup, 40, 44, 46, 54, 57
Four-week exercise plan for inner strength, outer beauty, 146-148
Four-week figure-firming plan, 149-155
Fragrance, 123, 131
Frames, eyeglasses, 68-69
Freckles, 91
French seam, 18
Frown lines, 73, 80

G

Gel-tint makeup, 43, 46
Gloves, 106, 115
Golden Door, 130, 137, 138
Grooming, 17-18, 119, 120-131
    aids, 122-123
    bath, 120
    checklist, 130-131
    guide to good, 120
    hair, 17-18
    shower, 119

H

Hair, 4-39, 113, 124-125, 131
    ash-blond, 51, 52
    black, 51
    body, 124-125
    body in, 6
    brittle, 6
    coarse, 7, 34
    color, 51-52, 113
    color-treated, 7, 37
    cowlick, 7
    cripple, how to avoid becoming, 31
    curl, strength of, 30
    curly, 6
    curved part, 7
    damaged, 31, 34
    dandruff, 33
    dry, 7
    easy-to-wave, 34
    fine, 7, 34
    golden blond, 51
    gray, 51
    grooming, 17-18
    hand-drying, 18
    hard-to-manage, 7
    hard-to-wave, 34
    hidden wave, 6-7
    length, 20
    light brown, 51
    limp, 34
    long, 20-21, 34
    loss of, 33
    lustrous, 6
    medium long, 20
    normal, 34
    oily, 7
    outer arms, 127
    porous, 7
    protection, 33
    removal, 122
    short, 20, 24
    straggly, 51
    straight, 6
    straightening, 35
    structure, 31
    texture, 7
    thin, 6
    type, 4-7
    white, 51
Hair care, 31-34
    acid rinse, 32
    afterpermanent, 35
    body permanent, 6
    brushing, 17
    color-treated, shampoo for, 31
    combing, 17
    conditioner, 32-33
    creme rinse, 32
    dandruff shampoo, 31
    dandruff treatment, 33
    detergent shampoo, 31
    dry shampoo, 31
    dry-hair shampoo, 31
    egg shampoo, 32
    hand driers, 18
    helps, 33
    herbal shampoo, 31
    home permanent, 34-35
    hot-oil treatment, 32-33
    lemon rinse, 32
    massage, 31
    moneysavers, 34
    normal-hair shampoo, 31
    oily-hair shampoo, 31
    permanent wave, 34-35
    rinse, 32
    setting-lotion conditioner, 32
    shampoo for hair type, 31
    shampoo, how to, 32
    soap shampoo, 31
    spray, 18
    straightening, 35
    swatch test, 34-35
    teasing, 17
    treatment, dandruff, 33
    vinegar rinse, 32
    washing and rinsing, 31-32
    winding, permanent 35
Hair coloring, 36-39
    certified color, 38
    chemistry of, 38
    choosing a hair color, 36
    color crayon, 37
    color rinse, 37
    developer, 38
    double blonding, 37
    drabbing drops, 38
    foam-in, 37
    frosting, 38
    highlight shampoo, 37
    lightener, 37, 38
    lotion tint, 37
    metallic dyes, 38
    one-process blonders, 37
    one-process permanent color, 37
    patch test, 36
    precautions, 38
    preparations, 37-38
    semipermanent, 37
    semipermanent color rinse, 37, 38, 39
    shampoo-in tint, 37
    skin tones related to, 39
    special effects, 38
    spray-on powder, 37
    strand test, 36
    streaking, 38
    sunlighteners, 37
    temporary, 36, 37
    three-week rinse, 37
    tint, 38
    tipping, 38
    toner, 38
    toners, 37-38
    two-process permanent, 37-38
    vegetable dyes, 38
Haircutting, 8-11
    all-one-length haircut, 10, 11
    blunt cut, 11
    bowl, 8
    cap cut, 18-19
    carefree, 8
    layered cut, 10-11
    no-set, 18-19
    shag, 10, 11
    windblow, 18-19, 28
Hairpieces, 21-22
    braid, figure-8, 22
    braided chignon, 22
    braids, 22
    chignon, 22
    curls, pin-on, 22
    fall, 22
    ponytail, 21, 22
    switch, 21, 22
    wiglet, 21
    wiglet, barrette, 21, 22
    wigs, 22-23
Hair styles, 12-15, 24, 25, 26, 27, 28-29, 68, 69, 112, 113
    angel cut, 29
    balance your face, 26
    best-liked, 28-29
    brush cut, 28
    cap coif, 28
    cap cut, 18-19
    cheekbones, for high, 27
    cheeks, for plump, 27
    chignon, 22
    chin, for small, 27
    curly Afro, 29
    diamond-shape face, for, 24-25
    dimension, 26
    direction, 26
    double ponytail, 20-21
    ears, hairdo to cover, 27
    eyeglasses, hairdo with, 68, 69
    face shape, analyze, 24
    face shapes, hairdos for, 24-25
    fall hairpiece, 22
    fat face, for, 27
    features, for irregular, 27
    flip, 29
    forehead, 26-27
    full-bang bob, 28
    full throat, hairdo for, 27
    glamour bob, 29
    hairpiece hairdos, 21-22
    heart-shape face, 24
    high cheekbones, hairdo for, 27
    high forehead, hairdo for, 26-27
    how-tos, 14-15
    irregular features, hairdo for, 27
    jutting jaw, hairdo for, 27
    large face, for, 26
    large nose, hairdo for, 26
    length, 26
    lily pad, 20-21
    long face, 24-25, 26

long-hair hairdos, 20-21
long neck, hairdo for, 26, 27
low forehead, hairdo for, 26-27
mass, 26
mini-hairdo, 55
no-set hairdos, 18-19
oriental elegance, 21
outline, 26
oval face, 24
pageboy, 29
plain face, 26
plump cheeks, hairdo for, 27
ponytail, double, 20-21
pouf, 28-29
problems, hairdos that solve, 26
round face, 24
sculpture wreath, 20-21
short neck, hairdo for, 27
small chin, hairdo for, 27
small face, hairdo for, 26
square face, hairdo for, 24
square jaw, hairdo for, 27
straight-line look, 29
strong jaw, hairdo for, 27
throat, 27
updo, 21
wide face, 24
width, 26
windblow, 18-19
wind-blown, 28
Hair styling, 6, 17-18, 30-32
  back-brushing, 17
  back-combing, 6, 17
  clip curls, 30, 31
  cotton, 30
  French seam, 18
  French twist, 18
  hairset, how to revive, 18
  hand driers, 18
  hand-drying hair, 18
  hot curlers, 30
  how to set hair, 30
  pin curls, 30, 31
  rollers, 30
  setting-lotion conditioner, 32
  tape, 30
  teasing, 17
  wave set, 30
  winding rollers, 30
Hair removal, 122
Hair type, 4-7
Hand care, 127
Hand creams and lotion, 127
Hand driers, 18
Hand grace, 115
Hand problems, 127
Hand protectors, 127
Hands, 112, 115, 127, 131
Hearing aids, 71
Heart, 155
Height, 108-109
Highlight, 40, 50
Hips, 138, 146, 152
Home permanent, 34-35
Hot curlers, 30
Hot-oil treatment, 32-33
House guest, 55
How to choose and use makeups, 43
How-tos, hair styles, 14-15
Hypoallergenic makeup, 46

I

Irrigator, mouth, 123
Isometric exercise, 76-77, 78-79

J

Jaw, 27, 66
Jaw line, 66

K

Keloids, 99
Klinger, Georgette, Salon, 99
Knees, 144, 145, 147, 148

Krane, Jessica, 100

L

Legs, 51, 105, 115, 129, 147, 154, 155
  beauty, 115
  dance of, 147
  exercises, 147, 154, 155
  heavy, 105
  makeup, 129
Light touch, handle skin with 84-87
Lights and shades, 40
Lines, deep, 82
Lip brush, 46
Lip color, 47
Lip gloss, 57
Lip liner, 43
Lips, plastic surgery, 72
Lips, thick, 72
Lipsticks, 43, 47, 51, 54
Loewendahl, Evelyn, 138
Long-hair hairdos, 20-21
Long-line look, 107
Look of beauty, 104-114
Lungs, 155

M

Makeup, 40-69, 112, 113
  ash blonde, 51
  base, 50
  black, 53
  black hair, 51
  blemish covers, 46
  blonde, 52
  blusher, 46, 50, 54, 57
  broad nose, makeup for, 64-65
  brow color, 47
  brow pencil, 54
  brows, 42, 43, 50, 57, 59-60, 68-69
  brows, shaping, 59-60
  brows, well-groomed, 66, 67
  brunette, 51, 52
  cheek color, 47
  colors, choose your, 58
  compact powder, 54
  complexion, cosmetics for, 46
  contour creams, 42
  contouring, 42, 46, 50, 113
  cover-up, 43
  daylight, 52-53
  daytime, 54
  double chin, makeup for, 65
  evening, 49-50
  eyebrow pouches, 60
  eyebrows, 69, 113
  eyeglasses, 68-69
  eyelashes, 54, 68-69
  eye liner, 42, 47
  eye shadow, 42, 47, 54, 57, 60
  eye shape, improving, 60
  eyes, 42, 50, 57, 67, 113
  eyes, close together, 60, 61
  eyes, highlight, 50
  eyes, protruding, 60, 61
  eyes, round, 60, 61
  eyes, small, 60
  face balance, 58-63
  face-changers, 66-67
  face-freshening, 51
  "face lift", 50
  face shape, 64-65, 66
  false lashes, 46, 57, 62-63, 68-69, 113
  famous salons, how they do new, 44
  foundation, 40, 46, 54, 57
  gel tint, 43, 46
  golden blonde, 51
  gray hair, 51
  hair color as a key, 51
  highlight, 40, 50
  hollow cheeks, 65
  how to choose and use new, 43
  hypoallergenic, 46
  judging, 43
  lash lengthener, 57
  lashes, 50

  lashes, false, 46, 57, 62-63, 68-69, 113
  light-brown hair, 51
  lights and shades, 40
  lip brush, 46
  lip color, 47
  lip gloss, 57
  lip liner, 43
  lip makeup, 47, 51
  lipsticks, 43, 54
  magic touch, 40-43
  mascara, 42, 47, 54, 57, 60, 61, 68
  medicated, 46
  mini-makeup, 55
  moisture base, 57
  mouth, 58-59, 67, 74, 75, 113
  mouth balance, 58-59
  mouth lines, 65
  mouth shaping, 58-59
  narrow nostrils, 65
  neck and throat, 42
  nightlight, 49
  "nose bob", 66, 67
  nose, high-bridge, 65
  nose, long, 64, 65
  nose, small, 66
  outdoor, 56
  party face fresheners, 50-51
  powder, 42, 46, 50, 54, 57
  receding chin, 65
  redhead, 51, 53
  removal, 83
  rouge, 42, 57
  round face, 64, 65
  salon, 44
  shading, 42, 50
  shadow, 42
  shape your face with, 64
  shaping brows, 59, 60
  skin tones and, 47
  square jaw, 64, 65
  thin face, 64
  throat, 42
  translucent, 43, 46
  waterproof, 46, 55, 57
  white hair, 51
  wide face, 64
Manicure, 126-127
Manicure needs, 126
Manzoni, Pablo, 104
Mascara, 42, 44, 47, 54, 57, 60, 61, 68
Mask, facial, 86-87, 88, 93
Massage, foot, 130
Massage, scalp, 31
Measurements, body, 108
"Medical Specialists, Directory of", 71
Mini-hairdo, 55
Mini-makeup, 55
Miss Craig's instant-thinning plan, 116-117
Miss Craig's tension-freeing exercise, 140-141
Moisturizer, 40, 57, 13
Moles, 99
Moneysavers, 34
Mouth, 67, 74, 75, 82, 85, 113
  balance, 58-59
  freshness, 122-123
  lines, 65
  makeup, 58-59
  shaping, 58-59
Mouthwash, 122

N

Nail biting, 127
Nail hardeners, 126
Nail patching, 126
Nail polish, 127
Nail shaping, 126
Nails, artificial, 127
Nails, breaking, 127
Natural cosmetics, 99
Neck, 26, 27, 82, 105, 144, 145, 153
  exercises, 144, 145, 153
  long, 26, 27, 105
  short, 106, 107

Neck and throat, makeup, 42
Neckline, 106
Neck stretching, 106
Night cream, 87
Nightlight, look your best in, 49
Nose, 26, 27, 64-65, 66, 67, 71, 74, 82, 85
    broad, 64-65
    high-bridge, 65
    large, 26, 27
    long, 64, 65
    narrow nostrils, 65
    reshaping, 71
    small, 66
"Nose bob", 66, 67
No-set hairdos, 18-19
Nude beauty, 124

O

Optometrist, 68, 70
Outdoor beauty, 56-57
Outdoor makeup, 56

P

Party face fresheners, 50-51
Patch test, 36
Pedicure, 130
Perfume, 99, 123
    type, 123
Permanent, home, 34-35
Perspiration, 91, 122
Petroleum jelly, 57
Photographs, 71, 110-111
Picking things up, 115
Pickups, preparty, 51
Picture, how to look prettier in, 110-111
Pill, skin problems on, 99
Pimples, 82
Pin curls, 30-31
Plastic surgeon, 71
Plastic surgery, 71-73, 99
Pollution, air, 91, 97
Ponytail, 21, 22
Pores, enlarged, 82
Portraits, 110
Posture, 110, 114-115, 116-117
Powder, 42, 44, 46, 50, 54, 57, 122
    compact, 54
    deodorant, 122
    loose, 42
    pressed, 46
    translucent, 44, 57
Powers, John Robert, Charm School, 114
Pregnancy, 99
Preparty pickups, 51
Problems, skin, 99
Proportions, 108
Protection, skin, 80, 83
Prudden, Bonnie, 132, 148
Psychology of beauty, 104

R

Relaxation, 80, 110, 112
Rouge, 42, 46, 57
Round face, 64, 65
Runge, Senta Maria, 76

S

Sachet, 123
Safety razor, 125
Salon facial, 91, 92-93
Salon makeup, 44
Sand rashes, 125
Scalp massage, 31
Scars, 70, 71, 72, 73, 99
Sensitivity, skin, 91
Setting-lotion conditioner, 32
Shading, 42, 50
Shadows, under-eye, 51
Shag haircut, 10, 11
Shampoo, 31-32
    detergent, 31
    dry, 31
    dry hair, 31
    egg, 32
    herbal, 31
    how to, 32
    normal hair, 31
    oily hair, 31
    soap, 31
Shape your face with makeup, 64
Shaving, 122
Shower bath, 51, 112, 119
Silhouette, 106, 109
Silicone foam, 70
Silicone implants, 71, 72, 73
Sitting, 114-115, 142, 144-145
Skin, 46, 50, 54, 74, 80-100, 112-113, 125
    acne, 70, 72-73, 82, 99
    aging, 90, 95
    analysis chart and key, 82
    any-age care, 90
    beauty guide, 80
    birthmarks, 99
    blackheads, 82
    bleach for facial hair, 70
    blemish covers, 46
    brown spots, 99
    care, 83-90, 112, 113
    chapping, feet, 130
    cleaning, 83, 86
    cleanser, deep-pore, 83, 88
    cleansers, stimulating, 83
    cleansing and relaxation, 92
    cleansing grains, 83
    combination skin, 90, 94-95
    complexion, 67, 131
    complexion, normalize, 97
    condition, 80
    conditioning, 83, 93, 98-99
    cover cream, 54
    cream removal, 86-87
    cream, structured, technique, 103
    creams, 90, 97, 98, 99, 103
    day care, 86
    deep cleansing, 92
    deep-pore cleansing, 83, 88
    dermabrasion, 71
    dry, 82, 90, 94, 112
    elbows, 127
    face, how to clean, 83
    facial, fast, 87
    facial, home, 88
    facial, salon, 91, 92-93
    facial, water, 90
    handling, 84-87
    irritation, 125
    light touch, 84-87
    lines, deep, 82
    makeup removal, 83
    mask, facial, 86-87, 88, 93
    mask treatment, 86-87
    moisturizer, 40, 57, 113
    natural cosmetics, 99
    night care, 86
    night cream, 87
    normal, 90, 97
    oily, 90, 94
    outdoor care, 90-91
    perspiration, 91, 122
    pimples, 82
    pores, enlarged, 82
    problems, 99
    protection, 80, 83
    salon facial, 91, 92-93
    sensitivity, skin, 91
    soother, 119
    stimulating cleansers, 83
    stimulation, 93
    sunburn, 91, 124
    tanning, 91
    toning, 83, 93, 98
    troubled, 90, 95
    type, 94-95
    warts, 127
    water facial, 90
    weathering, 97
    wrinkles, 70, 74-75, 82, 113
    wrinkles, how to stroke away, 100-103
Slim-and-trim eye-foolers, 107
Slim while you sit, 144-145
Snapshots, 110
Soap, 83
Soap-and-water wash, 83
Soaps, deodorant, 122
Sponge, 57
Sports, 47
Stairs, 114
Stand, how to, 107
Standing, 110-111, 115, 116-117
Straightening, hair, 35
Strand test, 36
Sunburn, 91, 124
Sunglasses, 54, 55, 70
Sunlighteners, 37
Swatch test, 34-35
Switch, 21, 22

T

Tan, instant, 129
Tanning, 91
Teeth, 113, 122-123
Temperature, bath, 118
Tension, 80, 140-141
Tension-freeing exercise, 140-141
Thighs, 105
Thompson, Roger, 10
Throat, 42, 85, 106, 113
Throat-stretcher, 67
Time, 131
Tissue, flabby, 82
Toenails, ingrown, 130
Toilet water, 123
Tooth brushing, 122-123
Total look, 104-116
Tourist, 54
Translucent makeup, 43, 46
Traveler, beauty for, 54-55
Tweezing, 122

U

Underarms, 112
Under-eye circles, 76-77
Under-eye puffiness, 51
Under-eye shadows, 50, 51, 76-77, 113
Underwear, 131

V

Valmy, Christine, Salon, 91
Veins, 130
Vidal Sassoon International, 10
Vision, 68, 69, 113
Vitality, 131
Vito, Victor, 7

W

Waist, 106, 138, 148, 150
Walking, 114
Wardrobe, 112
Warts, 127
Water facial, 90
Waterproof makeup, 46, 55, 57
Wave set, 30
Waxing, 122
Weathering, skin, 90, 97
Weight, 134
Weights, desirable, 135
Wiglet, 21, 22
Wigs, 22-23
Windblow, 18-19
Wind-blown hairdo, 28
"Woo" position, 102
Working wife, beauty for, 112
Wrinkles, 70, 74, 75, 82, 100-103, 113
    forehead, 73, 74
    how to stroke away, 100-103

Y

Yoga, 144-145, 146-147
Yoga, perfect posture, 148

159

ACKNOWLEDGMENTS

Page

8 (left) and 9—Hairstyle by Philip Mason,
creative director, Vidal Sassoon, New York.
8 (right)—Hairstyle by Roger Thompson,
creative director, Vidal Sassoon International.
12-13—Hairstyles by 1 Michel Kazan.
2 Henri Bendel. 3, 5, 6, 7, 8, 9 Christiaan.
4 Maury Hopson. 10 Jason Croy of Antenna.
11, 12 Pierre Henri, Saks Fifth Avenue Salons.
19-20—"No-set Hairdos" by Benjamin of Cinandre.
40, 42—"Give Your Makeup a Magic Touch" by
Mildred Simpson, Tourneur Salons.
41, 44-45—Makeup by Don Nelson.
48-49, 52-53—Makeup by Stan Place.
84—"Daytime Makeup that Lasts All Day" by Hal King.
82—"Skin-analysis Chart and Key" from
Georgette Klinger Salons.
84-87—"Handle Your Skin with a Light Touch"
by Don Nelson.
90—"Any-age Skin Care" by Margrit Ehrlich,
Ernest & Josephine Hair Design, Mamaroneck, New York.
92-93—"Salon Facial" by Mme. Bilan, New York.
96—Makeup by Marie Irvine.
76-79—"Under-Eye Circles and How To Relieve Them"
and "To Eliminate Crow's Feet" adapted from
"Face Lifting by Exercise" by Mme. Senta Maria Rungé
© 1961, 1970.
100-103—"How To Stroke Wrinkles Away"
adapted from "How To Use Your Hands To Save Your
Face" by Jessica Krane, Avon Books © 1969, 1972.
104-106—"Total Look of Beauty" by Pablo Manzoni,
creative director, Elizabeth Arden.

Page

116-117—"Miss Craig's Instant Thinning Plan
for Abdomen and Waist" adapted from "Miss Craig's
21-Day Shape-up Program for Men and Women" by
Majorie Craig. Copyright © 1968 by Random House, Inc.
Reprinted by permission of the publisher.
126-127—"Professional Manicure To Do
At Home" from Revlon.
135—"Basic Diet Pattern" from
"Family Circle Diet & Exercise Guide" © 1966, 1972 by
The Family Circle Inc.

PHOTO CREDITS

Cover, 1—Rik Van Glintenkamp
4-5, 8-9—Mort Mace
12-13—Rik Van Glintenkamp (Nos. 1, 2, 6, 7, 8, 9)
12-13—George K. Nordhausen (Nos. 3, 4, 5, 11, 12)
12-13—Ben Swedowsky (No. 10)
16—Emeric Bronson
41, 44-45, 48-49—Rik Van Glintenkamp
52-53—Victor Skrebneski
56—Rik Van Glintenkamp
81—Les Carron
84-85—Jim Dorrance
88-89—George K. Nordhausen
92-93—Rik Van Glintenkamp
96—Skylar Robins
121, 124-125, 128-129—Rik Van Glintenkamp
132-133—John Engstead
136—Bob Willoughby